Oral Complications of Cancer and its Management

Oral Complications of Cancer and its Management

Edited by

Dr Andrew N. Davies
Consultant in Palliative Medicine
Royal Marsden Hospital
UK

Prof Joel B. Epstein
Professor of Oral Medicine
Otolaryngology and Head and Neck Cancer
University of Illinois at Chicago
USA

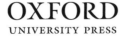
OXFORD
UNIVERSITY PRESS

OXFORD

UNIVERSITY PRESS

Great Clarendon Street, Oxford, OX2 6DP,
United Kingdom

Oxford University Press is a department of the University of Oxford.
It furthers the University's objective of excellence in research, scholarship,
and education by publishing worldwide. Oxford is a registered trade mark of
Oxford University Press in the UK and in certain other countries

Published in the United States of America by Oxford University Press
198 Madison Avenue, New York, NY 10016, United States of America

British Library Cataloguing in Publication Data

Data available

Library of Congress Cataloging in Publication Data

Data available

ISBN 978-0-19-954358-8

Preface

Globally, oral and pharyngeal cancers are leading sites of disease, and overall they make up the eighth most common site in men. In the United States of America, there are about 1.5 million new cases of cancer diagnosed each year, and more than 35 000 of these cancers involve the oral and pharyngeal sites. In spite of advances in surgery, radiation therapy, and chemotherapy, the overall 5-year survival rate has not significantly improved over recent years (~59%). The reason for the relatively poor survival is the often advanced presentation of the disease, stemming from the often delayed diagnosis of the problem. In an attempt to improve survival, treatments have become even more aggressive, frequently resulting in ever more complex and/or more severe oropharyngeal complications.

Similar issues of tumour control occur in cancers of other systems, and, not surprisingly, similar strategies have been adopted in the management of these cancers, i.e. the use of more aggressive treatments in an attempt to improve survival rates. Indeed, many patients with more common malignancies now undergo extremely toxic chemotherapy, and even a bone marrow or stem cell transplant, in an attempt to arrest or 'cure' the tumour. Many of these systemic treatments can cause a variety of oral complications. A common and critical adverse effect is oral mucositis, which is associated with physical problems (e.g. pain, impaired nutritional intake), psychological problems, decreased quality of life, and at times can even be life threatening. Furthermore, oral mucositis is associated with increased healthcare expenditure (e.g. more medications, longer hospital stays).

This unique book serves as an outstanding resource for the many oral complications of cancer and its treatment. It is written by international authorities in their respective specialties, and includes contributions from all of the members of the multi-professional oncology team. The book comprises 30 chapters, and includes extensive tables, figures, clinical photographs, and references to aid the understanding of the text. It covers topics such as oral anatomy and physiology, oral assessment and oral hygiene, as well as the more common oral complications of cancer and its treatment. Surgical, radiation therapy, and chemotherapy responses are detailed in overview chapters, whilst specific problems are discussed in detail in separate chapters (e.g. oral mucositis, osteonecrosis of jaw bones). Other chapters focus on oral infections, and oral symptoms experienced by patients with cancer (e.g. xerostomia, taste disturbance). Furthermore, there are chapters addressing the needs of specific groups of patients (paediatric patients, geriatric patients, patients with advanced cancer), and the health economic impact of oral complications.

It is envisaged that the availability of this comprehensive, evidence-based (when available), practical reference text will help facilitate all healthcare professionals involved in the care of patients with cancer to provide the most appropriate care for the oral complications of cancer and its treatment. It is a welcome addition to the available resources in this area of practice.

Prof Sol Silverman
Professor of Oral Medicine
University of California, San Francisco,
USA

Contents

Contributors *ix*

1 Introduction *1*
Andrew Davies and Joel Epstein

2 The oral cavity *11*
Anita Sengupta and Anthony Giles

3 Oral assessment *21*
Michael Brennan and Peter Lockhart

4 Common oral conditions *27*
Katherine Webber and Andrew Davies

5 Pretreatment screening and management *35*
Peter Stevenson-Moore, Debbie Saunders, and Joel Epstein

6 Oral hygiene *43*
Petrina Sweeney and Andrew Davies

7 Oral cancer *53*
Crispian Scully and Jose Bagan

8 Other tumours of the oral cavity *65*
Barbara Murphy, Jill Gilbert, and Anderson Collier III

9 Overview of complications of oral surgery *79*
Antonia Kolokythas and Michael Miloro

10 Overview of complications of radiotherapy (radiation therapy) *89*
Kate Newbold and Kevin Harrington

11 Trismus *99*
Pieter Dijkstra and Jan Roodenburg

12 Post-radiation osteonecrosis (osteoradionecrosis) of the jaws *117*
Fred Spijkervet and Arjan Vissink

13 Overview of complications of systemic chemotherapy *123*
Douglas Peterson and Rajesh Lalla

14 Oral complications of haematopoietic stem cell transplantation *129*
Sharon Elad, Judith Raber-Durlacher, and Michael Y. Shapira

15 Oral mucositis *141*
Stephen Sonis and Nathaniel Treister

16 Bisphosphonate-related osteonecrosis of the jaws *151*
James Sciubba and Joel Epstein

17 Oral infections – introduction *163*
Susan Brailsford and David Beighton

18 Oral fungal infections *171*
Lakshman Samaranayake and Mohaideen Sitheeque

19 Oral bacterial infections *185*
Anthony Chow

20 Oral viral infections *195*
Deborah Lockhart and Jeremy Bagg

21 Salivary gland dysfunction *203*
Andrew Davies

22 Taste disturbance *225*
Carla Ripamonti and Fabio Fulfaro

23 Halitosis *233*
Stephen Porter

24 Orofacial pain *241*
Paul Farquhar Smith and Joel Epstein

25 Miscellaneous oral problems *253*
Andrew Davies

26 Oral care in paediatric cancer patients *261*
Alessandra Majorana and Fulvio Porta

27 Oral supportive care and the geriatric oncology patient *271*
Ira R. Parker, Joanne E. Mortimer, and Joel Epstein

28 Oral care in advanced cancer patients *279*
Andrew Davies

29 Quality of life and health economics *291*
Jennifer Beaumont, David Cella, and Joshua Epstein

30 Sources of information *301*
Andrew Davies and Joel Epstein

Index *305*

Contributors

Dr Jose Bagan
Professor of Oral Medicine,
Valencia University, Valencia,
Spain

Prof Jeremy Bagg
Professor of Clinical Microbiology,
University of Glasgow Dental School,
Glasgow,
UK

Dr Jennifer Beaumont
Department of Medical Social Sciences,
Northwestern University Feinberg School
of Medicine, Chicago,
USA

Prof David Beighton
Professor of Oral Microbiology,
KCL Dental Institute, London,
UK

Dr Susan Brailsford
Consultant in Epidemiology and
Health Protection,
NHS Blood and Transplant,
London
UK

Dr Mike Brennan
Department of Oral Medicine,
Carolinas Medical Center, Charlotte,
USA

Prof David Cella
Department of Medical Social Sciences,
Northwestern University Feinberg School
of Medicine, Chicago,
USA

Prof Anthony Chow
Division of Infectious Diseases
(Faculty of Medicine),
University of British Columbia, Vancouver,
Canada

Dr Anderson Collier III
Assistant Professor of Pediatric
Hematology/Oncology,
Vanderbilt-Ingram Cancer Center, Nashville,
USA

Dr Andrew Davies
Consultant in Palliative Medicine,
The Royal Marsden Hospital, Sutton,
UK

Prof Pieter Dijkstra
Professor of Clinical Epidemiology,
University Medical Center Groningen,
Groningen,
The Netherlands

Dr Sharon Elad
Department of Oral Medicine,
The Hebrew University-Hadassah School
of Dental Medicine, Jerusalem,
Israel

Prof Joel Epstein
Professor of Oral Medicine,
Otolaryngology and Head and Neck Cancer
University of Illinois at Chicago, Chicago,
USA

Dr Joshua Epstein
Manager Medical Outcomes Research
and Economics,
Baxter Bioscience,
Westlake Village,
USA

Dr Paul Farquhar-Smith
Consultant Anaesthetist,
The Royal Marsden Hospital, Sutton,
UK

Dr Fabio Fulfaro
Department of Surgery and Oncology,
University of Palermo, Palermo,
Italy

Dr Jill Gilbert
Assistant Professor of Medicine,
Vanderbilt-Ingram Cancer Center,
Nashville,
USA

Mr Anthony Giles
General Dental Practitioner,
Tetbury Dental Practice,
Tetbury,
UK

Dr Kevin Harrington
Consultant in Clinical Oncology,
The Royal Marsden Hospital,
London,
UK

Dr Antonia Kolokythas
Assistant Professor of Oral and
Maxillofacial Surgery,
University of Illinois at Chicago,
USA

Dr Rajesh Lalla
Department of Oral Health and Diagnostic
Sciences, School of Dental Medicine,
University of Connecticut Health Center,
Farmington,
USA

Miss Deborah Lockhart
Specialist Registrar in Oral Microbiology,
Glasgow Dental Hospital and School,
Glasgow,
UK

Dr Peter Lockhart
Department of Oral Medicine,
Carolinas Medical Center,
Charlotte,
USA

Prof Alessandra Majorana
Dental Clinic,
Universita degi Studi di Brescia,
Brescia,
Italy

Prof Michael Miloro
Professor of Oral and Maxillofacial Surgery,
University of Illinois at Chicago,
USA

Prof Joanne E. Mortimer
Division of Medical Oncology and
Experimental Therapeutics,
City of Hope Comprehensive Cancer Center,
Duarte,
USA

Dr Barbara Murphy
Associate Professor of Medicine
(Hematology/Oncology),
Vanderbilt-Ingram Cancer Center, Nashville,
USA

Dr Kate Newbold
Consultant in Clinical Oncology,
The Royal Marsden Hospital, Sutton,
UK

Prof Ira R. Parker
Division of Geriatric Medicine,
University of California, San Diego,
USA

Prof Douglas Peterson
Department of Oral Health and Diagnostic
Sciences, School of Dental Medicine,
University of Connecticut Health Center,
Farmington,
USA

Dr Fulvio Porta
Department of Paediatrics,
Universita degi Studi di Brescia,
Brescia,
Italy

Prof Stephen Porter
Professor of Oral Medicine,
UCL Eastman Dental Institute,
London,
UK

Dr Judith Raber-Durlacher
Department of Haematology,
Leiden University Medical Center, Leiden,
The Netherlands

Dr Carla Ripamonti
Rehabilitation and Palliative Care
Operative Unit,
National Cancer Institute of Milan,
Milan,
Italy

Prof Jan Roodenburg
Department of Oral Diseases,
Oral Surgery and Special Dentistry,
University Medical Center Groningen,
Groningen,
The Netherlands

Prof Lakshman Samaranayake
Professor Oral Microbiology,
University of Hong Kong,
Hong Kong

Dr Debbie Saunders
Medical Director,
Department of Dental Oncology,
Sudbury Regional Cancer Program,
Ontario,
Canada

Prof James Sciubba
Professor of Otolaryngology,
Head and Neck Surgery,
Greaater Baltimore Medical Center,
Baltimore,
USA

Prof Crispian Scully
Professor of Oral Medicine,
Pathology and Microbiology,
UCL Eastman Dental Institute,
London,
UK

Dr Anita Sengupta
Specialist Registrar in Dental and
Maxillofacial Radiology,
University Dental School of Manchester,
Manchester,
UK

Dr Michael Y. Shapira
Bone Marrow Transplantation and Cancer
Immunotherapy Department,
Hadassah University Hospital, Jerusalem,
Israel

Prof Sol Silverman
Professor of Oral Medicine,
University of California, San Francisco,
USA

Prof Mohaideen Sitheeque
Professor in Oral Medicine,
University Dental Hospital,
Peradeniya,
Sri Lanka

Prof Stephen Sonis
Department of Oral Medicine and Dentistry,
Brigham and Women's Hospital,
Boston,
USA

Prof Fred Spijkervet
Department of Oral and
Maxillofacial Surgery,
University Medical Center Groningen,
Groningen,
The Netherlands

Dr Peter Stevenson-Moore
Consultant in Oral Oncology,
British Columbia Cancer Agency,
Vancouver,
Canada

Dr Petrina Sweeney
Clinical Senior Lecturer in Adult
Special Care Dentistry,
University of Glasgow Dental School,
Glasgow,
UK

Dr Nathaniel Treister
Department of Oral Medicine and Dentistry,
Brigham and Women's Hospital,
Boston,
USA

Prof Arjan Vissink
Professor of Oral and Maxillofacial Surgery,
University Medical Center Groningen,
Groningen,
The Netherlands

Dr Katherine Webber
Research Fellow in Palliative Medicine,
The Royal Marsden Hospital,
Sutton,
UK

Chapter 1

Introduction

Andrew Davies and Joel Epstein

'to cure sometimes
to relieve often
to comfort always'
(Anonymous, 15th Century A.D.)

Introduction

Oral problems are common in cancer patients, and are a significant cause of morbidity and impaired quality of life in this group of patients[1]. Moreover, in some patients they can prevent administration of potentially life-saving treatment, whilst in other patients they can themselves cause potentially life-threatening complications.

Oral problems are usually predictable, and may be prevented or ameliorated by appropriate interventions[1]. However, even when it is not possible to prevent the oral problem, it is usually possible to treat/palliate the oral problem (and so to prevent or ameliorate the associated complications).

This chapter aims to provide an introduction to the oral complications of cancer and its management, and particularly to highlight the importance/relevance of these problems for patients with cancer.

Epidemiology

The World Health Organization (WHO) and the International Union Against Cancer (UICC) have estimated that in 2002 there were 10.9 million new cases of cancer, 6.7 million deaths from cancer, and 24.6 million people 'living with cancer' worldwide[2]. Furthermore, the WHO and the UICC have predicted that over the next 10–15 years there will be a significant increase in these statistics in all countries, and particularly in newly industrialized and developing countries[2].

The statistics vary from country to country, and often vary within an individual country. For example, the Office of National Statistics (UK) reports that, at present, approximately one in three people will develop cancer during their lifetime, and approximately one in four people will die from cancer in the United Kingdom[3]. However, people living in Scotland have a higher (~15% higher) incidence of cancer, and, not surprisingly, a higher (~15% higher) mortality rate[3].

The Surveillance Epidemiology and End Results Program of the National Cancer Institute (USA) estimates that, in 2008, there will be 1.44 million new cases of cancer, and 0.57 million deaths from cancer in the United States of America (USA)[4]. However, the statistics vary depending on age, gender, and race/ethnicity. For example, older people have a much higher incidence of cancer, and thus a much higher mortality rate. Indeed, the median age at diagnosis is 67 years, and the median age at death is 73 year (Figure 1.1)[4].

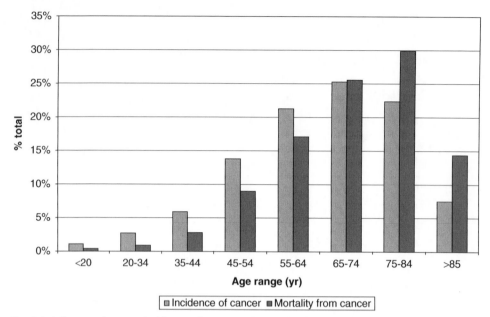

Fig. 1.1 Influence of age on incidence of cancer and mortality from cancer in United States of America.

The epidemiology of oral problems is discussed in the next section of this chapter, and also in the relevant sections of other chapters in the book.

Aetiology

Oral problems may develop in response to a variety of individual factors, or a combination of factors (Box 1.1). Thus, oral problems may develop in patients with any type of cancer, with any stage of disease, and receiving any type of cancer treatment (or no cancer treatment).

Effect of the cancer

Oral problems may result from a direct effect of the tumour (i.e. tumour within the oral cavity or surrounding tissues), or, more commonly, from an indirect effect of the tumour (i.e. tumour distant from the oral cavity or surrounding tissues). Moreover, oral problems may sometimes represent paraneoplastic syndromes, i.e. 'pathological conditions that are caused by a cancer but not brought about directly by local infiltration or metastatic spread'[5]. Examples, of relevant paraneoplastic syndromes, include bullous pemphigoid (associated with non-Hodgkin's lymphoma and chronic lymphocytic leukaemia)[6], and salivary gland dysfunction (associated with non-Hodgkin's lymphoma)[7].

Primary tumours of the oral cavity and surrounding tissues are relatively uncommon in the developed world (see Chapters 7 and 8). Such tumours may develop from any tissue, and usually represent a localized malignant process, although sometimes they represent a more generalized malignant process (e.g. acute myeloid leukaemia, non-Hodgkin's lymphoma). Secondary tumours of the oral cavity and surrounding tissues (with the notable exception of the lymph nodes) are extremely uncommon throughout the world[8].

Box 1.1 Aetiology of oral problems in patients with cancer.

- Direct effect of the cancer*
- Indirect effect of the cancer**
- Direct effect of the cancer treatment*
- Indirect effect of the cancer treatment**
- Direct/indirect effect of supportive care interventions*/**
- Related to coexistent oral condition
- Related to coexistent other physical condition
- Related to coexistent psychological condition
- Direct/indirect effect of interventions for other condition */**
- Combination of factors

* 'Local' effect
** 'Systemic' effect

Cancer can cause oral problems via a number of indirect mechanisms. For example, bone marrow infiltration may result in pancytopenia, which may manifest as gingival haemorrhage (secondary to thrombocytopenia), and/or mucosal infection (secondary to leucopenia)[1]. Moreover, cancer-related physical disabilities (e.g. fatigue, pain) may affect the patient's ability to undertake routine oral hygiene measures, which, in turn, may lead to a variety of oral problems[1].

Effect of the cancer treatment

A number of different modalities are used in the management of cancer, including surgery, radiotherapy (radiation therapy), chemotherapy, hormone therapy, and biological therapy. All of these modalities can produce oral complications, although some are more relevant than others (e.g. chemotherapy, head and neck radiotherapy). Indeed, the National Cancer Institutes estimates that 10% of patients receiving adjuvant chemotherapy, 40% of patients receiving primary chemotherapy, 80% of patients receiving myeloablative chemotherapy (i.e. during haematopoietic stem cell transplantation), and all patients receiving head and neck radiotherapy will develop oral complications[1].

The common oral complications of conventional chemotherapy are shown in Table 1.1, and discussed in more detail in Chapter 13. The oral complications of chemotherapy may be secondary to a local effect and/or a systemic effect of the treatment. For example, oral infections can be related both to the local effects of chemotherapy (i.e. mucositis), and also to the systemic effects of the chemotherapy (i.e. leucopenia)[1]. The common oral complications of head and neck radiotherapy are shown in Table 1.2, and discussed in more detail in Chapter 10. The oral complications of radiotherapy are invariably the result of a local effect of the treatment. Interestingly, the new 'targeted' therapies are also associated with oral side effects (Tables 1.3 and 1.4)[9].

Effect of supportive care interventions

Many drugs are associated with oral complications[10], including many supportive care/palliative care drugs (e.g. bisphosphonates, analgesics)[11,12]. Indeed, some of the drugs used

Table 1.1 Oral complications of chemotherapy [1].

Complication	Comment
Oral mucositis	Acute complication
Oral infections ♦ viral ♦ fungal ♦ bacterial	Acute complication
Taste disturbance	Acute complication
Salivary gland dysfunction	Acute complication
Neuropathy	Acute complication Jaw pain may occur with vinca alkaloids
Haemorrhage	Acute complication Haemorrhage may occur with oral mucositis, oral infections and/or thrombocytopenia
Dental/skeletal developmental problems	Chronic complication Occurs in paediatric patients
Induction of second malignancy	Chronic complication

to manage oral problems can themselves cause other oral problems. For example, chlorhexidine may cause discolouration of the tongue, discolouration of the teeth (dental restorations/dental prostheses), taste disturbance, 'burning' sensation of the tongue, oral desquamation, and swelling of the parotid glands (very uncommon)[9]. Similarly, palifermin, which is recommended for the prevention of oral mucositis in patients undergoing autologous haematopoietic stem cell transplantation[13], may cause taste disturbance (>10% patients), thickening or discolouration of the tongue/oral mucosa (>10% patients), and oedema of the tongue/oral mucosa (very uncommon)[9].

Table 1.2 Oral complications of head and neck radiation therapy [1].

Complication	Comment
Oral mucositis	Acute complication
Oral infections ♦ fungal ♦ bacterial	Acute/chronic complication
Taste disturbance	Acute/chronic complication
Salivary gland dysfunction	Acute/chronic complication
Osteonecrosis	Chronic complication
Soft tissue necrosis	Chronic complication
Soft tissue fibrosis	Chronic complication Trismus may result from fibrosis of muscles of mastication and/or temporomandibular joint
Dental/skeletal developmental problems	Chronic complication Occurs in paediatric patients
Induction of second malignancy	Chronic complication

Table 1.3 Oral complications of selected novel chemotherapy agents [9].

Drug	'Very common' side effects (≥ 1/10 patients)	'Common' side effects (≥ 1/100–1/10 patients)	'Uncommon' side effects (≥ 1/1000–1/100 patients)	Comments
Bortezomib – proteasome inhibitor	–	Mucositis Oral ulcers Taste disturbance Xerostomia	Oral pain Jaw pain Gingival haemorrhage Coated tongue Discoloured tongue Hypersalivation	
Dasatinib – protein kinase inhibitor	(Superficial oedema)	Mucositis Taste disturbance	–	Superficial oedema is very common problem, including oral oedema.
Erlotinib – protein kinase inhibitor	Mucositis	–	–	
Imatinib – protein kinase inhibitor	–	Taste disturbance Xerostomia	Mucositis Oral ulcers	
Sorafenib – protein kinase inhibitor	(Pain)	Mucositis (Xerostomia) (Glossodynia)	–	Pain is very common problem, including oral pain. Xerostomia and glossodynia were included in 'stomatitis' subcategory.
Sunitinib – protein kinase inhibitor	Mucositis Taste disturbance Glossodynia	Xerostomia Oral pain	–	

Table 1.4 Oral complications of selected novel biological agents [9].

Drug	'Very common' side effects (≥ 1/10 patients)	'Common' side effects (≥ 1/100–1/10 patients)	'Uncommon' side effects (≥ 1/1000–1/100 patients)	Comments
bevacizumab – monoclonal Ab against VEGF	Mucositis Taste disturbance	(Haemorrhage)	–	Haemorrhage is common problem, including gingival haemorrhage
Cetuximab – monoclonal Ab against EGFR	Mucositis	–	–	
Trastuzumab – monoclonal Ab against HER2	Mucositis Taste disturbance	Xerostomia	–	
Alemtuzumab – monoclonal Ab against CD52 Ag (B & T lymphocytes)	–	Mucositis Taste disturbance Oral candidosis Oral oedema	Xerostomia Oral discomfort Gingivitis Gingival haemorrhage Tongue ulcers	
Rituximab – monoclonal Ab against CD20 Ag (B lymphocytes)	–	Mucositis	Taste disturbance	

Ab = antibody

Ag = antigen

VEGR = vascular endothelial growth factor

EGFR = epidermal growth factor receptor

HER2 = human epidermal growth factor receptor 2

Effect of co-existent oral conditions

Patients with cancer may have co-existent oral conditions, which may predispose/aggravate cancer-related oral problems (e.g. poor oral hygiene, dental caries)[1]. Indeed, clinical guidelines invariably recommend the treatment of pre-existing oral conditions prior to the initiation of chemotherapy or head and neck radiotherapy[1].

Effects of co-existent physical conditions

Many patients with cancer will have co-existent physical conditions, which may predispose/ aggravate cancer-related oral problems. For example, diabetes mellitus is associated with various oral infections (e.g. oral candidosis, periodontal disease)[14]. Physical conditions may also impact on the patient's ability to undertake oral hygiene measures, and many drugs used to treat these conditions are themselves associated with oral complications[10].

Effects of co-existent psychological/psychiatric conditions

Many patients with cancer will also have co-existent psychological problems, which again may predispose/aggravate cancer-related oral problems. For example, depression is associated with salivary gland dysfunction[15]. Psychological/psychiatric conditions may also impact on the patient's interest or ability to undertake oral hygiene measures[15], and many drugs used to treat these conditions are themselves associated with oral complications[10].

Combination of factors

In many patients, there is more than one factor responsible for the development/maintenance of the relevant oral problem.

Clinical features

Oral problems cause morbidity *per se*, although the impact of oral problems varies from individual to individual[16]. Thus, some oral problems are short lived, mild in intensity, and not associated with significant distress. However, other oral problems are long-lasting, severe in intensity, and associated with significant distress (e.g. radiotherapy-related salivary gland dysfunction). Importantly, some mundane oral problems (e.g. taste disturbance) can have as much/greater impact than some dramatic oral problems (e.g. oral mucositis). It should be noted that patients frequently do not report the presence of oral problems, even if these oral problems are the source of significant morbidity[17].

Oral problems also cause morbidity through the development of various complications. For example, salivary gland dysfunction is associated with a number of physical (e.g. taste disturbance), psychological (e.g. low mood), and social complications (e.g. social isolation)[12,18]. Oral problems can also result in mortality through the development of serious complications. For example, oral infection can, in certain circumstances, progress to systemic infection[19]. In addition, oral problems may lead to reduction, prolongation, and/or discontinuation of the anticancer treatment, and so ultimately may lead to a reduction in the success of the anticancer treatment[20].

The clinical features of the various oral problems are discussed in detail in the following chapters.

Management

The standard of care in the management of cancer, and the management of cancer-related oral problems, involves the utilization of multi-disciplinary teams (MDTs) and the adoption of evidence-based guidelines. Certain cancer patients are at particular risk of oral complications, and these cancer patients tend to receive intensive oral care support (e.g. patients receiving myeloablative chemotherapy, patients receiving head and neck radiotherapy). However, all cancer patients are at risk of oral complications, and so all cancer patients should be given appropriate oral care support.

Oral care should be the concern of all members of the MDT, although some members will have specific roles in the prevention/management of oral problems (e.g. dentists, dental hygienists). It is vital that experienced oral care specialists are involved in the training of non-specialists, and, importantly, in the development of understandable local care pathways and treatment guidelines. (Studies suggest that oncology specialists receive little training in oral care/oral problems, and so have limited confidence in providing oral care/treating oral problems)[21,22].

Prophylaxis is as important an aspect of management as treatment. Thus, patients should be assessed by members of the MDT for pre-existing oral problems that may compromise cancer treatment and/or exacerbate the oral complications of cancer treatment[1]. Furthermore, patients should be given appropriate instructions on how to maintain oral hygiene, and when and how to report new oral problems. Nevertheless, patients should be routinely re-assessed by members of the MDT for new oral problems.

The management of cancer-related oral problems should (whenever possible) be based upon evidence-based, cancer-specific oral care guidelines. However, individual patients require individualized treatment, and informed decision-making about treatment depends on good communication within the MDT (i.e. between the oncology team and the dental/oral medicine team), and also between the MDT and the patient and their carers. Thus, the decision to undertake a specific intervention depends on a variety of cancer-related factors (type of cancer, stage of cancer), cancer treatment-related factors (type of treatment, date of treatment), and patient-related factors (e.g. performance status, likelihood of adherence).

The management of the various oral problems is discussed in detail in the following chapters.

References

1 National Cancer Institute (2008). Oral complications of chemotherapy and head/neck radiation. Health Professional Version. Available from NCI website: http://www.cancer.gov/cancertopics/pdq/supportivecare/oralcomplications/healthprofessional

2 World Health Organization and International Union Against Cancer (2005). Global action against cancer. Available from WHO website: http://www.who.int/topics/cancer/en/

3 Office for National Statistics (UK) website: http://www.statistics.gov.uk/

4 Surveillance Epidemiology and End Results Program of the National Cancer Institute (USA) website: http://www.seer.cancer.gov/

5 Smith IE, de Boer RH (2002). Paraneoplastic syndromes other than metabolic, in Souhami RL, Tannock I, Hohenberger P, Horiot J-C (eds) Oxford Textbook of Oncology, 2nd edn, pp. 933–58. Oxford University Press, Oxford.

6 Helm TN, Camisa C, Valenzuela R, Allen CM (1993). Paraneoplastic pemphigus. A distinct autoimmune vesiculobullous disorder associated with neoplasia. Oral Surg Oral Med Oral Pathol, 75(2), 209–13.

7 Folli F, Ponzoni M, Vicari AM (1997). Paraneoplastic autoimmune xerostomia. Ann Intern Med, 127(2), 167–8.

8 Zachariades N (1989). Neoplasms metastatic to the mouth, jaws and surrounding tissues. J Craniomaxillofac Surg, 17(6), 283–90.

9 Electronic Medicines Compendium (UK) website: http://emc.medicines.org.uk

10   Smith RG, Burtner AP (1994). Oral side-effects of the most frequently prescribed drugs. *Spec Care Dentist*, 14(3), 96–102.

11   Migliorati CA, Siegel MA, Elting LS (2006). Bisphosphonate-associated osteonecrosis: a long-term complication of bisphosphonate treatment. *Lancet Oncol* 7(6), 508–14.

12   Davies AN, Broadley K, Beighton D (2002). Salivary gland hypofunction in patients with advanced cancer. *Oral Oncol*, 38(7), 680–5.

13   Keefe DM, Schubert MM, Elting LS (2007). Updated clinical practice guidelines for the prevention and treatment of mucositis. *Cancer*, 109(5), 820–31.

14   Skamagas M, Breen TL, LeRoith D (2008). Update on diabetes mellitus: prevention, treatment, and association with oral diseases. *Oral Dis*, 14(2), 105–14.

15   Friedlander AH, Mahler ME (2001). Major depressive disorder. Psychopathology, medical management and dental implications. *J Am Dent Assoc*, 132(5), 629–38.

16   Portenoy RK, Thaler HT, Kornblith AB, et al. (1994). The Memorial Symptom Assessment Scale: an instrument for the evaluation of symptom prevalence, characteristics and distress. *Eur J Cancer*, 30A(9), 1326–36.

17   Shah S, Davies AN (2001). Medical records vs. patient self-rating. *J Pain Symptom Manage*, 22, 805–6.

18   Rydholm M, Strang P (2002). Physical and psychosocial impact of xerostomia in palliative cancer care: a qualitative interview study. *Int J Palliat Nurs*, 8(7), 318–23.

19   Meurman JH, Pyrhonen S, Teerenhovi L, Lindqvist C (1997). Oral sources of septicaemia in patients with malignancies. *Oral Oncol*, 33(6), 389–97.

20   Rosenthal DI (2007). Consequences of mucositis-induced treatment breaks and dose reductions on head and neck cancer treatment outcomes. *J Support Oncol*, 5(9Suppl4), 23–31.

21   Ohrn KE, Wahlin YB, Sjoden PO (2000). Oral care in cancer nursing. *Eur J Cancer Care*, 9(1), 22–9.

22   Southern H (2007). Oral care in cancer nursing: nurses' knowledge and education. *J Adv Nurs*, 57(6), 631–8.

Chapter 2

The oral cavity

Anita Sengupta and Anthony Giles

Introduction

The boundaries of the oral cavity comprise the lips anteriorly, the cheeks laterally, the pillars of fauces posteriorly, the hard and soft palate superiorly, and the floor of mouth inferiorly (Figure 2.1). The contents of the oral cavity include the alveolar processes, the teeth, the tongue, and the ducts of the major and minor salivary glands. The anatomy of these structures will be discussed in more detail in the following sections. The major functions of the oral cavity are communication (verbal and non-verbal), nutrition, and respiration. The role of various structures in these major functions will also be discussed in greater detail in the following sections.

The pillars of fauces

The pillars of fauces (Figure 2.1) are musculo-mucosal folds connecting the soft palate to the root of tongue anteriorly (the palatoglossal fold), and to the wall of the pharynx posteriorly (the palatopharyngeal fold). The palatine tonsils are found in a triangular area (the tonsillar fossa) between the palatoglossal and palatopharyngeal folds. The palatine tonsils contain lymphoid tissue, are part of the lymphatic/immune system, and are thought to be involved in the regulation of infections of the pharynx and upper respiratory tract. The palatine tonsils are often simply referred to as the 'tonsils'.

The palate

The hard palate (Figure 2.1) is formed by the palatine processes of the maxillary bone and the horizontal plates of the palatine bones. It separates the oral cavity from the nasal cavity. The hard palate is involved in speech production. A small bulge of tissue (the incisive papilla) is present in the anterior midline of the hard palate, and represents the site where the nasopalatine nerve exits the base of skull. Either side of the midline are a number of raised projections called rugae, which provide additional areas for grinding of food during mastication.

The soft palate is formed by the tendinous aponeurosis of tensor palati muscle, fibres of the tensor palati/levator palati muscles, and lymphatic tissue. It separates the oral cavity from the nasopharynx. The soft palate is involved in swallowing function (closes off the nasal passages), speech production, and also the 'gag reflex'. The muscular uvula hangs in the midline between left and right pillars of fauces. There are many normal variations in the shape of the vault of the palate. However, a high arched palate is a characteristic feature of Marfan's syndrome.

The alveolar processes

The maxilla and mandible have bony extensions that provide sockets for the teeth (the dental alveoli). The individual dental alveoli fuse together to form a continuous alveolar process (Figure 2.1).

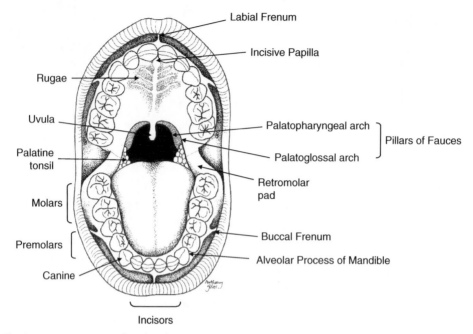

Fig. 2.1 Gross anatomy of oral cavity.

The soft tissue behind the last molar tooth in the lower alveolar process (the mandibular dental arch) is called the retromolar pad. The upper alveolar process (the maxillary dental arch) expands posteriorly into the maxillary tuberosity. The alveolar processes are called alveolar ridges in edentulous patients. (The alveolar processes start to resorb when permanent teeth are lost/removed.)

The alveolar processes divide the oral cavity into the vestibule/sulcus (located outside the alveolar processes), and the oral cavity proper (located inside the alveolar processes). The vestibule is interrupted by frena/frenula: these are cords of mucous membrane, which sometimes contain muscle fibres, which extend from the lips or cheeks onto the alveolar processes. Frena may cause spacing between teeth (diastema), and are susceptible to trauma (e.g. from overzealous toothbrushing).

The teeth

There are four different morphological types of tooth in the human dentition: (1) incisors; (2) canines; (3) premolars; and (4) molars. The first two types are used for tearing food, whilst the latter two types are used for grinding food.

Humans have evolved two sets of dentition: a deciduous or primary ('baby') set, which is fully replaced by a larger permanent or secondary ('adult') set by the age of 12 years. The deciduous dentition comprises two incisors, one canine, and two molars in each quadrant of the jaws (i.e. 20 teeth in total). There are an additional two premolars and one molar (third molar – 'wisdom tooth') in the adult quadrants (i.e. 32 teeth in total). A variety of teeth-numbering schemes are in clinical use, including the FDI World Dental Federation notation, the Palmer notation/Zsigmondy system (especially in the UK), and the Universal numbering system (especially in the USA).

The third molar tooth is frequently missing from the dental arcade. It may have failed to develop, or be partially erupted or impacted in the jawbone. Other teeth that are often missing are the upper second incisors, and the lower second premolars. In such instances, the deciduous predecessors may have been retained. Hypodontia is a condition in which even fewer teeth have erupted, and may be associated with certain congenital syndromes. Supernumerary (additional) teeth may occur sporadically, or again be associated with certain congenital syndromes. Such teeth may resemble normal teeth (supplemental), or have a disordered morphology.

The crown of the tooth is visible in the oral cavity, whilst the root of the tooth is contained within the alveolar bone (Figure 2.2). Most teeth have a single root, but molars have two or three roots. The tooth narrows between crown and root at the cervix ('neck'). The gingiva (gum) is the soft tissue above the alveolar bone, and there is a small (2–3 mm in depth) crevice/sulcus between it and the tooth. The periodontal ligament is the specialized connective tissue that attaches the tooth to the alveolar bone. The periodontal ligament is a proprioceptive organ, and has an important role in the regulation of mastication. Deepening of the gingival crevice, or bleeding from it, indicates active inflammation of the gingiva (gingivitis) or of the periodontal ligament (periodontitis).

The bulk of the tooth is made up of dentine, which is composed of tubules that provide the tooth with its strength and resilience (Figure 2.2). The dentine is a living mineralized tissue, and the cells (odontoblasts) reside at the bottom of each tubule within the dental pulp. The dental pulp is the soft-tissue component of the tooth, and contains the blood vessels, lymphatics, and nerves. The pulp cavity extends into the root of the tooth (to form the root canal). In the crown, the dentine is covered by enamel. Enamel is a non-living tissue, which is highly mineralized (95%), and so is very tough in nature. In the root, the dentine is covered by a thin layer of cementum.

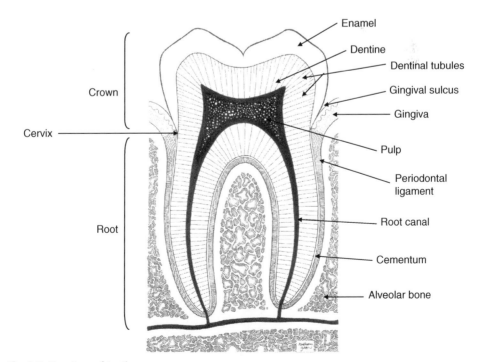

Fig. 2.2 Structure of teeth.

Cementum is another living mineralized tissue, which contains fibres that hold the tooth in the alveolar bone.

The floor of mouth

In the midline, a prominent frenum (the lingual frenum) extends from the alveolar process to the floor of mouth, and from there to the ventral surface of the tongue (Figure 2.3). The mucosa of the floor of mouth is raised on either side by the sublingual folds, which contain the two sublingual salivary glands, which drain through a series of ducts on the summit of the sublingual fold. Similarly, the mucosa of the floor of mouth is raised on either side of the lingual frenum by the sublingual papillae, which contain the ducts of the submandibular glands (the Wharton ducts). Saliva pools in the floor of mouth, and so the mucosa of the floor of mouth should be moist and glistening (at normal salivary flow rates).

The tongue

The ventral surface of the tongue reveals the deep lingual veins, and more laterally the fimbriated (fringed) folds (Figure 2.3). The deep lingual veins often develop varicosities with increasing age.

The dorsal surface of the tongue is divided into the body or anterior two-thirds, and the base or posterior third (Figure 2.4). The boundary is seen as a 'V'- shaped line called the sulcus terminalis. At the apex of the 'V' is a depression (the foramen caecum), which is the site of origin of the thyroid gland prior to its descent into the neck. In a small percentage of people, functional thyroid tissue remains at this site ('lingual thyroid').

The mucosa of the anterior two-thirds of the tongue is not smooth, but is covered in tiny projections known as papillae. The thread-like (filiform) papillae are scattered widely and provide a 'rasping' surface to aid mastication. The other papillae carry taste buds: (1) fungiform papillae – these pale-red, mushroom-shaped papillae are less numerous, and are loosely scattered between the filiform papillae; (2) foliate papillae – these leaf-shaped papillae appear as ridges on the posterior edges of the tongue; and (3) circumvallate papillae – these rampart-shaped papillae appear as large circular structures anterior to the sulcus terminalis.

The innervation of the tongue is complicated, as it is formed from different embryological structures, each supplied by a different cranial nerve (Table 2.1).

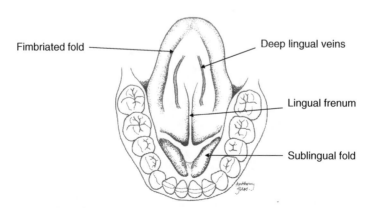

Fig. 2.3 Gross anatomy of floor of mouth.

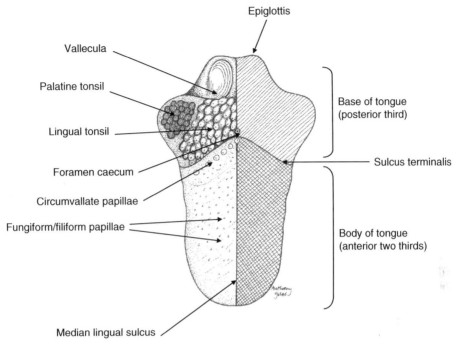

Fig. 2.4 Gross anatomy of dorsum of tongue.

Salivary glands

The mouth is covered with secretions from the three pairs of major salivary glands (parotid, submandibular, and sublingual) located within the head and neck area, and the numerous minor salivary glands located within the oral mucosa. The physiology of the salivary glands, the composition of saliva, and the functions of saliva are discussed in detail in Chapter 21.

The ducts of minor salivary glands may become blocked, resulting in retention of the secretions and swelling of the gland. These swellings are known as mucocoeles, and occur frequently in the lips and floor of mouth.

Nervous innervation of oral cavity

The sensory innervation to the oral mucosa and teeth is provided by branches of the trigeminal (Vth cranial) nerve. Figure 2.6 shows the regional innervation of the oral cavity. The trigeminal nerve also innervates the muscles of mastication (e.g. masseter, medial pterygoid).

Table 2.1 Nervous innervation of the tongue

Area of tongue	Normal sensation (touch, pain, and temperature)	Special sensation (taste)	Motor function
Anterior two-thirds	Lingual nerve (branch of V cranial nerve)	Chorda tympani (VII cranial nerve via lingual nerve)	Hypoglossal nerve (XII cranial nerve)
Posterior third	Glossopharyngeal nerve (IX cranial nerve)	Vagus nerve (X cranial nerve)	Hypoglossal nerve (XII cranial nerve) except palatoglossus muscle (IX and X cranial nerves)

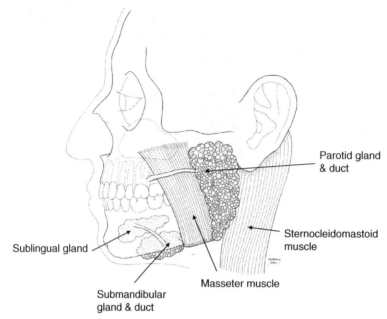

Fig. 2.5 Gross anatomy of major salivary glands.

Parotid gland & duct

Sternocleidomastoid muscle

Masseter muscle

Submandibular gland & duct

Sublingual gland

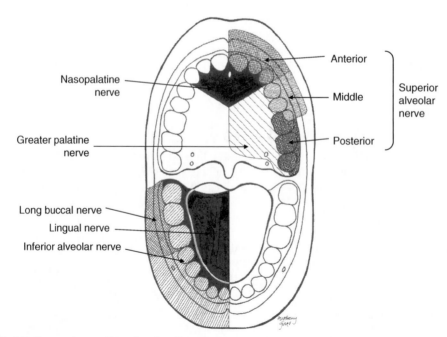

Fig. 2.6 Nervous innervation of oral cavity.

Anterior

Middle

Posterior

Superior alveolar nerve

Nasopalatine nerve

Greater palatine nerve

Long buccal nerve

Lingual nerve

Inferior alveolar nerve

Table 2.2 Anatomy of the salivary glands

Salivary gland	Location	Location of intraoral duct	Pre-ganglionic nerve	Post-ganglionic nerve	Type of secretion
Parotid glands (2)	Side of face (anterior to tragus of ear).	Parotid duct connects via parotid papilla (in the cheek, opposite the upper second molar tooth)	Glossopharyngeal (IX) nerve	Trigeminal (V) nerve	Mainly serous (90%)
Submandibular glands (2)	Submandibular triangle of neck (around mylohyoid muscle)	Wharton's duct connects via sublingual papilla (in the floor of mouth, behind lower incisor teeth).	Facial (VII) nerve	Trigeminal (V) nerve	Mucinous + serous
Sublingual glands (2)	Floor of mouth	Numerous ducts connect via sublingual folds. Wharton's duct also collects some sublingual secretions.	Facial (VII) nerve	Trigeminal (V) nerve	Mainly mucinous
Minor salivary glands (numerous)	Distributed throughout oral mucosa	Secrete directly/locally into oral cavity.	Facial (VII) nerve	Trigeminal (V) nerve	Mucinous

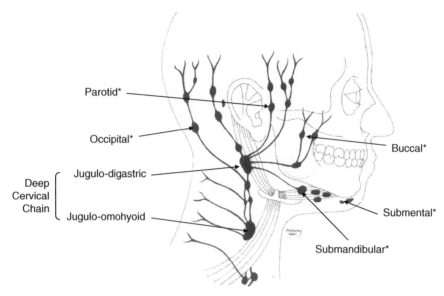

Parotid*
Occipital*
Buccal*
Jugulo-digastric
Deep Cervical Chain
Jugulo-omohyoid
Submental*
Submandibular*

*Superficial group of lymph nodes

Fig. 2.7 Lymphatic drainage of head and neck region.

Special sensory innervation, such as taste sensation, is supplied by the facial (VIIth cranial) nerve 'hitch-hiking' in branches of the trigeminal nerve. The facial nerve also innervates the muscles of facial expression (e.g. buccinator, orbicularis oris).

The parasympathetic nervous supply to the salivary glands is shown in Table 2.2. The sympathetic nervous supply to the salivary glands (and other intraoral tissues) is derived from the cervical sympathetic chain.

Vasculature/lymphatic drainage of the oral cavity

The arterial system of the oral cavity is via branches of the lingual, facial, and maxillary arteries, which in turn are all branches of the external carotid artery.

Extracellular fluid (ECF) from the superficial tissues passes through the superficial group of lymph nodes, through the deep cervical lymph nodes (deep cervical chain), and then into the systemic circulation via the right and left jugular trunks (Figure 2.7). ECF from the deep tissues passes directly through the deep cervical lymph nodes, and then into the systemic circulation via the right and left jugular trunks.

The posterior-third of the tongue contains raised mounds of lymphatic tissue (the lingual tonsil) (Figure 2.4). This is one of the four lymphatic elements, collectively known as Waldeyer's ring, that encircle the entrance to the oropharynx. The other elements are the palatine tonsils, pharyngeal tonsils (the adenoids), and tubal tonsils found at the entrance of the auditory tube.

References

1 Berkovitz BK, Holland GR, Moxham BJ (2002). *Oral Anatomy, histology and embryology*, 3rd edn. Mosby, London.
2 Ellis H (2006). *Clinical anatomy*, 11th edn. Blackwell Publishing, Oxford.

3 Nanci A (2007). *Ten Cate's oral histology: development, structure, and function*, 7th edn. Mosby, London.

4 Sinnatamby CS (2006). *Last's anatomy: regional and applied*, 11th edn. Churchill-Livingstone, Edinburgh.

5 Scully C (2008). *Oral and maxillofacial medicine: the basis of diagnosis and treatment*, 2nd edn. Churchill-Livingstone, Edinburgh.

6 Edgar WM, O'Mullane DM (1996). *Saliva and oral health*, 2nd edn. British Dental Association, London.

Chapter 3

Oral assessment

Michael Brennan and Peter Lockhart

Introduction

Oral assessment is fundamental to the management of patients with cancer. Thus, oral problems may occur in any patient with cancer, although they especially occur in patients with selected cancers (e.g. head and neck cancer)[1]. Oral problems may be related to the cancer itself, the cancer treatment, a concomitant condition, or a combination of these factors.

Assessment of the health of the oral cavity should be performed on an ongoing/regular basis, i.e. before, during, and following any cancer therapy. Indeed, oral problems can occur at any stage of the disease, and can even occur in patients 'cured' of the disease. All members of the multi-disciplinary team have a role to play in the assessment of oral problems, with oral specialists being involved in the assessment of patients with specific oral problems.

Oral assessment involves taking a detailed history, performing a thorough examination, and the use of appropriate investigations[2]. The aim of assessment is to identify both established oral problems and treatable factors associated with the development of oral problems (e.g. poor oral hygiene). Thus, the early identification of oral problems, and initiation of appropriate treatment strategies, may minimize the impact of such oral problems.

It is important that oral assessments are performed in a suitable location, and in an appropriate manner. The patient should be afforded a degree of privacy, made comfortable prior to the assessment, and made aware of the nature of the assessment (and provide verbal consent for the assessment). Universal infection control measures should be employed, with healthcare professionals wearing gloves when performing intraoral examinations, including when handling intraoral prostheses[3].

Oral history

The history should include questions about the most common oral symptoms (Table 3.1). However, patients may experience other oral symptoms. Thus, patients should be encouraged to report 'any other problems' relating to the oral cavity. Patients with oral prostheses should be asked specifically about associated problems (i.e. discomfort, poor fitting).

It is insufficient to simply ask about the presence of a symptom. The format of additional questioning will depend on the nature of the symptoms. For example, if a patient presents with pain, then the following parameters are useful to establish a diagnosis: CHaracter, Location, Onset, Radiation, Intensity, Duration, and Exacerbating factors ('CHLORIDE' mnemonic).

In addition to assessing current oral symptoms, it is important to determine previous oral/dental problems (and treatments). Similarly, enquiries should be made concerning factors that may influence the development of oral problems (e.g. current/proposed anticancer treatment, concurrent medical conditions, concurrent medical treatments)[1].

Table 3.1 Common oral symptoms in patients with cancer

- Oral discomfort/pain
- Dry mouth (xerostomia)
- Taste disturbance
- Difficulty chewing (dysmasesia)
- Difficulty swallowing (dysphagia)
- Difficulty speaking (dysphonia)
- Bleeding
- Bad breath (halitosis)
- Difficulty opening mouth (trismus)

Oral examination

A systematic examination of the extra- and intraoral tissues is necessary to fully assess oral diseases and cancer treatment-related oral complications.

Extraoral examination

A thorough examination includes inspection for asymmetry, swelling, or skin lesions in the head and neck region. Similarly, it includes palpation of the lymph nodes, the salivary glands, neck muscles, and the temporomandibular joint and muscles of mastication. Cranial nerve function should also be evaluated.

Lymph nodes in the submental, submandibular, and cervical chains should be assessed for the presence of tenderness, texture, and mobility or fixation. A non-tender and fixed lymph node is a common finding in metastatic head and neck tumours, while tender and freely movable nodes are more likely to represent an infectious or inflammatory process.

Salivary glands should be palpated for tenderness or masses. The parotid glands are located below the ear near the angle of the mandible, while the submandibular and sublingual glands are located between the inferior borders of the mandible (see Chapter 2, Figure 2.5). The submandibular and sublingual gland can be evaluated by bimanual palpation with one finger over the floor of the mouth and the other finger under the mandible.

Table 3.2 Terminology of oral mucosal lesions [2]

Term	Description
Erythema	Red colouration
Erosion	Partial thickness loss of epithelium (underlying connective tissue not exposed)
Ulcer	Full thickness loss of epithelium (underlying connective tissue exposed)
Papule	Small, well-defined, elevated area
Plaque	Large, well-defined, elevated area
Vesicle	Well-defined accumulation of fluid within/beneath epithelium (<5mm in diameter)
Bulla	Well-defined accumulation of fluid within/beneath epithelium (>5mm in diameter)
Sinus	Blind-ending tract
Fistula	Connecting tract (between two epithelial surfaces)

The temporomandibular joint should be evaluated for the presence of clicking, pain to palpation, and limitations or deviations in jaw opening.

Intraoral examination

The intraoral examination includes a thorough inspection of the soft tissues, saliva, hard tissues (i.e. teeth), periodontal tissues, and any removable prostheses.

The examination includes a systematic inspection of the following soft-tissue locations: lips, buccal mucosa, floor of mouth, tongue, palate, and oropharynx (Figure 3.1, see colour plate section). Areas of erythema, white patches, erosions, ulcers, haemorrhages, masses, or other lesions should be noted (Table 3.2). Maxillary and mandibular tori are common findings and represent a variation of normal anatomy (Figure 3.2, see colour plate section). Tongue mobility should also be evaluated.

The presence, colour, and consistency of saliva expressed from the major salivary gland orifices should be assessed. A thick, cloudy, or purulent discharge may represent a bacterial infection of the relevant salivary gland.

An assessment of the dentition should include an examination for presence of plaque, calculus ('tartar'), fractures, mobility, dental caries, restorations ('fillings'), and any swellings or draining sinuses adjacent to restorations (most likely related to dental infection) (Figure 3.3, see colour plate section).

Periodontal health is represented by a pink gingiva with no evidence of plaque or calculus (Figure 3.3). On the other hand, poor periodontal health is usually represented by an erythematous, 'boggy' gingiva that bleeds easily with manipulation. Periodontal disease is commonly associated with the presence of plaque or calculus, and mobility of the teeth.

Removable prostheses are commonly used to restore oral function in patients who have lost teeth. A full denture replaces all remaining teeth in an edentulous (without any teeth) maxillary or mandibular arch, while a partial denture will restore function to a partially edentulous arch. The retention, stability, and tissue health under removable appliances should be evaluated.

Investigations

A wide range of investigations is used in Oral Medicine[2]. The decision to perform an investigation will depend on the nature of the problem, the nature of the investigation (i.e. non-invasive or not), the likely outcome of the investigation (i.e. management altered or not), and the condition of the patient. The role of specific investigations is discussed in subsequent chapters.

Radiographic examination

Dental radiographs (X-rays) are a vital test to evaluate dental and periodontal disease. Ideally, the dentist should have imaging of the complete dental structure including the supporting bone of the teeth. This may involve a full-mouth series (FMS) of radiographs or a panoramic radiograph (OPG: orthopantogram).

Microbial testing

The need and type of microbial testing will depend on the clinical suspicion of the type of infection:

- ♦ Bacterial infection – the presence of swelling and purulence would be suggestive of a bacterial infection, and aerobic and anaerobic cultures of purulent discharge will help determine the appropriate antibiotic regimen.

- Fungal infections – can have the following clinical appearances: a plaque that can be rubbed off with gauze (pseudomembranous candidosis); a red lesion (erythematous candidosis); a white lesion that does not rub off (hyperplastic candidosis); or redness and cracking at the corners of mouth (angular cheilitis). Diagnostic tests for fungal infections include cytology smears, culture, or biopsy[4]. Certain oral infections, such as pseudomembranous candidosis, are often treated on the basis of a clinical diagnosis, with diagnostic tests only undertaken for non-responsive lesions.
- Viral infection – can appear as blistering and/or ulcerated, erythematous lesions. Testing for viral infection may include cytology smears and cultures. Biopsy is less commonly used for herpes simplex virus and varicella zoster virus, but may be required for diagnosis of cyto-megalovirus or Epstein–Barr virus infection[4,5].

Salivary flow-rate measurement

In certain circumstances, it may be appropriate to measure salivary flow rates ('sialometry'), and even analyse saliva composition ('sialochemistry'). However, salivary gland hypofunction can invariably be elicited by asking questions such a: Do you sip liquids to aid in swallowing dry foods? Does your mouth feel dry when eating a meal? Do you have difficulties swallowing any foods? Does the amount of saliva in your mouth seem to be too little or too much – or don't you notice it?[6].

The technique for measuring unstimulated whole salivary flow rate involves spitting all saliva produced during a 5-min period into a pre-weighed test tube. Due to diurnal variations in saliva flow, collections are usually completed in the morning hours. In addition, patients are asked to refrain from any oral stimulation (e.g. food, drink, oral hygiene) for 1.5 h prior to saliva collection. An unstimulated whole salivary flow of less than 0.12–0.16 ml/min is

Table 3.3 The Oral Assessment Guide [adapted from reference 8]

Category	Numerical and descriptive ratings		
	1	**2**	**3**
Voice	Normal	Deeper or raspy	Difficulty talking or painful
Swallow	Normal swallow	Some pain on swallow	Unable to swallow
Lips	Smooth and pink and moist	Dry or cracked	Ulcerated or bleeding
Tongue	Pink and moist and papillae present	Coated or loss of papillae with a shiny appearance with or without redness	Blistered or cracked
Saliva	Watery	Thick or ropy	Absent
Mucous membranes	Pink and moist	Reddened or coated (increased whiteness) without ulcerations	Ulcerations with or without bleeding
Gingiva	Pink and stippled and firm	Oedematous with or without redness	Spontaneous bleeding or bleeding with pressure
Teeth or dentures (or denture bearing area)	Clean and no debris	Plaque or debris in localized areas (between teeth if present)	Plaque or debris generalized along gum line or denture bearing area

considered low/abnormal [7]. The technique for measuring stimulated whole salivary flow rate involves a similar procedure with the addition of a suitable stimulus to secretion (e.g. chewing paraffin wax).

Assessment tools

Oral assessment tools are commonly used in clinical practice, although there are concerns surrounding the validity/appropriateness of many of these tools. Thus, many of the tools have not been properly validated, or only validated in specific situations (e.g. Oral Assessment Guide and oral mucositis [8]). Furthermore, some tools only assess certain oral problems, whilst other tools use inappropriate methods to assess oral problems (e.g. consistency of saliva and salivary gland dysfunction). Indeed, the use of oral assessment tools does not preclude the use of the aforementioned clinical assessment methods.

The Oral Assessment Guide (OAG) is one of the most commonly used assessment tool in Oncology[8]. The OAG was developed to more accurately assess mucositis and other relevant oral complications in oncology patients undergoing chemotherapy. This tool assesses eight variables: voice, swallow, lips, tongue, saliva, mucous membranes, gingiva, and teeth or dentures (Table 3.3). The main advantage of this scale is ease of use in a patient care setting. However, the OAG does not assess other important oral manifestations of cancer therapy, such as pain, xerostomia, taste disturbance, and oral infection.

References

1 National Cancer Institute (2008). Oral complications of chemotherapy and head/neck radiation. Health Professional Version. Available from NCI website: http://www.cancer.gov/cancertopics/pdq/supportivecare/oralcomplications/healthprofessional

2 Birnbaum W, Dunne SM (2000). *Oral diagnosis: the clinician's guide.* Wright, Oxford.

3 Bagg J (1996). Common infectious diseases. *Dent Clin North Am*, 40(2), 385–93.

4 Jontell M, Holmstrup P (2008). Red and white lesions of the oral mucosa, in Greenberg MS, Glick M, Ship JA (eds) *Burket's Oral Medicine*, 11th edn, pp. 77–106. BC Decker, Hamilton.

5 Woo SB, Greenberg MS (2008). Ulcerative, vesicular, and bullous lesions, in Greenberg MS, Glick M, Ship JA (eds) *Burket's Oral Medicine*, 11th edn, pp. 41–75. BC Decker, Hamilton.

6 Fox PC, Busch KA, Baum BJ (1987). Subjective reports of xerostomia and objective measures of salivary gland performance. *J Am Dent Assoc*, 115(4), 581–4.

7 Navazesh M, Christensen C, Brightman V (1992). Clinical criteria for the diagnosis of salivary gland hypofunction. *J Dent Res*, 71(7), 1363–9.

8 Eilers J, Berger AM, Petersen MC (1988). Development, testing, and application of the oral assessment guide. *Oncol Nurs Forum*, 15(3), 325–30.

Chapter 4

Common oral conditions

Katherine Webber and Andrew Davies

Racial pigmentation [1,2]

- *Epidemiology* – Common. Occurs in people with dark complexions, such as those of African, Asian, and Southern European descent.
- *Clinical features* – Asymptomatic. The most common site is the gingivae (Figure 4.1, see colour plate section). Other common sites include the buccal mucosa and the palatal mucosa; less common sites include the lips, the tongue, and the floor of mouth. The areas of pigmentation are variable in size, but are usually symmetrical in distribution. Over time, the lesions may darken in colour.
- *Management* – No treatment is required (reassurance).

Oral varicosities (varices or venous lakes) [1,3]

- *Epidemiology* – Common. Occurs in older people (>50 years).
- *Aetiology* – The lesions are due to dilatation of superficial veins.
- *Clinical features* – Asymptomatic. The most common sites are the lips and the ventral surface of the tongue. However, they can occur elsewhere within the oral cavity. On the lips they appear as blue/purple swellings, which blanch on pressure (Figure 4.2, see colour plate section); on the tongue they appear as dilated, tortuous veins. Over time, the lesions may become more conspicuous. Oral varicosities occasionally thrombose, but rarely haemorrhage.
- *Management* – Usually, no treatment is required (reassurance). Sometimes, treatment is given for aesthetic reasons for lesions on the lips, i.e. excision, cryotherapy, or laser therapy.

Fissured tongue (scrotal tongue) [1,4]

- *Epidemiology* – Relatively common (0.5–5% of the population). May be associated with Down's syndrome and Melkersson–Rosenthal syndrome.
- *Aetiology* – Developmental anomaly. The cause is unknown. May be familial.
- *Clinical features* – Generally asymptomatic, although some patients complain of discomfort. There are multiple fissures on the dorsal surface of the tongue (Figure 4.3, see colour plate section). The fissures are variable in number, size, and depth, but are usually symmetrical in distribution. Fissured tongue may coexist with geographic tongue (see below).
- *Management* – None required unless symptomatic measures necessary.

Geographic tongue (benign migratory glossitis or erythema migrans) [1,5]

♦ *Epidemiology* – Relatively common (1–2% of the population). May be associated with psoriasis.

♦ *Aetiology* – The lesions are due to desquamation of the filiform papillae. The cause is unknown. May be familial.

♦ *Clinical features* – Generally asymptomatic, although patients sometimes complain of discomfort. There are multiple, irregularly shaped patches on the dorsal surface of the tongue: the patches have a narrow, raised, white edge, and a smooth, flat, erythematous centre (Figure 4.4, see colour plate section). Geographic tongue is a dynamic condition: patches appear then disappear; patches change size and/or shape. Similar lesions may rarely occur on the lateral/ventral surface of tongue, and on the remaining oral mucosa ('geographic stomatitis'). Geographic tongue is frequently intermittent, and often resolves spontaneously (weeks to years). Geographic tongue may coexist with fissured tongue.

♦ *Management* – None required unless symptomatic measures necessary.

Black hairy tongue (hairy tongue or brown hairy tongue) [1,6]

♦ *Epidemiology* – Relatively common.

♦ *Aetiology* – The lesions are due to hypertrophy/elongation of the filiform papillae. The discolouration may be due to overgrowth of chromogenic bacteria, or to pigments derived from eating/smoking. The cause is usually unknown, although it is associated with poor oral hygiene, salivary gland dysfunction, smoking, antibiotic use, and other drug use (e.g. ferrous sulphate).

♦ *Clinical features* – Generally asymptomatic, although some patients complain of discomfort/taste disturbance. There is a 'hairy' patch in the central, posterior part of the dorsal surface of the tongue. The 'hairs' are yellow, brown, or black in colour (Figure 4.5, see colour plate section).

♦ *Management* – Treatment involves oral hygiene measures, including tongue cleaning (brushing and scraping). Associated factors should be discontinued/avoided.

Oral ulceration

The term 'ulcer' is used to describe a full-thickness loss of epithelium with exposure of the underlying connective tissue[7]. (The term 'erosion' is used to describe a partial thickness loss of epithelium.) There are a number of causes of ulceration in patients with cancer, including specific causes (i.e. related to the cancer/cancer treatment) and non-specific causes (i.e. related to other factors). The most common causes of oral ulceration in the general population are shown in Table 4.1[8].

The assessment of oral ulceration involves basic clinical skills (i.e. taking a history, performing an examination), and use of appropriate investigations (e.g. microbiological testing, tissue biopsy). It is especially important to determine the number of ulcers, and the duration of ulceration[9]. Thus, a single ulcer that is persistent in nature suggests malignancy, chronic trauma, chronic infection (e.g. syphilis, tuberculosis), or mucocutaneous disease. Similarly, multiple ulcers that are persistent in nature suggest drugs, mucocutaneous disease, haematological disorders, or gastrointestinal disease. Multiple, transient lesions are usually due to aphthous ulcers, or viral infection.

Table 4.1 Common causes of oral ulceration in general population [adapted from reference 8]

Category	Examples
Local causes	
Trauma	Sharp teeth
	Sharp restorations
	Loose dentures
'Burns'	Heat
	Cold
	Chemical
Recurrent aphthous ulcers	Minor aphthous ulceration
	Major aphthous ulceration
	Herpetiform aphthous ulceration
Infection	Acute necrotizing ulcerative gingivitis (mixed organisms)
	Herpetic stomatitis (herpes simplex virus)
	Hand, foot, and mouth disease (Group A coxsackie virus)
Malignancy	Oral tumour
	Radiotherapy – oral mucositis
	Chemotherapy – oral mucositis
	Bisphosphonate therapy – simple ulceration, osteonecrosis of jaw
Drugs	Non-steroidal anti-inflammatory drugs
	Aspirin (local effect)
	Iron salts (local effect)
Systemic disease	
Mucocutaneous disease	Behcet's syndrome
	Epidermolysis bullosa
	Pemphigus vulgaris
Haematological disorders	Anaemia
	Neutropenia
	Myelodysplastic syndrome
Gastrointestinal disease	Coeliac disease
	Crohn's disease
	Ulcerative colitis

Recurrent aphthous ulcers (recurrent aphthous stomatitis or recurrent oral ulceration) [1,10]

◆ *Epidemiology* – Very common (10–30% population). More common in young adults, and in females.

◆ *Aetiology* – The cause is unknown. (Patients rarely have iron, folate, or vitamin B12 deficiency). Attacks may be precipitated by stress, trauma, and menstruation.

Table 4.2 Clinical features of recurrent aphthous ulcers [11]

Type	Site	Number	Size	Characteristics	Natural history	Other comments
Minor	Lip, buccal mucosa, tongue, mucolabial fold, mucobuccal fold	1–6	Medium (2–6mm)	Oval Narrow red margin Shallow base Whitish-yellow pseudomembrane	Persist for 5–7 days Often recur every few months	Most common type A 'burning' sensation may precede (24–48hr) the ulceration Very painful
Major	Lip, buccal mucosa, tongue, soft palate	1–5	Large (1–2cm)	Deep base Ulcers may heal by scarring	Persist for 3–6 weeks Often recur every few months	Very painful
Herpetiform	Anywhere in oral cavity	10–100	Small (1–2mm)	Shallow base Ulcers may coalesce to form larger lesions	Persist for 1–2 weeks Attacks recur over period of 1–3 yr	Very painful

♦ *Clinical features* – Recurrent aphthous ulcers have been classified into three main types: (1) minor (Figure 4.6, see colour plate section); (2) major; and (3) herpetiform. The clinical features of the different types of recurrent aphthous ulcers are shown in Table 4.2[11].

♦ *Management* – Various agents have been used to treat aphthous ulceration. Topical corticosteroids are the mainstay of treatment, whilst systemic corticosteroids are reserved for treatment of severe/refractory cases. Other therapeutic agents that have been used include, tetracycline mouthwashes, and (in selected cases) thalidomide. Symptomatic management involves avoidance of aggravating factors, coating agents, topical analgesics, and systemic analgesics.

Neutropenic ulcers [1,12]

♦ *Epidemiology* – Common (in high-risk groups).

♦ *Aetiology* – The lesions are related to low neutrophil counts. However, in about one-third of cases, additional factors appear to be relevant (e.g. trauma, infection). The underlying cause of the neutropenia, include inherited disorders (e.g. cyclic neutropenia), and acquired disorders (e.g. bone marrow infiltration with cancer, bone marrow suppression with chemotherapy).

♦ *Clinical features* – Neutropenic ulcers are often painful, and may be associated with other oral symptoms (hypersalivation, difficulty eating, etc.). The ulcers vary in number (often multiple), in size (often large), and in site: the most common sites are the gingivae, the tongue, the palate, and the tonsils. The edge of the ulcer is usually well-demarcated, although there are few signs of surrounding inflammation. The base of the ulcer is usually covered with

Table 4.3 Causes of oral white lesions in general population [adapted from reference 13]

Category	Examples
Local causes	Debris from poor oral hygiene
	'Burns' – heat, chemical
	Keratoses – frictional keratosis, smoker's keratosis
Congenital	Fordyce spots (ectopic sebaceous glands)
	Leukoedema
	Inherited dyskeratoses
Inflammatory	
Infective	Fungal – oral candidosis
	Viral – oral hairy leukoplakia (EBV), warts/papillomas (HPV)
	Bacterial – syphilis
Non-infective	Oral mucositis – chemotherapy, radiotherapy
	Lichen planus
	Lupus erythematous
Pre-malignant/malignant	Leukoplakia
	Keratoses
	Carcinoma

Table 4.4 Causes of oral red lesions in general population [adapted from reference 14]

Localized lesions	Generalized lesions
Oral candidosis – erythematous candidosis, denture stomatitis	Oral candidosis – erythematous candidosis, denture stomatitis
Erythroplasia	Iron deficiency
Purpura	Avitaminosis B
Telangiectases – hereditary haemorrhagic telangiectasia, systemic sclerosis	Oral mucositis – chemotherapy, radiotherapy
Angiomas	Lichen planus
Kaposi's sarcoma	Mucosal atrophy
Burns	Polycythaemia
Lichen planus	
Lupus erythromatosus	
Avitaminosis	

a grey-white/yellow pseudomembrane. Neutropenic ulcers are often associated with other relevant oral pathology (gingivitis, mucositis, etc.).

◆ *Management* – The management of neutropenic ulcers is essentially symptomatic (good oral hygiene, topical corticosteroids, topical analgesics, etc.). Improvement in the neutrophil count is associated with improvement in the ulceration. Granulocyte-colony stimulating factors may be useful in treating neutropenia secondary to bone marrow suppression with chemotherapy.

Oral white lesions

The causes of oral white lesions in the general population are shown in Table 4.3[13]. The assessment of oral white lesions is similar to that of oral ulceration. Focal lesions are often due to keratoses, whilst multifocal lesions are often due to oral candidosis or lichen planus[13]. (Lichen planus is characterized by striated lesions). Diffuse lesions are often due to keratoses (any site), leucoedema (buccal mucosa), or lichen planus (buccal mucosa). Pain may be a feature of white lesions caused by burns, oral candidosis, lichen planus, or lupus erythematosus.

Oral red lesions

The causes of oral red lesions in the general population are shown in Table 4.4[14]. The assessment of oral red lesions is similar to that of oral ulceration[15].

References

1 Sengupta A, Eveson J (2005). Miscellaneous oral problems, in Davies A, Finlay I (eds) *Oral Care in Advanced Disease*, pp.145–55. Oxford University Press, Oxford.

2 Amir E, Gorsky M, Buchner A, Sarnat H, Gat H (1991). Physiologic pigmentation of the oral mucosa in Israeli children. *Oral Surg Oral Med Oral Pathol*, 71(3), 396–8.

3 del Pozo J, Pena C, Garcia Silva J, Goday JJ, Fonseca E (2003). Venous lakes: a report of 32 cases treated by carbon dioxide laser vaporization. *Dermatol Surg*, 29(3), 308–10.

4 Leston JM, Santos AA, Varela-Centelles PI, Garcia JV, Romero MA, Villamor LP (2002). Oral mucosa: variations from normalcy, part II. *Cutis*, 69(3), 215–7.

5 Assimakopoulos D, Patrikakos G, Fotika C, Elisaf M (2002). Benign migratory glossitis or geographic tongue: an enigmatic oral lesion. *Am J Med*, 113(9), 751–5.

6 Sarti GM, Haddy RI, Schaffer D, Kihm J (1990). Black hairy tongue. *Am Fam Physician*, 41(6), 1751–5.

7 Birnbaum W, Dunne SM (2000). *Oral diagnosis: the clinician's guide.* Wright, Oxford.

8 Scully C, Felix DH (2005). Oral medicine – update for dental practitioner. Aphthous and other common ulcers. *Br Dent J*, 199(5), 259–64.

9 Scully C, Felix DH (2005). Oral medicine – update for dental practitioner. Mouth ulcers of more serious connotation. *Br Dent J*, 199(6), 339–43.

10 Ship JA, Chavez EM, Doerr PA, Henson BS, Sarmadi M (2000). Recurrent aphthous stomatitis. *Quintessence Int*, 31(2), 95–112.

11 Laskaris G (1994). *Colour atlas of oral diseases.* 2nd edn. Georg Thieme Verlag, Stuttgart.

12 Barrett AP (1987). Neutropenic ulceration. A distinctive clinical entity. *J Periodontol*, 58(1), 51–5.

13 Scully C, Felix DH (2005). Oral Medicine – update for the dental practitioner. Oral white patches. *Br Dent J*, 199(9), 565–72.

14 Scully C, Porter S (2000). ABC of oral health: swellings and red, white, and pigmented lesions. *Br Med J*, 321(7255), 225–8.

15 Scully C, Felix DH (2005). Oral Medicine – update for the dental practitioner. Red and pigmented lesions. *Br Dent J*, 199(10), 639–45.

Chapter 5

Pretreatment screening and management

Peter Stevenson-Moore, Debbie Saunders, and Joel Epstein

Introduction

Oral complications of treatment are a major cause of morbidity in patients with cancer[1]. Each treatment modality is associated with a slightly different spectrum of potential oral complications. The subsequent chapters discuss these oral complications in detail (Chapter 9 – head and neck surgery; Chapter 10 – radiotherapy/radiation therapy; and Chapter 13 – chemotherapy). The frequency of oral complications varies, although standard estimates help in determining the importance of targeting groups for pretreatment oral care (i.e. 10% patients receiving adjuvant chemotherapy, 40% patients receiving primary chemotherapy, 80% patients receiving myeloablative chemotherapy, and 100% patients receiving head and neck radiotherapy [1]). It should be noted that some patients will receive more than one type of treatment. For example, in head and neck cancer, radiotherapy is often used in combination with systemic chemotherapy, and with targeted biological therapies (e.g. cetuximab – a monoclonal antibody to epidermal growth factor receptor).

In the case of head and neck radiotherapy, these complications include rampant tooth decay as the result of chronic hyposalivation (and the consequent lack of defence to demineralization caused by overgrowth of acidogenic bacteria such as *Streptococcus mutans* and lactobacilli). This condition has been referred to as 'radiation caries', but should more accurately be referred to as 'caries secondary to radiation-induced salivary gland hypofunction'[2,3]. Dental caries is discussed in detail in Chapter 19. Investigators have also demonstrated changes in the structure of radiated teeth that result from exposure to radiation in excess of 4500 cGy (that may lead to biomechanical weakness)[4,5]. The combination of acid attack and weakened tooth structure can lead to a devastating decline in the integrity of tooth structure, precipitating the need for extraction of the affected teeth. However, the extraction of teeth from irradiated bone may lead to the often devastating occurrence of post-radiation osteonecrosis of the jaws (PRON). PRON is discussed in detail in Chapter 12.

The response of host tissues to both chemotherapy and radiotherapy is highly individual. Thus, the tissues of some subjects appear to show very little response, while the tissues of other subjects will sometimes demonstrate such severe degrees of inflammation that treatment must be interrupted or discontinued. (This has implications for the outcome of the cancer treatment.) These reactions may be more severe in patients with pre-existing oral infection and/or inflammation. Importantly, the severity of oral complications can be reduced significantly when an aggressive approach to stabilizing oral health is initiated prior to cancer treatment[6,7]. The lack of this knowledge often results in the under-treatment of the mouth prior to cancer treatment. Thus, some healthcare providers are so concerned about the cancer (and starting treatment for the cancer) that they ignore pre-existing conditions that would benefit from management.

Lack of knowledge may also result in over-treatment of the mouth prior to cancer treatment. Hence, some healthcare professionals are so keen to do as much as possible to assist their patients that they may undertake unnecessary procedures as a result of anticipating risks that are insignificant or non-existent. The involvement of a dental team experienced in oral oncology is extremely helpful in determining the appropriate level of treatment in this group of patients.

This chapter will outline the necessary steps in assessing a cancer patient prior to the initiation of treatment with head and neck radiotherapy, primary chemotherapy and adjuvant chemotherapy, and/or radiotherapy with haematopoietic stem cell transplantation. The overall goal of a pretreatment oral screening is to develop/complete a comprehensive oral care plan, which stabilizes or eliminates oral disease that could produce complications during these cancer treatments [8]. Achieving this goal will reduce the patient's risk for oral toxicities (with consequent reduced risk for systemic sequelae), enhance the patient's quality of life during treatment, reduce the overall cost of patient care, and improve of the cancer-treatment outcome[9]. It is important to recognize that the full range of recommended precautions is only necessary for patients undergoing head and neck radiotherapy when the radiation impacts directly on the oral structures, and when the radiation is of sufficient intensity to cause permanent damage. A radiation dosage of >4500 cGy is often considered to be the threshold above which permanent damage can be expected, although there will be some patients in whom irreversible changes are encountered at lower dosage levels.

Pretreatment assessment

The actual information that one assembles during the pretreatment examination of a cancer patient is similar to that which is obtained during the pretreatment examination of a regular patient in dental practice. However, there are some details that may be accumulated in greater depth in order to assist in the determination of treatment need prior to the initiation of cancer treatment, and to provide a baseline to which all later observations can be compared. It is assumed that the demographic data, medical history, dental history, family history, social history, and history of smoking and alcohol abuse have been obtained prior to patient examination (Table 5.1). In addition, it is essential to have accumulated some information regarding the type and extent of disease, the proposed cancer treatment, and the tissues directly/indirectly at risk of the proposed cancer treatment.

The pretreatment screening examination will establish a baseline to which later assessments can be compared. Observations should be standardized, so that they remain comparable during the lifetime of the patient[3].

Examination of the tissues of the head and neck

Head and neck examination is useful in appreciating an existing diagnosis of head and neck cancer, and in checking that additional disease has not been missed. (In head and neck cancer, there is a real possibility that second primary lesions will be discovered.) Examination of the tissues of the head and neck is discussed in detail in Chapter 3.

Intraoral examination of the tissues of the mouth and oropharynx

A detailed assessment should be made of the hard and soft tissues of the mouth. The dental examination should be recorded on an odontogram, and include notations about the presence/absence of teeth, and the presence of restorations (and the materials of which they are made). In addition, information should be recorded about periodontal probings, gingival recessions, and tooth mobilities. An assessment of oral hygiene is important for determining the patient's ability to maintain the integrity of dentition in a compromised oral environment. It is important that original records remain intact, and that they not be altered as changes occur in oral status. Examination of the tissues of the mouth and oropharynx is discussed in detail in Chapter 3.

Table 5.1 Pre-treatment assessment (history).

History	Details
Demographic information	
Presenting complaint(s)	Oral problems – in detail
	Systemic problems – as above
Medical history	Past medical history
	Current medical problems
	Current medications
	Drug allergies
	Other allergies
Cancer history	Site of cancer
	Histology of cancer
	Stage of cancer
	Impact of cancer
	Previous treatment – type, dose, intention (i.e. curative, palliative)
	Current treatment – as above
	Planned treatment – as above
Dental history	Current dental problems – in detail
	Current soft tissue problems – as above
	Dental prostheses
	Previous dental problems/treatment
	Previous soft tissue problems/treatment
	Frequency visits dentist/dental hygienist
Family history	
Social history	Tobacco usage – present, past
	Alcohol usage – present, past

Photography provides a useful record of current oral status, and of specific oral presentations (e.g. facial view, upper and lower standard occlusal views). Study models/casts are useful as a permanent record of baseline tooth position, and useful for the construction of fluoride gel carriers (see below).

Imaging

Imaging provides data important to treatment planning, and to the assessment of future complications resulting from cancer therapy. Panoramic, cone-beam, or computed tomography (CT) radiography is used to give an overall assessment of the orofacial complex. All of these methodologies are capable of providing excellent screening images. Three-dimensional imaging is likely to replace two-dimensional imaging as the method of choice, but many dentists are more accustomed to interpreting the more detailed two-dimensional images. Periapical views are used to provide additional detail about the teeth (Figure 5.1).

Supplementary radiography

Ideally, simulator films describing the tumour volume, and the planned radiation treatment volume, should be reviewed prior to determining the dental treatment plan. These images may be useful in determining the risks associated with the long-term effects of radiotherapy (and so the necessity for tooth extractions).

Copies of the two- or three-dimensional data used by the radiation oncologist and the radiation physicist in planning treatment must be kept on record. The absence of this information can

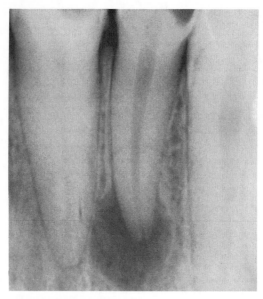

Fig. 5.1 Periapical X-ray showing dental abscess.

significantly compromise the ability to make appropriate treatment planning decisions if/when complications occur some years after the original treatment has been completed.

Measurement of resting and stimulated salivary output

The casual observation of salivary output is somewhat unreliable. Thus, formal measurement of resting and stimulated salivary output should be undertaken. In normal patients, unstimulated saliva output primarily represents the output of the submandibular glands (60% of the total), with additional contributions from the parotid (25%), sublingual (7–8%), and minor salivary glands (7–8%)[10]. The unstimulated saliva output is the most important output for tooth protection. Stimulated salivary output primarily represents the increased output from parotid glands (50% of the total) with eating/related stimuli, with additional contributions from the submandibular (35%), sublingual (7–8%), and minor salivary glands (7–8%)[10]. It should be noted that self-reporting by patients of salivary output is extremely unreliable (particularly during the post-treatment period). Measurement of salivary flow rates is discussed in detail in Chapter 3.

Laboratory investigations

Laboratory investigations may be required for certain patients undergoing invasive procedures (e.g. full blood count, clotting screen).

Pretreatment management

Decisions concerning the preparation of the oral cavity for cancer treatment are modified by the type of disease, the extent of the disease, and the proposed treatment of the disease. The determination of appropriate management strategies prior to the initiation of cancer treatment must take into account both the short-term and long-term effects of the cancer treatment. For example, when surgical treatment of a cancer of the head and neck is planned, there is less urgency for preparation of the mouth than is required for treatment involving radiotherapy or systemic chemotherapy.

(Surgery is unlikely to affect the integrity of the oral tissues and their supporting structures, and delayed interventions are not contraindicated by the effects of surgical interventions.)

For treatment to proceed, the first consideration will be the elimination of conditions that may interfere with the delivery of cancer therapy. The treatment objectives include: (1) the management of foci of infection (gingival, periodontal, and periapical); (2) the elimination of teeth with severe infection; (3) the extraction of unrestorable teeth; (4) the elimination of rough or sharp surfaces on teeth that could irritate oral tissues; and (5) the assessment of removable prostheses (with a view to improving fit and/or removing rough or sharp surfaces, so as to minimize the development of trauma-induced mucosal lesions). Other interventions may be necessary in some patients, including treatment of pre-existing oral mucosal disorders/infections, salivary gland dysfunction, temporomandibular joint disorders, and myofacial pain syndromes.

Some decision-making will be determined by the patient's past oral care performance and related assessments: (1) does the patient understand the effects of cancer treatment on the oral tissues?; (2) does the patient demonstrate skills appropriate to the maintenance of oral health?; and (3) can the patient access sufficient resources to prepare the mouth for cancer treatment, and to maintain the mouth following the completion of cancer treatment? Patients who have had limited past dental care, have poor oral hygiene, and show evidence of past dental/periodontal disease may require more aggressive pretreatment dental management.

It is important that no patient be regarded as a statistic at any time during management. It is true that less favourable treatment outcomes are frequently associated with more advanced disease status. However, decisions made on the basis that life expectancy is short, can frequently lead to management strategies that are later found to be inappropriate (when the patient survives for an unexpected length of time). Many cancer centres have found it beneficial to retain dental practitioners, who have the necessary experience in making these sorts of decision.

The management of children is somewhat different, since children have a remarkable capacity for recovery following radiotherapy. Thus, children may recover sufficient salivary function to maintain adequate protection of the dentition. The integrity of the radiated soft tissues and bones will also be less compromised. Hence, the later extraction of teeth from radiated bone is not associated with the same incidence of compromised healing and osteoradionecrosis as in adults. Consequently, the need for tooth extraction prior to radiotherapy must be viewed differently in children. For example, incomplete development of the teeth should not precipitate pretreatment extraction of these teeth.

Tooth extractions

The teeth in high-dose radiation fields that should be extracted prior to radiotherapy are: (1) those that are unrestorable; (2) those that require significant restorative, periodontal, endodontic, or orthodontic intervention that cannot be satisfactorily managed prior to radiotherapy; and (3) those with moderate to severe periodontal disease (i.e. pockets >5 mm, advanced recession). The recommendation for tooth extraction is frequently not willingly accepted. Patients with serious periodontal problems may have been unaware that they had anything wrong with the teeth, while others may have invested heavily in the placement of sophisticated restorations that they are reluctant to lose.

There is some urgency required in performing tooth extractions prior to the onset of radiotherapy or chemotherapy. Extractions must be carried out as atraumatically as possible, with the minimum amount of damage to both soft and hard tissues. The intention is to achieve primary closure of the extraction site without tension in the tissues. This will frequently require that a significant alveolectomy be undertaken. Ideally, the healing of extraction sites should be complete prior to commencing the cancer therapy (although frequently the ideal is impractical). Some dentists have recommended that a minimum healing period of 6 weeks be allowed, but many oncologists will not be willing to delay treatment for so long. However, experienced providers agree that shorter healing periods are generally acceptable (i.e. 1–2 weeks) [11]. The actual healing period required is best determined on an individual basis, with attention being given to the presence of co-morbid factors that may affect healing such as diabetes mellitus, neutropenia or neutrophil dysfunction, and immunosuppression.

A minimum of 14 days is required for the initial stages of healing to be completed. Thus, a period of only 48 h may be sufficient prior to initiation of radiation therapy, since healing should continue to take place during the first 10–12 days of radiotherapy (provided that conservative techniques have been utilized, and that wound closure is stable at 48 h). Maturation of the extraction site will occur over a much longer period than would normally be expected, although tissue integrity should be maintained provided that no unnecessary stress is imposed on the extraction site. Frequently, this will require adjustment of an existing prosthesis, and sometimes confiscation of the prosthesis, in order to avoid trauma to the wound. It should be noted that longer healing periods are required if primary closure of the extraction site has not been achieved.

There are occasions when the oncologist will not be prepared to allow any waiting period following tooth extraction. In such cases, antibiotic coverage may be needed in order to minimize the risks of starting cancer treatment.

Implants

There is no reported incidence of the loss of integration of implants due to the effects of radiotherapy. Indeed, once an implant has integrated with the surrounding bone, there would seem to be no reason that the inflammation associated with radiotherapy could cause destruction of the bone-to-implant interface. However, a recently placed implant may take longer to integrate than normal; loading of a recently placed implant should be delayed in order to allow integration to become optimal. If an implant has very recently been placed, with no expectation that any degree of integration has yet been achieved, then the implant should be removed from bone that will be in the high-dose volume of radiation. It is generally accepted that the intensity of incident radiation must exceed 4500 cGy before a significant level of risk to integration is encountered. (Implants that are not in the high-dose volume experience no increased level of risk to integration.)

Restorations

Metallic restorations can significantly complicate the imaging of oral structures. The problem results from a phenomenon known as backscatter, where radioactive particles reflect from metallic surfaces with an intensity that is proportional to the atomic number of the relevant material.

There is concern that metal objects included in the treatment volume will cause backscatter capable of intensifying the treatment dose on one side of the metallic object, and diminishing the dose on the opposite side of the object (that being the side that might be considered to be in the 'shadow' of the metallic object). This will only be of any significance in the high-dose treatment volume. The attenuation of energy occurs within a few millimetres of the surface of the object from which the energy is reflected.

It should be noted that two opposing beams of radiation create the same amount of incident and reflected radiation intensity. Hence, the effect of backscatter from one beam is largely cancelled out by the shadow effect of the opposing beam. It is thought that more sophisticated schemes of dose distribution can effectively ameliorate the contribution of backscatter at any particular site (e.g. intensity-modulated radiation therapy: IMRT).

Additional precautions are possible to minimize the effects of backscatter. Thus, the creation of a flexible mouthguard with significant thickness can deflect mobile soft-tissue structures away from reflective metallic surfaces. The use of such guards will be particularly helpful where interstitial forms of radiotherapy are used (such as implants to the tongue or floor of the mouth), or where external radiotherapy with unilateral fields are used (including acutely angled wedged pair fields).

Mouth-guard material built to a thickness in excess of 6 mm can achieve the necessary separation between soft tissue and metal (and without compromising the patient's ability to wear the device for the duration of radiation treatment). Processed resin devices, some containing a material that attenuates radiation (such as Cerrobend low-fusing metal), have also been used, although the bulk of such devices is frequently objectionable to patients.

From the foregoing discussion it may be understood that, under most circumstances, even extensive fixed metallic restorations can be left in place in the mouth without the expectation of significant adverse consequences. However, removable prostheses containing metal should be taken out during the actual delivery of radiotherapy.

Ongoing management

The use of simple techniques to reduce the colonization of normal and pathogenic organisms may be effective in reducing the overall levels of mucosal inflammation during cancer therapy. The measures used to reduce the colonization of normal and pathogenic organisms are similar to those used for the maintenance of soft and hard tissue health in normal patients (see Chapter 6, Table 6.1). These measures must be modified to reflect the increasing fragility of tissues during cancer treatment, and may eventually have to be discontinued if the inflammatory response becomes too severe. Oral hygiene measures are discussed in detail in Chapter 6.

Remineralizing strategies are required in all patients, and are dependent on the degree to which saliva output is reduced. Gel carriers constructed from flexible thermoplastic material are used to apply neutral sodium fluoride or remineralizing gel to the teeth (Figure 5.2). The carriers must overlap the gingival margins of the teeth in order to adequately enclose the teeth (but avoid

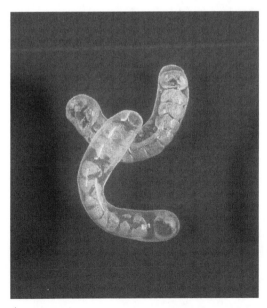

Fig. 5.2 Fluoride gel carrier.

unnecessary contact with the soft tissues). Carriers are preferred to mouth rinses for the application of fluoride. The frequency of usage varies from after each meal (3 times a day) to once a week, depending upon the degree of suppression of saliva output. Applications are for 1 min, with rinsing permitted after usage.

Some time must be allocated to teaching the patient about the expected changes in the oral tissues, and the methods that must be employed to maintain oral health. In addition, it is helpful to provide an indication of the changes that will require further professional intervention. It is important that patients undergoing cancer treatment can call upon their healthcare providers to offer additional support (according their areas of expertise). Such support will include professional cleaning of the oral cavity to replace home-care techniques, the prescription of bacteriostatic and bactericidal agents, and the prescription of topical and systemic analgesics. Research has demonstrated that patients require repetition, reinforcement, and follow-up in order to ensure that the prescribed preventative home-care measures are maintained. For example, some patients may mistakenly assume that the home application of fluoride gel ceases when the first bottle prescribed has been finished.

References

1 National Cancer Institute (2008). Oral complications of chemotherapy and head/neck radiation. Health Professional Version. Available from NCI website: http://www.cancer.gov/cancertopics/pdq/supportivecare/oralcomplications/healthprofessional

2 Pernot M, Luporsi E, Hoffstetter S, et al. (1997). Complications following definitive irradiation for cancers of the oral cavity and the oropharynx (in a series of 1134 patients). *Int J Radiat Oncol Biol Phys,* 37(3), 577–85.

3 Vissink A, Jansma J, Spijkervet FK, Burlage FR, Coppes RP (2003). Oral sequelae of head and neck radiotherapy. *Crit Rev Oral Biol Med,* 14(4), 199–212.

4 Kielbassa AM, Beetz I, Schendera A, Hellwig E (1997). Irradiation effects on microhardness of fluoridated and non-fluoridated bovine dentin. *Eur J Oral Sci,* 105(5 Pt 1), 444–7.

5 Kielbassa AM, Munz I, Bruggmoser G, Schulte-Mönting J (2002). Effect of demineralization and remineralization on microhardness of irradiated dentin. *J Clin Dent,* 13(3), 104–10.

6 Sonis S, Kunz A (1988). Impact of improved dental services on the frequency of oral complications of cancer therapy for patients with non-head-and-neck malignancies. *Oral Surg Oral Med Oral Pathol,* 65(1), 19–22.

7 Sonis ST, Woods PD, White BA (1990). Oral complications of cancer therapies. Pretreatment oral assessment. *NCI Monogr,* (9), 29–32.

8 Stevenson-Moore P (1990). Oral complications of cancer therapies. Essential aspects of a pretreatment oral examination. *NCI Monogr,* (9), 33–6.

9 Beck SL (1990). Prevention and management of oral complications in the cancer patient, in Hubbard SM, Greene PE, Knobf MT (eds) *Current Issues in Cancer Nursing Practice,* pp. 27–38. J.B. Lippincott Company, Philadelphia.

10 Whelton H (2004). Introduction: the anatomy and physiology of salivary glands, in Edgar M, Dawes C, O'Mullane D (eds) *Saliva and Oral Health,* 3rd edn, pp. 1–13. British Dental Association, London.

11 Cramer CK, Epstein JB, Sheps SB, Schechter MT, Busser JR (2002). Modified Delphi survey for decision analysis for prophylaxis of post-radiation osteonecrosis. *Oral Oncol,* 38(6), 574–83.

Chapter 6

Oral hygiene

Petrina Sweeney and Andrew Davies

Introduction

Maintenance of good oral hygiene is important for all patients with cancer, and especially for patients receiving systemic chemotherapy and/or head and neck radiotherapy[1]. Poor oral hygiene is associated with morbidity *per se* (e.g. halitosis)[2], as well as the development of other oral problems (e.g. periodontal disease) [3] and certain systemic problems (e.g. aspiration pneumonia)[4]. Moreover, poor oral hygiene can lead to associated psychosocial consequences. For example, poor oral hygiene may cause halitosis, which may result in the patient becoming depressed, and also in the family/friends becoming more distant[5]. Poor oral hygiene is also associated with morbidity from anti-cancer treatment (e.g. oral mucositis)[6], and indirectly with mortality from anti-cancer treatment (e.g. septicaemia)[7]. Hence, maintenance of good oral hygiene is important for maintenance of good quality of life in patients with cancer.

Maintenance of oral hygiene

Maintenance of good oral hygiene depends on adequate assessment, appropriate treatment, and adequate re-assessment. All cancer patients should have an initial oral assessment, which should include an appraisal of oral hygiene, and the ability to undertake necessary oral hygiene measures. Oral assessment is discussed in detail in Chapter 3. Oral hygiene measures will vary from patient to patient, and may vary within the same patient over time. Nevertheless, there are some basic principles of care, which are applicable to most patients with cancer, and indeed to most patients with chronic illness (see below). All cancer patients should equally have regular oral re-assessments, which should again include an appraisal of oral hygiene, and the ability to continue to undertake necessary oral hygiene measures.

In most instances the patient will be able to perform their own oral hygiene measures, although they often require support from generic healthcare professionals, and occasionally input from oral healthcare professionals (e.g. dentists, dental hygienists). It is important that patients not only understand how to maintain good oral hygiene, but that they understand the rationale for maintaining good oral hygiene. Thus, patients are more likely to adhere to oral hygiene regimens if they understand the importance of good oral hygiene, and the consequences of poor oral hygiene. In addition, patients need to be encouraged to have regular dental reviews, and to report the development/deterioration of oral problems.

However, in some instances the patient will require assistance to perform oral hygiene measures, and this assistance may involve family members when the patient is at home, and healthcare professionals when the patient is in hospital (or a similar institution). Again, it is important that such surrogates not only understand how to maintain good oral hygiene, but that they understand the rationale for maintaining good oral hygiene. Family members invariably need advice about providing such care, but even many healthcare professionals also need advice about providing such care[8]. Oral healthcare professionals are ideally suited to providing oral care training, and devising appropriate oral hygiene regimens[9].

It is important that healthcare professionals undertake oral care in a suitable location, and in an appropriate manner. Thus, patients should be afforded a degree of privacy, made comfortable before the procedure, made aware of the nature of the procedure (and provide verbal consent), and, if necessary, be allowed to pause/discontinue the procedure. Universal infection-control measures should be employed, with healthcare professionals wearing gloves when undertaking oral care, including when handling oral prostheses[10].

Dental care

Toothbrushing

The single most important oral hygiene measure is toothbrushing, which should be undertaken at least twice daily.

A wide range of toothbrushes is available commercially, including powered toothbrushes ('electric toothbrushes'). It is recommended that a small-headed brush, which has soft-to-medium texture bristles, is used. 'Ultra soft' toothbrushes can be used for patients whose mouth is sore. These toothbrushes include baby brushes and specialist brushes (e.g. TePe® Special Care toothbrush). Attention should also be paid to the handle, which can be easily adapted to allow a firmer grip for those with problems of manual dexterity.

A recent systematic review has reported that many powered toothbrushes are no better at removing plaque than manual toothbrushes[11]. However, powered toothbrushes with a rotation–oscillation action do appear to be better at removing plaque than manual toothbrushes[11]. Patients with disability/fatigue that experience difficulties in maintaining oral hygiene with a manual toothbrush may have fewer difficulties in maintaining oral hygiene with a powered toothbrush.

The recommended life span of a toothbrush is approximately 3 months, but it should be replaced sooner if the filaments of the brush become softened and/or misshapen. (At this stage

Table 6.1 Oral care procedures for dentate patients

Procedure	Comments
Clean teeth at least twice daily	Use a suitable/personalized toothbrush and a fluoridated toothpaste Use suitable interdental cleaning aid Carers should undertake tooth brushing in dependent patients
Consider chemical plaque control	Chlorhexidine mouthwash (or similar) may be used in patients unable to adequately clean their teeth
Maintain cleanliness of oral mucosa	Rinse mouth regularly, and particularly after meals to remove any oral debris Carers should undertake mucosal cleaning in dependent patients (with a water-moistened gauze or a foam stick)
Clean any partial denture at least daily	See Table 5.1
Maintain complex dental work	The dental team should provide advice on oral hygiene for patients with complex restorations (e.g. implants, bridges)

the brush is no longer effective at removing dental plaque.) Toothbrushes should be replaced sooner if the patient is immunosuppressed/receiving chemotherapy. Furthermore, toothbrushes should be replaced immediately if the patient has experienced any type of oral infection.

There are many types of toothpaste available commercially. Patients should use toothpaste containing at least 1000 ppm fluoride. (Patients with radiation-induced salivary gland dysfunction should use specialist toothpaste containing 5000 ppm fluoride)[12]. Most toothpaste contains a foaming agent, which may prove problematic for those patients who have difficulty swallowing (and who are at risk of aspiration). In these cases, a non-foaming alternative should be used (e.g. Biotene® toothpaste, chlorhexidine gel)[13]. If patients cannot tolerate the use of toothpaste (due to oral discomfort), then patients can simply use water during toothbrushing.

Whilst a number of toothbrushing techniques have been described, a controlled gentle 'scrub' is recommended, with emphasis placed on gentle pressure and small movements[14]. No more than two teeth should be cleaned at a time, and a systematic approach should be adopted, which ensures that all the surfaces of all the teeth are included. Cleaning someone else's teeth is completely different from cleaning one's own teeth. Appropriate techniques are illustrated in Figure 6.1. It is usually easier to provide assisted toothbrushing from behind the patient. The head should be cradled and supported by the arm and hand of the carer. If access from behind is not possible, or proves too uncomfortable for the patient, then an approach from the side should be adopted.

Interdental cleaning

Interdental aids are designed to remove dental plaque from the areas between teeth that cannot be reached by a toothbrush. Ideally, some form of interdental cleaning should be used on a daily basis, though this may not be achievable/appropriate for some patients. The types of cleaning aids available include dental floss, dental tape, wood sticks, and interdental brushes. Interdental cleaning aids may cause damage to the oral tissues if used inappropriately.

Chemical plaque control

For some patients, mechanical plaque control is extremely difficult because of their level of debilitation and/or the presence of oral pathology. In such cases chemical plaque control may be considered for maintenance of oral hygiene.

At present, the most effective anti-plaque agent is chlorhexidine[15]. The chlorhexidine molecule has a positive charge at either end, and binds readily to negatively charged sites on the dental enamel pellicle, mucosal cells, and bacterial cells. Chlorhexidine is slowly released from such surfaces, so maintaining its antimicrobial activity (a property known as substantivity). In view of this property, there are no indications for using chlorhexidine more than twice a day[16]. Chlorhexidine exerts its antimicrobial effect by damaging the microbial cell membrane and precipitating the microbial cell contents. It also inhibits microbial adherence.

It is important to realize that chlorhexidine will not remove established plaque. Thus, established plaque must initially be physically removed by a dentist/dental hygienist. Chlorhexidine is used most commonly as a 0.12–0.2% mouthwash (10–15 ml twice a day), but it is also available as a 1% gel and a 0.2% spray in certain countries.

The most common side effect associated with long-term use of chlorhexidine is staining of the teeth and the dorsal surface of the tongue. This does not happen in all patients, and is related to the intake of tannin from tea and coffee[17]. These tooth stains can easily be removed by a dentist/dental hygienist. Other problems include the taste of the mouthwash, and the alcohol content of the mouthwash (which may cause mucosal discomfort). These problems may be overcome by diluting the mouthwash with up to an equivalent volume of water[18].

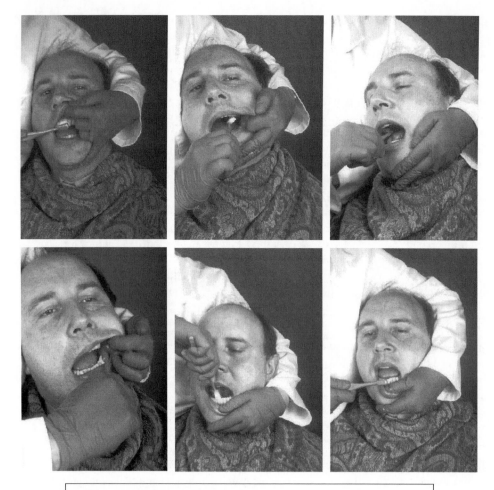

- Patient should be seated comfortably
- Clothes/pyjamas protected
- Patient's head must be well supported by operator
- The operator approaches from behind
- The lower jaw should be supported at all times
- Soft tissues are carefully retracted
- Follow a systematic approach to ensure that all tooth surfaces are cleaned

Figure 6.1 Procedure for cleaning the teeth of a dependent patient with one operator.
Source: Reproduced with permission from Davies A and Finlay I (2005), Oral Care in Advanced Disease. Oxford University Press, Oxford

Denture care

Dentures are readily colonized with microorganisms, acting as reservoirs of infection and predisposing to denture stomatitis (a variant of oral candidosis involving the alveolar margin and hard palate) (Figure 18.2, see colour plate section). It is, therefore, essential that a high level of denture hygiene is maintained.

Removal and insertion of complete dentures

The removal and insertion of dentures is an essential part of mouth care. If at all possible, patients should remove and insert their own dentures. However, this may be difficult for debilitated patients, and so healthcare professionals and other caregivers must become proficient at removal and insertion of dentures. The technique for denture removal is illustrated in Figure 6.2. The lower denture should be removed first to reduce any risk of aspiration of denture-related debris. The insertion of a denture essentially entails a reversal of the procedure for the removal of the denture (Figure 6.3).

Removal and insertion of partial dentures

Most partial dentures are easy to remove and insert, but for some it is necessary to follow specific paths of removal and insertion. The patient should be aware of the best way to remove and insert the partial denture, but if difficulties are encountered advice may be sought from the dental team. (Small partial dentures are easily broken if excess force is applied.) If removal and insertion of the denture proves difficult and/or distressing for the patient, then a decision should be made to leave the denture out of the mouth either temporarily or permanently depending on the circumstances.

Denture hygiene

Denture hygiene must be carried out regularly and should be incorporated into a daily oral care routine (Table 6.2). It should is done at least once per day (preferably at night). Cleaning a denture is not difficult, and it should take no more than a few minutes to achieve a satisfactory result. All dentures must be cleaned outside the mouth, and the soft tissues of the mouth cleaned separately (see below).

Dentures, particularly acrylic dentures, are somewhat fragile. Hence, they should always be cleaned over water, so that if dropped they will not be damaged. The denture should first be held under running water to remove debris, and then be brushed thoroughly with a large toothbrush, denture brush, or personal nailbrush to dislodge any remaining debris or plaque. Commercial products are available for cleaning dentures, but soap and water, or water on its own, is usually satisfactory. Ordinary toothpaste should not be used, because they are quite abrasive and may damage the polished surface of the denture. The denture should be rinsed well before placing it back in the patient's mouth. Ultrasonic baths are available to aid denture cleaning.

Dentures should ideally be rinsed under running water after every meal, and the lining of the mouth checked for food debris before re-inserting the dentures. Calculus ('tartar') may form on the smooth surfaces of a denture as a result of deposition of calcium from the saliva. Calculus may irritate/damage the underlying oral mucosa, and should be professionally removed as soon as it is noticed.

In order to maintain a healthy oral mucosa, it is advisable to leave dentures out of the mouth at night. If patients are reluctant to leave their dentures out at night, then they should be encouraged to remove them for at least an hour during the day. Plastic dentures should be soaked overnight in a dilute solution of sodium hypochlorite (e.g. 1 part Milton® 1% to 80 parts of water). This allows disinfection of the denture, and reduces the likelihood of denture stomatitis. The denture should be rinsed well before being returned to the patient's mouth. For those dentures with metal parts (cobalt-chrome dentures), sodium hypochlorite should not be used, as it can cause discolouration/ damage of the metal parts of the denture. Instead, the denture should be soaked in chlorhexidine gluconate (0.12–0.2% solution). It should be noted that while commercially available products

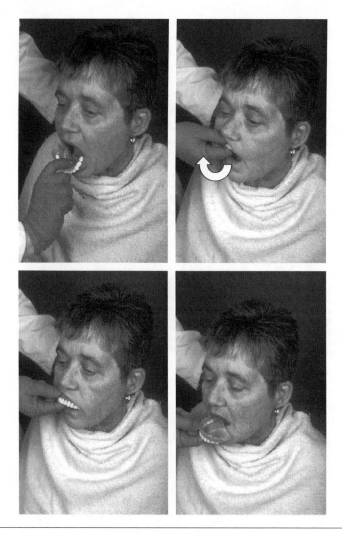

- The lower denture is removed first by grasping it firmly in the midline, lifting it upwards, and gently rotating it out of the mouth
- The upper denture is removed by grasping it firmly in the midline, breaking the seal with the palate, dropping it downwards, and gently rotating it out of the mouth. The seal is broken by tilting the denture forward while applying upper pressure on the front teeth, and supplying support to the back of the head

Figure 6.2 Procedure for removal of a complete denture.
Source: Reproduced with permission from Davies A and Finlay I (2005), Oral Care in Advanced Disease. Oxford University Press, Oxford

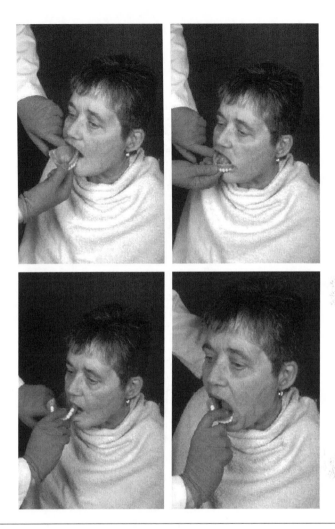

- The upper denture is inserted first by rotation, and seated firmly in place
- The lower denture is inserted by rotation, and seated firmly in place

Figure 6.3 Procedure for insertion of a complete denture.
Source: Reproduced with permission from Davies A and Finlay I (2005), Oral Care in Advanced Disease. Oxford University Press, Oxford

may be very effective in cleaning dentures, they might not be as effective in actually disinfecting dentures.

Dentures can be marked with the patient's name. The decision to mark dentures depends on the individual circumstances. However, it is a good idea to mark the dentures of dependent patients, particularly if they are resident for any length of time in a care institution (hospital, nursing home, etc.). Denture marking kits are available from dental-supply companies.

Table 6.2 Oral care procedures for edentulous patients

Procedure	Comments
Clean denture at least daily	Use a suitable/personal brush and soap and water (Clean dentures over water) Dentures should be rinsed after meals Carers should undertake denture cleaning for dependent patients
Remove/sterilize dentures at night	Plastic dentures may be soaked in either dilute sodium hypochlorite, or chlorhexidine Dentures with metal parts should be soaked in chlorhexidine Dentures should be rinsed after sterilization
Maintain cleanliness of oral mucosa	Rinse mouth regularly, and particularly after meals to remove any oral debris Carers should undertake mucosal cleaning in dependent patients (with a water-moistened gauze or a foam stick)
Consider marking denture with owner's name (e.g. hospital inpatients, care home residents)	Denture marking kits are commercially available
Maintain dentures	Check dentures regularly for sharp edges, cracks, and missing teeth

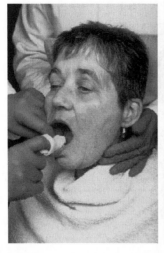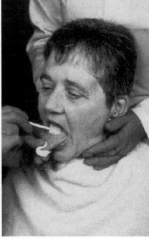

- The head is supported by a second operator
- A moistened piece of gauze wrapped around finger or a moistened foam swab is used to remove food and other debris from the oral mucosa
- The tongue should always be cleaned from back to front. (Cleaning the tongue is easier if the tongue is held/immobilised using a piece of gauze.)

Figure 6.4 Procedure for maintaining cleanliness of the oral mucosa.
Source: Reproduced with permission from Davies A and Finlay I (2005), Oral Care in Advanced Disease. Oxford University Press, Oxford

Care of the oral mucosa

The oral mucosa should be cleaned 3–4 times per day, ideally following each meal. For those patients who are able, rinsing the mouth with water is adequate to remove any debris. For those who are unable to rinse, the mucosa should be cleaned mechanically with a water-moistened gauze or foam stick (Figure 6.4). The tongue should be cleaned from back to front to reduce the risk of aspiration of any debris.

References

1 National Cancer Institute (2008). Oral complications of chemotherapy and head/neck radiation. Health Professional Version. Available from NCI website: http://www.cancer.gov/cancertopics/pdq/supportivecare/oralcomplications/healthprofessional

2 Porter SR, Scully C (2006). Oral malodour (halitosis). *Br Med J*, 333(7569), 632–5.

3 Petersen PE, Ogawa H (2005). Strengthening the prevention of periodontal disease: the WHO approach. *J Periodontol*, 76(12), 2187–93.

4 Li X, Kolltveit KM, Tronstad L, Olsen I. Systemic diseases caused by oral infection. *Clin Microbiol Rev 2000*, 13: 547–58.

5 Shorthose K, Davies A (2005). Halitosis, in Davies A, Finlay I (eds) *Oral Care in Advanced Disease*, pp. 125–31. Oxford University Press, Oxford.

6 McGuire DB, Correa ME, Johnson J, Wienandts P (2006). The role of basic oral care and good clinical practice principles in the management of oral mucositis. *Support Care Cancer*, 14(6), 541–7.

7 Meurman JH, Pyrhonen S, Teerenhovi L, Lindqvist C (1997). Oral sources of septicaemia in patients with malignancies. *Oral Oncol.* 33(6), 389–97.

8 Sweeney P (2005). Oral hygiene, in Davies A, Finlay I (eds) *Oral Care in Advanced Disease*, pp.21–35. Oxford University Press, Oxford.

9 Davies A (2005). Introduction, in Davies A, Finlay I (eds) *Oral Care in Advanced Disease*, pp.1–6. Oxford University Press, Oxford.

10 Bagg J (1996). Common infectious diseases. *Dent Clin North Am*, 40(2), 385–93.

11 Robinson PG, Deacon SA, Deery C, et al. (2005). Manual versus powered toothbrushing for oral health. *Cochrane Database of Sys Rev*, Issue 2, Art No.: CD002281.

12 Tavss EA, Mellberg JR, Joziak M, Gambogi RJ, Fisher SW (2003). Relationship between dentifrice fluoride concentration and clinical caries reduction. *Am J Dent*, 16(6), 369–74.

13 Griffiths J, Boyle S (1993). *Colour guide to holistic oral care: a practical approach.* Mosby, London.

14 Levine RS (1985). The scientific basis of dental health education. A Health Education Council policy document. *Br Dent J*, 158(6), 223–6.

15 Jones CG (1997). Chlorhexidine: is it still the gold standard? *Periodontol 2000*, 15, 55–62.

16 Loe H, Schiott CR (1970). The effect of mouthrinses and topical application of chlorhexidine on the development of dental plaque and gingivitis in man. *J Periodontal Res*, 5(2), 79–83.

17 Leard A, Addy M (1997). The propensity of different brands of tea and coffee to cause staining associated with chlorhexidine. *J Clin Periodontol*, 24(2), 115–18.

18 Axelsson P, Lindhe J (1987). Efficacy of mouthrinses in inhibiting dental plaque and gingivitis in man. *J Clin Periodontol*, 14(4), 205–12.

Chapter 7

Oral cancer

Crispian Scully and Jose Bagan

Introduction

Oral cancer is a major public health problem throughout the world. In most cases (90%), the tumour is an oral squamous cell carcinoma (OSCC), although a variety of other types of tumour can be found within the oral cavity. This chapter will focus on OSCC, whilst Chapter 8 will focus on the other types of tumour found within (and around) the oral cavity.

Epidemiology

Worldwide, OSCC is the sixth most common cancer for both sexes[1], with 350–400 000 new cases identified each year.

Geographical factors

The incidence varies widely between countries and geographical areas[1], but is generally more common in 'developing' countries. These variations have traditionally been explained by the exposure of these groups of people to specific risk factors (e.g. tobacco, alcohol, betel use), although other factors such as genetics, environmental factors (especially infective agents) and socioeconomic factors may also be at play[2].

Two out of three cases in males, and three out of four cases in females, are in the developing world. OSCC is the third most common cancer in developing nations, and it is particularly common in south-central Asia, where approximately 58% of the cases are concentrated[3]. In most regions of India, oral cancer is the most common cancer in men, and the third most common cancer in women. In Karachi (Pakistan), which has one of the highest reported incidences in the world, oral cancer is the second commonest malignancy amongst both males and females[4].

In the United States, OSCC is the tenth most common cancer amongst males[5]. Central and East European countries (Croatia, Hungary, Lithuania, Russia, Slovenia, and Ukraine) have high rates at over seven cases per 100 000 of the population; intermediate rates at 6–7 cases per 100 000 are seen in Germany, Italy, Poland, Spain, and Switzerland; and low rates at less than four cases per 100 000 are found in England and Wales, Greece, the Netherlands, and some Nordic countries[6]. However, the highest recorded incidence worldwide of OSCC has been reported in parts of France, such as Bas-Rhin (up to 55 cases per 100 000)[6,7].

Other factors

The incidence of OSCC increases with age, with a steep increase beginning in the 60–64-year age group[8]. However, there have been increases in OSCC in the younger generations, which appear to be mainly related to lifestyle habits (i.e. tobacco, alcohol, and betel use).

The male-to-female ratio is greater than 2:1 for OSCC[9]. The gender difference in OSCC rates has been decreasing over time, presumably due to the equalizing in tobacco and alcohol consumption[10].

Mortality

OSCCs are routinely discovered late, and have one of the lowest 5-year survival rates of any major cancer site (i.e. 53%). The 5-year survival rate has not changed in the past 30 years[11]. Not surprisingly, localized cancers have the highest 5-year survival rates (79%), those with regional disease have intermediate figures (42%), and those with distant metastases have the lowest 5-year survival rates (19%)[12].

A recent review of the SEER (The Surveillance Epidemiology and End Results Program of the National Cancer Institute) database showed that disease specific mortality from cancer of the tongue increases with age[13], which may be a reflection of increasing co-morbidities with increasing age. OSCC is also associated with the potentially lethal development of second primary tumours (up to a 20 times higher risk than controls)[14].

Aetiology

Carcinogenesis is the result of disturbed growth control arising from DNA damage (mutation), which can arise spontaneously, but may also be precipitated by a range of mutagens[15]. OSCC arises as a consequence of multiple DNA mutations, and seems to gradually evolve from normal epithelium through precursor lesions to full-blown malignancy.

Tobacco, alcohol, and betel are the main risk factors for OSCC. The results of many studies of lifestyle factors have been summarized by the International Agency for Research on Cancer (IARC)[16–18]. However, significant numbers of younger patients with OSCC deny any of the known risk factors[19–21].

Tobacco

Tobacco contains addictive components (e.g. nicotine), and releases many carcinogens including polycyclic aromatic hydrocarbons (e.g. benzopyrene), nitrosamines (e.g. nitrosonornicotine), and aldehydes (e.g. formaldehyde).

Cigarette smokers appear to be about 5 times more likely to develop OSCC than are non-smokers. Compared to non-smokers, the risk of oral cancer to low/medium-tar cigarette-smokers was 8.5 times, and for high tar cigarette mokers the risk was significantly greater at 16.4 times in one European study[22].

Other types of tobacco usage/smoking are also associated with an increased risk of OSCC, including:

- Bidi smoking (South Asia) [23] – these unfiltered cigarettes contain a small amount of flaked tobacco.

- Cigar smoking [24]

- Pipe smoking [25]

- Reverse smoking (India, Philippines, Taiwan, and South America) [24] – reverse smoking involves holding the burning end of cigarettes or cigars within the mouth. Reverse smoking is strongly associated with OSCC.

- Use of smokeless tobacco products [24] – these diverse products contain tobacco and a variety of other constituents (dependent on the geographical region).

- Snuff [25] – these finely powdered materials principally contain tobacco (and are used orally or nasally). The risks are mainly in snuff users, who also use other tobacco products[26].

It should be noted that oral cancer risk shows a clear decline after stopping tobacco use[27].

A review of two cohort studies, and 14 case-control studies, showed a possible association between marijuana use and cancer risk[28], although users of marijuana are often also heavy cigarette smokers.

Alcohol

Increased consumption of alcohol-containing beverages is associated with an increased risk of OSCC[29,30]. The risk decreases after stopping alcohol use, but the effects appear to persist for several years[31]. The risk is greatest amongst the heaviest drinkers of alcohol[32,33]. The type of alcoholic beverage appears to influence the risk, with hard liquors ('spirits') conferring a higher risk[32,33]. Epidemiological studies suggest that the impact of alcohol on OSCC has increased in recent years[33,34].

The combined effect of alcohol and tobacco is far greater than the sum of the two effects (Tables 7.1 and 7.2)[35–38].

The risk of OSCC amongst users of mouthwashes with high alcohol content (≥25%) is increased by 40% in men, and by 60% in women[39]. However, it appears as if the effect of alcohol from mouthwash could be similar to that of alcohol used for drinking, although in terms of attributable risk, the contribution of mouthwash use to OSCC must be very small[40].

Betel leaves and areca nut

Areca nut wrapped in betel leaves ('betel nut') is chewed in many cultures, and produces a mild stimulant effect (*cf.* drinking coffee). Betel nut is probably used by 20% of the world population. Chewing betel nut is associated with OSCC[41,42], and this may be exacerbated by the addition of tobacco to the combination.

Genetic factors

A case-control study in Brazil showed the risk for cancer in the head and neck to be raised for those who reported cancer at any site in a first-degree relative, with a greater risk if the relative had cancer in the head and neck[43]. It has been suggested that such familial clustering of cancer points to a possible genetic component in the development of OSCC.

Table 7.1 Effects of cigarette smoking and alcohol use on risk of cancer of the upper GI tract [35]

Consumption tobacco (number cigarettes/day)	Relative risk of cancer
Never smoked	1
Ex-smoker	1.52
<20	2.74
>20	9.02
Consumption alcohol* (g alcohol/day)	**Relative risk of cancer**
0	1
>0 – 30	1.21
>30 – 60	3.17
>60	9.22

* Mean lifelong consumption of alcohol

Table 7.2 Effects of combined cigarette smoking and alcohol use on risk of cancer of the upper GI tract [35]

| | | Consumption tobacco (number cigarettes/day) | | |
		Non smoker	<20	>20
Consumption alcohol (g alcohol/day)	>0 – 30	RR – 1	RR – 2	RR – 6.8
	>30 – 60	RR – 2.6	RR – 5.1	RR – 20.7
	>60	RR – 6.9	RR – 22	RR – 48.7

RR = relative risk

Socioeconomic status

Socioeconomic status plays an important role, with most OSCC being seen in people of low socioeconomic status[44,45]. In addition, a number of different manual occupations have been found to be associated with increased risk of oral cancer.

Diet

Fried foods and charcoal-grilled red meat have been implicated as risk factors for OSCC[46]. However, an increased consumption of fruits and vegetables is associated with a lower risk of OSCC[47].

Microorganisms

Microorganisms have been implicated in the aetiology of OSCC[48]. Thus, *Treponema pallidum*[49], *Candida albicans*[50], herpesviruses, and human papillomaviruses (HPV) [51] may be implicated in at least some cases of oral cancer.

Candidal leukoplakia are potentially malignant[50], and autoimmune polyendocrinopathy-candidiasis-ectodermal dystrophy (APECED), an autosomal recessive disease associated with a limited T-lymphocyte defect, seems to favour the growth of *Candida albicans* and predisposes to chronic stomatitis and OSCC[52].

Viral infections, particularly with oncogenic HPV subtypes, can have a tumourigenic effect[53]. Oropharyngeal cancer is significantly associated with oral HPV type 16, and also associated with a high lifetime number of vaginal-sex partners (>26), and oral-sex partners (≥6). In one study, HPV-16 DNA was detected in 72% tumour samples[54].

Oral health

Table 7.3 shows some oral lesions which can progress to OSCC.

Poor oral hygiene may be associated with an increased risk of OSCC, although not all workers agree about this association (and so further studies are required).

Systemic health

There is an increase in the incidence of OSCC in transplant recipients[55], and of tongue tumours in patients with systemic sclerosis[56]. Epidemiological studies also suggest an association between diabetes mellitus and oral cancer[57].

Table 7.3 Potentially pre-malignant oral lesions and conditions

Malignant potential	Lesion	Known aetiological factors	Main clinical features
Very high (≥ 85%)	Erythroplasia (erythroplakia)	Tobacco/alcohol	Velvety red plaque
High (≥ 30%)	Actinic cheilitis	Sunlight	White plaque/erosions
	Candidal leukoplakia	Candida albicans	White or speckled white and red plaque
	Dyskeratosis congenital	Genetic	White plaques
	Leukoplakia (non-homogeneous)	Tobacco/alcohol	Speckled white and red plaque or nodular plaque
	Proliferative verrucous leukoplakia	Tobacco/alcohol/human papillomavirus (HPV)	White or speckled white and red or nodular plaque
	Sublingual leukoplakia (sublingual keratosis)	Tobacco/alcohol	White plaque
	Submucous fibrosis	Areca nut	Immobile pale mucosa
	Syphilitic leukoplakia	Syphilis	White plaque
Low (< 5%)	Atypia in immuno-compromised patients	? Human papillomavirus (HPV)	White or speckled white and red plaque
	Leukoplakia (homogeneous)	Friction/tobacco/alcohol	White plaque
	Discoid lupus erythematosus	Autoimmune	White plaque/erosions
	Lichen planus	Idiopathic	White plaque/erosions
	Paterson-Kelly-Brown syndrome	Iron deficiency	Post-cricoid web

Radiation

Lip cancer is seen in people with chronic sun exposure [58]. (Ionizing radiation exposure is a possible risk factor for second primary cancers[59]).

Clinical features

Many OSCCs can be detected visually[60], although early OSCCs may be asymptomatic, and can be overlooked if the examination is not thorough enough[61]. Cancer must be suspected when there is a single oral lesion persisting for more than 3 weeks.

In the developed world, some 42% of OSCC affect the lip, with the majority of intraoral OSCC involving the floor of the mouth or lateral border of the tongue (22% the tongue and 17% the floor of mouth)[62]. However, in the developing world, tongue and buccal mucosal cancers are the most common[63].

OSCC may present variously as[64,65]:

♦ A lump – may be indurated and/or fixed (to mucosa, deeper tissues, or overlying skin); may have abnormal supplying blood vessels.

♦ An ulcer – may be indurated and/or fixed (to mucosa, deeper tissues, or overlying skin); may have fissured/raised exophytic margins.

- A red lesion (erythroplasia).
- A white or mixed white-and-red lesion.
- Loose teeth.
- A non-healing extraction socket.
- Pain.
- Sensory changes (e.g. numbness).
- Other local symptoms.
- Systemic symptoms.
- Cervical lymph node enlargement – especially if there is hardness or fixation. Enlarged nodes in a patient with oral carcinoma may be caused by infection, reactive hyperplasia, or metastatic disease. Occasionally (~5% cases) cervical lymph node enlargement is detected in the absence of any obvious primary tumour – the most likely site for the primary in order of predilection is the tongue base, tonsil, or nasopharynx (Figures 7.1 and 7.2, see colour plate section).

It should be noted that many of the classic features of OSCC such as ulceration, induration, bleeding, and cervical lymphadenopathy are features of advanced, not early stage, disease[66].

OSCC should be staged according to the TNM (tumour, node, metastasis) classification of the International Union against Cancer. This classification relates well to overall survival rate, i.e. the earlier the tumour, the better the prognosis (and the less complicated is the treatment)[67,68]. Prognosis is also influenced by the degree of differentiation of the tumour (i.e. the more differentiated the tumour the better the prognosis; see Table 7.4).

Oral cancers may have a multicentric origin[69]. Furthermore, dysplastic or malignant changes may be detectable in clinically normal mucosa at sites far removed from an OSCC ('field change') [70,71]. It is, therefore, hardly surprising that second primary tumours are seen in up to about one-third of patients within a five-year period (and are a crucial factor in treatment failure)[72].

Investigations

The reliable differentiation of benign lesions from malignant lesions is not possible by clinical inspection alone[64]. The only method currently available to reliably determine the diagnosis is a histopathological examination of a biopsy tissue sample[73]. Indeed, the golden rule is to biopsy any persistent mucosal lesion where there is not absolute confidence that the diagnosis is of a benign lesion. Thus, a biopsy is invariably indicated for a solitary lesion present for over 3 weeks. The early diagnosis (and treatment) of OSCC are the goals of such a strategy[67,68].

An incisional biopsy is invariably indicated and should be sufficiently large to include enough suspect and apparently normal tissue to give the pathologist a chance to make a diagnosis (and not to

Table 7.4 Stage versus prognosis of intraoral carcinoma [67,68]

Tnm stage	5 year survival (%)
T1 N0 M0	~ 85
T2 N0 M0	~ 65
T1-3 N1 M0 T3 N0 M0	~ 40
Any T4 Any N2-3 Any M1	~ 10

have to request a further specimen). Some authorities take several biopsies at the first visit in order to avoid a false-negative pathology report. An excisional biopsy should be avoided, since this is unlikely to have excised an adequately wide margin of tissue if the lesion is malignant. If the pathology report denies malignancy, and yet clinically this is suspected, then a re-biopsy is invariably indicated.

Toluidine blue staining is a simple diagnostic tool that uses a blue dye to highlight abnormal areas of mucosa. The reported sensitivity of positive staining in one meta-analytical study ranged from 93.5% to 97.8%, and the specificity ranged from 73.3% to 92.9%, in patients at high risk for OSCC[74]. In the highest risk population (i.e. patients with prior upper autodigestive tract cancer), toluidine blue staining has a higher sensitivity to detect carcinoma *in situ* and OSCC when compared to clinical examination (96.7% and 40%, respectively)[75]. False-positive staining (when lesions stain blue, but no carcinoma is identified) occurred in 8–10% of cases associated with keratotic lesions and the regenerating edges of ulcers and erosions[75].

In cases of confirmed OSCC, a variety of other investigations are invariably required, including specific staging investigations (e.g. radiological imaging) and non-specific pretreatment investigations (see Chapter 5). Many patients with OSCC have significant co-morbidities, and assessment of these co-morbidities is also required prior to initiation of cancer treatment.

Management

A variety of different modalities is used in the management of OSCC, including surgery, laser therapy, radiotherapy, chemotherapy, and biological therapy. Furthermore, in many cases, more than one modality is used to try and improve the control of the disease[76]. The choice of treatment is determined by a number of factors, including stage of the disease, performance status of the patient, preference of the patient, and availability of specific interventions. Unfortunately, developments in the treatment of oral cancer have not led to significant improvements in 5-year disease-specific survival over the decades.

Surgery

Surgery is the oldest form of treatment for oral cancer, and current surgical treatment has recently been reviewed[77,78]. Surgery may be used in a number of different ways:

- Diagnostic surgery.
- Staging surgery.
- Preventive (or prophylactic) surgery.
- 'Curative' surgery – is used to treat early-stage disease. It may be used along with radiotherapy and/or chemotherapy, which can be given prior to or following the operation. In some cases, radiotherapy is actually used during an operation (intraoperative radiotherapy).
- Debulking (or cytoreductive) surgery – is done in some cases when removing a tumour entirely would cause too much damage to an organ or surrounding area. Radiotherapy and/or chemotherapy are also typically used in such circumstances.
- 'Palliative' surgery – is used to treat the complications of advanced disease.
- Supportive surgery – is used to help with other types of treatment. For example, a vascular-access device, such as a catheter port, can be placed into a large vein to facilitate chemotherapy.
- Restorative (or reconstructive) surgery – is used to restore a person's appearance or the function of an organ or body part following primary surgery. Examples include the use of tissue flaps, bone grafts, or prosthetic materials. Dental and prosthetic rehabilitation are enhanced by successful surgical reconstruction[77].

Perioperative surgical complications are common, and occurred in 47% of patients with mouth cancer in one report from the UK (with an operative death rate of 3.2%)[79]. Factors predicting complications included the stage and differentiation of tumour; the nature, scale, and duration of surgery; pre-existing cardiovascular disease, respiratory disease, and alcohol consumption. The overall 30-day mortality rate was 3.83% in another European centre[80]. The risk factors for mortality in that study were old age (≥70 year), female gender, and current alcohol addiction (and laryngeal location). The postoperative mortality was 1.63% for patients without risk factors, and was 6.41% for those with one or two risk factors.

Transoral laser microsurgery is a new trend for resection of tumours, and is associated with good preservation of function.

Radiotherapy

Radiotherapy is commonly used to treat oral cancer (and other tumours of the head and neck region), and may also be used in a number of different ways[81]:

◆ 'Radical' radiotherapy

1. Primary treatment – radiotherapy may be used in isolation to treat patients with early ('curable') disease.

2. Adjuvant treatment – radiotherapy may be used following surgery to treat patients at high risk of recurrence (e.g. patients with positive surgical margins or positive lymph nodes)[82]. In some cases, chemotherapy is given in conjunction with the radiotherapy.

3. Neo-adjuvant treatment – radiotherapy may be used prior to surgery to 'down-size' the tumour. Again, in some cases, chemotherapy is given in conjunction with the radiotherapy.

◆ 'Palliative' radiotherapy

1. Primary treatment – radiotherapy may be used in isolation (or with chemotherapy) to treat patients with advanced ('incurable') disease.

2. Symptomatic treatment.

A variety of different modalities, techniques, and schedules may be employed in the management of OSCC. A detailed discussion of the various options is beyond the scope of this chapter, although these options are discussed in some detail in Chapter 10.

Chemotherapy

Chemotherapy is increasingly used to treat oral cancer (and other tumours of the head and neck region)[80]. Chemotherapy may be used in isolation (e.g. intra-arterial methotrexate for early SCC of lip)[81], or more commonly in combination with radiotherapy (chemoradiotherapy). In the latter instance, the chemotherapy may act as both an anti-neoplastic agent and a radiosensitizing agent.

Biological therapy

There is considerable interest in a range of so-called targeted therapies (biological therapies). One of the growth factors linked to oral cancers is epidermal growth factor. Cetuximab blocks epidermal growth factor receptors (EGFR), and has been approved by the Food and Drug Administration in the United States of America to use along with radiotherapy in people with advanced oral cancer[82]. Erlotinib also blocks EGFR, and also seems to help some patients with oral cancer.

A study of QOL changes from baseline to 6 and 12 months following treatment of patients with advanced OSCC treated with reconstructive surgery and adjuvant radiotherapy showed that most general quality-of-life issues (pain, constipation, insomnia, emotional functioning, etc.) did not to improve/change after treatment, and that head-and-neck-specific quality-of-life issues deteriorated immediately after treatment but returned to pretreatment levels at 12 months. The only exceptions were senses, opening mouth, sticky saliva, and coughing, which remained impaired in the long term. Tumour site and stage, extensive resections, and co-morbidity were significantly associated with adverse quality-of-life outcomes (as were age and marital status)[83].

References

1 Scully C, Moles D (2008). Oral cancer, in Heggenhougen KH, Quah S (eds) *International Encyclopedia of Public Health*, volume 4, pp. 668–77. Academic Press, San Diego.

2 Bagan JV, Scully C (2008). Recent advances in Oral Oncology 2007: epidemiology, aetiopathogenesis, diagnosis and prognostication. *Oral Oncol*, 44(2), 103–8.

3 Nair U, Bartsch H, Nair J (2004). Alert for an epidemic of oral cancer due to use of the betel quid substitutes gutkha and pan masala; a review of agents and causative mechanisms. *Mutagenesis*, 19(4), 251–62.

4 Bhurgri Y (2005). Cancer of the oral cavity – trends in Karachi South (1995–2002). *Asian Pac J Cancer Prev*, 6(1), 22–6.

5 Moore SR, Johnson NW, Pierce AM, Wilson DF (2000). The epidemiology of mouth cancer; a review of global incidence. *Oral Dis*, 6(2), 65–74.

6 Levi F, Lucchini F, Boyle P, Negri E, La Vecchia C (1998). Cancer incidence and mortality in Europe, 1988–92. *J Epidemiol Biostat*, 3, 295–361.

7 Blot WJ, McLaughlin JK, Devesa SS, Fraumeni JF, Jr (1996). Cancers of the oral cavity and pharynx, in Schottenfeld D, Fraumeni JF Jr (eds) *Cancer Epidemiology and Prevention*, 2nd edn, pp. 666–60. Oxford University Press, New York.

8 Espey DK, Wu XC, Swan J, et al. (2007). Annual report to the nation on the status of cancer, 1975–2004, featuring cancer in American Indians and Alaska Natives. *Cancer*, 110(10), 2119–52.

9 Ferlay J, Bray F, Pisani P, Parking DM (2001). *Globocan 2000. Cancer incidence, mortality and prevalence worldwide*. IARC Press, Lyon.

10 Tumino R, Vicario G (2004). Head and neck cancers: oral cavity, pharynx, and larynx. *Epidemiol Prev*, 28(2 Suppl), 28–33.

11 Swango PA (1996).Cancers of the oral cavity and pharynx in the United States: an epidemiologic overview. *J Public Health Dent*, 56(6), 309–18.

12 National Cancer Institute (1994). *SEER Cancer Statistics Review, 1973–1991*. National Cancer Institute, Bethesda.

13 Davidson BJ, Rook WA, Trock BJ (2001). Age and survival from squamous cell carcinoma of the oral tongue. *Head Neck*, 23(4), 273–9.

14 Cooper JS, Pajak TF, Rubin P, et al. (1989). Second malignancies in patients who have head and neck cancer: incidence, effect on survival and implications based on the RTOG experience. *Int J Radiat Oncol Biol Phys*, 17(3), 449–56.

15 Scully C, Field JK, Tanzawa H (2000). Genetic aberrations in oral or head and neck squamous cell carcinoma 3: clinico-pathological applications. *Oral Oncol*, 36(5), 404–13.

16 World Health Organization and International Agency for Research on Cancer (1986). *IARC Monographs on the evaluation of carcinogenic risks to humans. Volume 38: Tobacco smoking*. International Agency for Research on Cancer, Lyon.

17 World Health Organization and International Agency for Research on Cancer (1985). *IARC monographs on the evaluation of carcinogenic risks to humans. Volume 37: Tobacco habits other than smoking: betel-quid and areca-nut chewing; and some related nitrosamines*. International Agency for Research on Cancer, Lyon.

18 World Health Organization and International Agency for Research on Cancer (1988). *IARC monographs on the evaluation of carcinogenic risks to humans. Volume 44: Alcohol drinking.* International Agency for Research on Cancer, Lyon.

19 Mackenzie J, Ah-See K, Thakker N et al (2000). Increasing incidence of oral cancer amongst young persons: what is the aetiology? *Oral Oncol*, 36(4), 387–9.

20 Llewellyn CD, Linklater K, Bell J, Johnson NW, Warnakulasuriya KA (2003). Squamous cell carcinoma of the oral cavity in patients aged 45 years and under: a descriptive analysis of 116 cases diagnosed in the South East of England from 1990 to 1997. *Oral Oncol*, 39(2), 106–14.

21 Dahlstrom KR, Little JA, Zafereo ME, Lung M, Wei Q, Sturgis EM (2008). Squamous cell carcinoma of the head and neck in never smoker-never drinkers: a descriptive epidemiologic study. *Head Neck*, 30(1), 75–84.

22 La Vecchia C, Bidoli E, Barra S, et al. (1990). Type of cigarettes and cancers of the upper digestive and respiratory tract. *Cancer Causes Control*, 1(1), 69–74.

23 Rahman M, Sakamoto J, Fukui T (2005). Calculation of population attributable risk for bidi smoking and oral cancer in south Asia. *Prev Med*, 40(5), 510–14.

24 Shanks TG, Burns DM (1998). Disease consequences of cigar smoking, in Shopland DR (ed) *Smoking and Tobacco Control Monograph 9 – Cigars: Health Effects and Trends*, pp.105–58. National Cancer Institute, Bethesda.

25 Baric JM, Alman JE, Feldman RS, Chauncey HH (1982). Influence of cigarette, pipe, and cigar smoking, removable partial dentures, and age on oral leukoplakia. *Oral Surg Oral Med Oral Pathol*, 54(4), 424–9.

26 Axell T, Mornstad H, Sundstrom B (1978). [Snuff and cancer of the oral cavity - a retrospective study]. *Lakartidningen*, 75(22), 2224–6.

27 Accortt NA, Waterbor JW, Beall C, Howard G (2005). Cancer incidence among a cohort of smokeless tobacco users (United States). *Cancer Causes Control*, 16(9), 1107–15.

28 Hashibe M, Straif K, Tashkin DP, Morgenstern H, Greenland S, Zhang ZF (2005). Epidemiologic review of marijuana use and cancer risk. *Alcohol*, 35(3), 265–75.

29 World Cancer Research Fund and American Institute for Cancer Research (1997). *Food, nutrition and the prevention of cancer: a global perspective.* American Institute for Cancer Research, Washington DC.

30 World Health Organization and Food and Agriculture Organization (2003). *Diet, nutrition and the prevention of chronic diseases.* World Health Organization, Geneva

31 Franceschi S, Levi F, Dal Maso L et al (2000). Cessation of alcohol drinking and risk of cancer of the oral cavity and pharynx. *Int J Cancer*, 85(6), 787–90.

32 Barra S, Franceschi S, Negri E, Talamini R, La Vecchia C (1990). Type of alcoholic beverage and cancer of the oral cavity, pharynx and oesophagus in an Italian area with high wine consumption. *Int J Cancer*, 46(6), 1017–20.

33 Petti S, Scully C (2005). Oral cancer: the association between nation-based alcohol-drinking profiles and oral cancer mortality. *Oral Oncol*, 41(8), 828–34.

34 Hindle I, Downer MC, Moles DR, Speight PM (2000). Is alcohol responsible for more intra-oral cancer? *Oral Oncol*, 36(4), 328–33.

35 Boeing H (2002). Alcohol and risk of cancer of the upper gastrointestinal tract: first analysis of the EPIC data. *IARC Sci Publ*, 156, 151–4.

36 Blot WJ, McLaughlin JK, Winn DM, et al. (1988). Smoking and drinking in relation to oral and pharyngeal cancer. *Cancer Res*, 48(11), 3282–7.

37 Franceschi S, Talamini R, Barra S, et al. (1990). Smoking and drinking in relation to cancers of the oral cavity, pharynx, larynx, and esophagus in northern Italy. *Cancer Res*, 50(20), 6502–7.

38 Rodriguez T, Altieri A, Chatenoud L, et al. (2004). Risk factors for oral and pharyngeal cancer in young adults. *Oral Oncol*, 40(2), 207–13.

39 Winn DM, Blot WJ, McLaughlin JK, et al. (1991). Mouthwash use and oral conditions in the risk of oral and pharyngeal cancer. *Cancer Res*, 51(11), 3044–7.

40 Elmore JG, Horwitz RI (1995). Oral cancer and mouthwash use: evaluation of the epidemiologic evidence. *Otolaryngol Head Neck Surg*, 113(3), 253–61.

41 Nandakumar A, Thimmasetty KT, Sreeramareddy NM, et al. (1990). A population-based case-control investigation on cancers of the oral cavity in Bangalore, India. *Br J Cancer*, 62(5), 847–51.

42 Sankaranarayanan R, Duffy SW, Padmakumary G, Day NE, Krishan Nair M (1990). Risk factors for cancer of the buccal and labial mucosa in Kerala, southern India. *J Epidemiol Community Health*, 44(4), 286–92.

43 Foulkes WD, Brunet JS, Kowalski LP, Narod SA, Franco EL (1995). Family history of cancer is a risk factor for squamous cell carcinoma of the head and neck in Brazil; a case-control study. *Int J Cancer*, 63(6), 769–73.

44 Edwards DM, Jones J (1999). Incidence of and survival from upper aerodigestive tract cancers in the UK; the influence of deprivation. *Eur J Cancer*, 35(6), 968–72.

45 Greenwood M, Thomson PJ, Lowry RJ, Steen IN (2003). Oral cancer: material deprivation, unemployment and risk factor behaviour-an initial study. *Int J Oral Maxillofac Surg*, 32(1), 74–7.

46 Galeone C, Pelucchi C, Talamini R, et al. (2005). Role of fried foods and oral/pharyngeal and oesophageal cancers. *Br J Cancer*, 92(11), 2065–9.

47 Potter JD (1997).Cancer prevention: epidemiology and experiment. *Cancer Lett*, 114(1–2), 7–9.

48 Scully C, Prime SS, Cox M, Maitland NJ (1991). Infectious agents in the aetiology of oral cancer, in Johnson NW (ed) *Oral Cancer: Detection of Patients and Lesions at Risk*, pp. 96–113. Cambridge University Press, Cambridge.

49 Michalek AM, Mahoney MC, McLaughlin CC, Murphy D, Metzger BB (1994). Historical and contemporary correlates of syphilis and cancer. *Int J Epidemiol*, 23(2), 381–5.

50 Sitheeque MA, Samaranayake LP (2003). Chronic hyperplastic candidosis/candidiasis (candidal leukoplakia). *Crit Rev Oral Biol Med*, 14(4), 253–67.

51 Gillison ML, Koch WM, Shah KV (1999). Human papillomavirus in head and neck squamous cell carcinoma: are some head and neck cancers a sexually transmitted disease? *Curr Opin Oncol*, 11(3), 191–9.

52 Rautemaa R, Hietanen J, Niissalo S, Pirinen S, Perheentupa J (2007). Oral and oesophageal squamous cell carcinoma-a complication or component of autoimmune polyendocrinopathy-candidiasis-ectodermal dystrophy (APECED, APS-I). *Oral Oncol*, 43(6), 607–13.

53 Tsantoulis PK, Kastrinakis NG, Tourvas AD, Laskaris G, Gorgoulis VG (2007). Advances in the biology of oral cancer. *Oral Oncol*, 43(6), 523–34.

54 D'Souza G, Kreimer AR, Viscidi R et al. (2007). Case-control study of human papillomavirus and oropharyngeal cancer. *N Engl J Med*, 356(19), 1944–56.

55 Scheifele C, Reichart PA, Hippler-Benscheidt M, Neuhaus P, Neuhaus R (2005). Incidence of oral, pharyngeal, and laryngeal squamous cell carcinomas among 1515 patients after liver transplantation. *Oral Oncol*, 41(7), 670–6.

56 Derk CT, Rasheed M, Spiegel JR, Jimenez SA (2005). Increased incidence of carcinoma of the tongue in patients with systemic sclerosis. *J Rheumatol*, 32(4), 637–41.

57 Goutzanis L, Vairaktaris E, Yapijakis C, et al. (2007). Diabetes may increase risk for oral cancer through the insulin receptor substrate-1 and focal adhesion kinase pathway. *Oral Oncol*, 43(2), 165–73.

58 Luna-Ortiz K, Guemes-Meza A, Villavicencio-Valencia V, Mosqueda-Taylor A (2004). Lip cancer experience in Mexico. An 11-year retrospective study. *Oral Oncol*, 40(10), 992–9.

59 Hashibe M, Ritz B, Le AD, Li G, Sankaranarayanan R, Zhang ZF (2005). Radiotherapy for oral cancer as a risk factor for second primary cancers. *Cancer Lett*, 220(2), 185–95.

60 Sankaranarayanan R, Fernandez GL, Lence AJ, Pisani P, Rodriguez SA (2002). Visual inspection in oral cancer screening in Cuba: a case-control study. *Oral Oncol*, 38(2), 131–6.

61 Shugars DC, Patton LL (1997(. Detecting, diagnosing, and preventing oral cancer. *Nurse Pract*, 22(6), 105–15.

62 Krolls SO, Hoffman S (1976).Squamous cell carcinoma of the oral soft tissues: a statistical analysis of 14,253 cases by age, sex, and race of patients. *J Am Dent Assoc*, 92(3), 571–4.

63 Sankaranarayanan R (1990). Oral cancer in India; an epidemiologic and clinical review. *Oral Surg Oral Med Oral Pathol*, 69(3), 325–30.

64 Mashberg A, Merletti F, Boffetta P et al. (1989). Appearance, site of occurrence, and physical and clinical characteristics of oral carcinoma in Torino, Italy. *Cancer*, 63(12), 2522–7.

65 Mashberg A, Samit A (1995). Early diagnosis of asymptomatic oral and oropharyngeal squamous cancers. *CA Cancer J Clin*, 45(6), 328–51.

66 Mashberg A, Feldman LJ (1988). Clinical criteria for identifying early oral and oropharyngeal carcinoma: erythroplasia revisited. *Am J Surg*, 156(4), 273–5.

67 Woolgar J (1995). A pathologist's view of oral cancer in the north west. *Br Dent Nurs J*, 54(4), 14–16.

68 Sciubba JJ (2001). Oral cancer. The importance of early diagnosis and treatment. *Am J Clin Dermatol*, 2(4), 239–51.

69 Slaughter DP, Southwick HW, Smejkal W (1953). Field cancerization in oral stratified squamous epithelium; clinical implications of multicentric origin. *Cancer*, 6(5), 963–8.

70 Thomson PJ (2002). Field change and oral cancer: new evidence for widespread carcinogenesis? *Int J Oral Maxillofac Surg*, 31(3), 262–6.

71 Thomson PJ, Hamadah O (2007). Cancerisation within the oral cavity: the use of 'field mapping biopsies' in clinical management. *Oral Oncol*, 43(1), 20–6.

72 Lippman SM, Hong WK (1989). Second malignant tumors in head and neck squamous cell carcinoma: the overshadowing threat for patients with early-stage disease. *Int J Radiat Oncol Biol Phys*, 17(3), 691–4.

73 Lumerman H, Freedman P, Kerpel S (1995). Oral epithelial dysplasia and the development of invasive squamous cell carcinoma. *Oral Surg Oral Med Oral Pathol Oral Radiol Endod*, 79(3), 321–9.

74 Rosenberg D, Cretin S (1989). Use of meta-analysis to evaluate tolonium chloride in oral cancer screening. *Oral Surg Oral Med Oral Pathol*, 67(5), 621–7.

75 Epstein JB, Feldman R, Dolor RJ, Porter SR (2003). The utility of tolonium chloride rinse in the diagnosis of recurrent or second primary cancers in patients with prior upper aerodigestive tract cancer. *Head Neck*, 25(11), 911–21.

76 Preuss SF, Dinh V, Klussmann JP, Semrau R, Mueller RP, Guntinas-Lichius O (2007) Outcome of multimodal treatment for oropharyngeal carcinoma: a single institution experience. *Oral Oncol*, 43(4), 402–7.

77 Yao M, Epstein JB, Modi BJ, Pytynia KB, Mundt AJ, Feldman LE (2007). Current surgical treatment of squamous cell carcinoma of the head and neck. *Oral Oncol*, 43(3), 213–23.

78 Scully C, Bagan JV (2008). Recent advances in Oral Oncology 2007: imaging, treatment and treatment outcomes. *Oral Oncology*, 44(3), 211–15.

79 McGurk MG, Fan KF, MacBean AD, Putcha V (2007). Complications encountered in a prospective series of 182 patients treated surgically for mouth cancer. *Oral Oncol*, 43(5), 471–6.

80 Penel N, Amela E Y, Mallet Y, et al. (2007). A simple predictive model for postoperative mortality after head and neck cancer surgery with opening of mucosa. *Oral Oncol*, 43(2), 174–80.

81 National Comprehensive Cancer Network (NCCN) website: http://www.nccn.org

82 Blackburn TK, Bakhtawar S, Brown JS, Lowe D, Vaughan ED, Rogers SN (2007). A questionnaire survey of current UK practice for adjuvant radiotherapy following surgery for oral and oropharyngeal squamous cell carcinoma. *Oral Oncol*, 43(2), 143–9.

81 Wu CF, Chen CM, Chen CH, Shieh TY, Sheen MC (2007). Continuous intraarterial infusion chemotherapy for early lip cancer. *Oral Oncol*, 43(8), 825–30.

82 Astsaturov I, Cohen RB, Harari P (2007). EGFR-targeting monoclonal antibodies in head and neck cancer. *Curr Cancer Drug Targets*, 7(7), 650–65.

83 Borggreven PA, Aaronson NK, Verdonck-de Leeuw IM, et al. (2007). Quality of life after surgical treatment for oral and oropharyngeal cancer: a prospective longitudinal assessment of patients reconstructed by a microvascular flap. *Oral Oncol*, 43(10), 1034–42.

Chapter 8

Other tumours of the oral cavity

Barbara Murphy, Jill Gilbert, and Anderson Collier III

Introduction

Over 90% of tumours involving the oral cavity are epidermoid epithelial tumours[1]. The remaining 5–10% of tumours is composed of a wide array of benign and malignant histological types that arise from the epithelium, mesenchyme, vascular tissues, lymphoreticular system, and bone. The purpose of this chapter is to provide the reader with an overview of this heterogeneous group of tumours. Oral squamous cell carcinoma is discussed in detail in Chapter 7.

Salivary gland tumours

Salivary gland tumours are rare, occurring in 1–1.5 per 100 000 people in the US population. Salivary gland tumours represent a heterogeneous group of tumours. The majority of tumours are benign, and the vast majority of tumours arise within the parotid gland (70–80%). There is an inverse relationship between the size of the salivary gland and the probability of malignancy. Thus, tumours arising out of the parotid gland have an 80% chance of being benign versus 20% for tumours arising from the minor salivary glands. (Salivary gland tumours constitute ~5% of all head and neck cancers). There is a correlation between salivary gland tumours and low-dose radiation for treatment of benign diseases[2,3]. Radiation-induced tumours usually arise following a latent period of 15–20 years.

Benign salivary gland tumours

Pleomorphic adenoma

These are the single most common salivary gland tumours. They most frequently occur in the parotid gland. The peak incidence is in the 4th and 5th decade, and they exhibit a female predominance. Histologically, they have ductal epithelial and myoepithelial cells within a mesenchymal stroma[4]. Pleomorphic adenomas usually present as well-circumscribed lesions. They tend to be slow growing. Local recurrence following enucleation is common.

Warthin's tumour (papillary cystadenoma lymphomatosum)

These comprise ~6–10% of parotid tumours, and are usually located in the parotid tail[4]. They are most commonly found in men between the 4th and 7th decades of life. They are benign adenomas with lymphoid stroma, may be bilateral or multifocal, and tend to be slow growing. Malignant transformation is rare.

Oncocytoma

These are most commonly diagnosed in the parotid gland. The peak incidence is between the 7th and 8th decades, and they have a female predominance. They are composed of round cells with eosinophilic granules and small indented nuclei[4]. They are slow-growing, encapsulated tumours, which infrequently recur following surgical resection.

Malignant salivary gland tumours

Mucoepidermoid carcinoma

These comprise one-third of all malignant salivary gland tumours[5]. The most common primary site is the parotid followed by the palate. The peak incidence is in the 5th decade, and there is no gender predominance. The pathology consists of a mixed tumour with two main elements: epidermoid and mucus-producing cells[6]. A third cell type, the intermediate cell, is felt to be a progenitor cell that can give rise to the other two cell types[7]. The most common presenting symptom is a painless mass followed by pain, facial nerve weakness, and skin ulceration[8]. The behaviour of mucoepidermoid tumours is highly variable. Prognostic factors for a poor outcome include: age over 40, fixed tumours, higher tumour stage, and higher histological grade[9]. Low-grade tumours may behave in an indolent manner. However, high-grade tumours have a propensity to enlarge rapidly and metastasize to regional lymph nodes and to distant sites.

Adenoid cystic carcinoma

These comprise ~20% of malignant salivary gland tumours. The most common site is the palate[10]. The peak incidence is in the 6th and 7th decades, and there is a slight female predominance. There are three histological subtypes: solid, tubular/tubuloductal, and cribriform. (Patients with solid adenoid cystic carcinomas have a worse prognosis than cribriform subtypes[11]. Tubular or tubuloductal subtypes appear to behave in an intermediate fashion.) The most common presenting symptoms are asymptomatic swelling, pain, painful swelling, nasal mass, swelling in the neck, and voice change[10]. Adenoid cystic carcinomas are slow-growing tumours with a propensity for perineural spread. In addition, patients may develop metastatic disease, predominantly in the lungs. However, patients with metastases may survive for many years due to the slow rate of tumour growth. The 10-year disease-specific survival for patients with and without distant metastases is 72% and 48%, respectively[12]. Predictors for the development of distant metastatic disease include solid histological subtype and major salivary gland origin[12].

Acinic cell tumour

These are found most commonly within the parotid gland. These tumours have a wide age distribution, and a female predominance. They are histologically characterized by serous acinar cells, although other cell types may be present. Histological subtypes include solid, microcystic, papillary-cystic, and follicular[13]. Prognosis is best predicted by T-stage at diagnosis. In a series from the Mayo clinic, 44% patients developed local recurrence, and 19% patients developed metastatic disease following primary treatment[14]. (Patients with larger tumours are more likely to recur post-operatively).

Polymorphous low-grade adenocarcinoma

These are most commonly noted in the minor salivary glands with a predilection for the palate[15]. They present in the 6th to 8th decade, and are more commonly noted in women. The histology may include solid, tubular, and papillary variants. Overall, prognosis is good, although local regional failure, nodal spread, and distant metastases are commonly reported in patients with a significant component of papillary features.

Carcinoma ex pleomorphic adenoma

These are carcinomas that arise from a benign mixed tumour[4]. They are usually found within the parotid gland. They are most common in the 6th to 7th decade, with no gender predilection.

Patients typically present with rapid expansion of a previously stable or slow-growing mass. Histology reveals a circumscribed pleomorphic adenoma with an infiltrative component[16,17]. Prognosis is dependent on the extent of the invasive component. Patients with minimally invasive disease have a good prognosis. Conversely, patients with a large invasive component are more likely to develop nodal or distant disease.

'Adenocarcinoma not otherwise specified'

These represent a heterogeneous group of tumours. The behavior correlates with their site of origin along the salivary duct structure: tumours arising from the terminal ducts tend to be low grade as opposed to ductal carcinomas that tend to be high grade[18].

Minor salivary gland cancers of the oral cavity

A number of reports have centred on intraoral minor salivary gland tumours[19–22]. The frequency of histopatholgical subtypes varies amongst studies. This may be due to the changes in the classification systems over time, or variability due to racial or geographic characteristics[22,23].

Wang reported on 737 patients with intraoral minor salivary gland tumours treated in China[21]. The average age at presentation was 41 years. The female-to-male ratio was 1.1:1. Fifty-four percent of minor salivary gland tumours were malignant. Adenoid cystic carcinomas were the most common malignant tumour (36% of malignant tumours, and 19.4% of all tumours). Pleomorphic adenoma was the most common benign diagnosis (81.8% of benign tumours, and 37.3% of all tumours). The most common sites were the palate (67.4%), buccal mucosa (10.4%), and lip (7.1%).

Lopes reported the results of a retrospective analysis of 128 cases of minor salivary gland carcinomas involving the oral cavity[20]. Patients were treated over a protracted duration beginning in 1954 through to 1993. The median age at presentation was 49 years, and there were an equal number of men and women. The hard palate was the most common primary site (48.4%), followed by the tongue (12.5%) and the buccal mucosa (10.2%). The most common histological diagnoses were mucoepidermoid carcinoma (59%), adenoid cystic carcinoma (27%), and adenocarcinoma (7%). The T-stage at diagnosis was: T1 – 21.9%; T2 – 32.8%; T3 – 12.5%; and T4 – 32.8%. Nodal or distant metastatic disease was uncommon at presentation. The overall 5- and 10-year survival was high at 80.4% and 62.5%, respectively. In a multivariate analysis, predictors for survival included N-stage, histology, bone involvement, type of surgery, and gender.

The cornerstone of therapy for patients with salivary gland tumours is surgical resection. Patients with clinically evident nodal metastatic disease at the time of diagnosis should undergo neck dissection. In cases without clinical evidence of nodal metastases, elective neck dissection should be considered for those patients at high risk for occult nodal disease. The risk of development of nodal metastases is dependent on the primary site, the T-stage, and the histological type. (The site, stage, and histopathology have been combined to allow risk estimation for the presence of nodal metastases[24]).

Although largely retrospective, available data would indicate that post-operative radiation therapy improves outcomes in high-risk patients[25–27]. In the Dutch Head and Neck Oncology Cooperative Group study, the relative risk for local recurrence and regional recurrence was 9.7 and 2.3, respectively, for surgery alone compared to surgery followed by radiation[26]. Similarly, Mendenhall reported an overall increase in local control (42% vs. 90%), and regional control (40% vs. 81%), with the addition of post-operative radiation therapy[27]. High-risk features include patients with large tumors (T3 and T4), close or incomplete margins of resection, perineural invasion, and bone involvement. Patients with recurrent disease are also considered at high risk.

Radiation therapy may be considered as primary treatment for those patients who are deemed inoperable, those patients who refuse surgical resection, and those patients with metastatic disease who require palliation of local or regional disease. The cure rate for patients with unresectable disease treated with single-modality radiation therapy is ~20%[28]. Outcomes with radiation therapy alone are better for patients with earlier stage disease[29]. Salivary gland tumours may be considered for treatment with neutron beam therapy. The data would indicate that there is a potential improvement in local control for patients treated with neutron beam therapy (compared with conventional radiation therapy)[30]. However, this may be at the expense of increased toxicity. Furthermore, a survival advantage has yet to be demonstrated.

Although surgery with or without adjuvant radiation therapy is effective for disease control in many patients, a cohort of patients will develop locally recurrent or metastatic disease. Of note, recurrences may occur up to two decades following the initial surgery[31]. Palliative chemotherapy is only modestly effective in salivary gland tumours. Adriamycin has long been considered the most effective single agent for the treatment of salivary gland tumours. However, the studies supporting its use are methodologically flawed. Targeted agents are being investigated, but their role has yet to be defined.

Odontogenic tumours

Odontogenic tumours represent a rare, heterogeneous group of neoplasms of the oral cavity. Odontogenic tumours are derived from elements of the developing tooth, and are most commonly found in the mandible or maxilla. The majority of these tumors are 'benign', although even benign subtypes can be locally destructive[35]. The literature suggests that only 0–6% of odontogenic tumors are classically malignant[32]. Whilst tumours may only demonstrate epithelial origin, most benign tumour types demonstrate a combination of epithelial and ectomesenchymal origin[33–35].

Benign tumours

Ameloblastoma

The ameloblastoma is the second most common ondotogenic tumour (after the odontoma). The ameloblastoma has an epithelial cell of origin. Six different histopathological subtypes are described: follicular, acanthomatous, granular cell, basal cell, desmoplastic, and plexiform. Subtypes are based on the predominant pattern present. However, several critical histological features are noted amongst all the subtypes: background stroma of fibrous connective tissue; parallel orientation of the nuclei of the fibroblastic stromal cells; disconnected islands, strand, and cords of the epithelial component; budding growth pattern; characteristic pallisading pattern of nuclei; peripheral layer of tall columnar cells with hyperchromasia, reverse polarity of the nuclei, and subnuclear vacuole formation[36,37].

The average age of presentation of ameloblastoma is between 33 and 39 years. Ameloblastomas occur most often in the mandible (80%), especially in the molar–angle–ramus area. The majority of the other lesions originates in the maxilla (and may occur in slightly older individuals). Clinically, these lesions often present as a painless swelling in the jaw, although pain may be a feature in a minority of cases. Ulceration of the overlying mucosa may occur, or patients may complain of loose teeth, malocclusion, or failure of tooth eruption. Orthopantogram films classically demonstrate a radiolucent, multilocular appearance, although computed tomography (CT) scans demonstrate that the lesions are actually unilocular with a scalloped border.

Whilst the majority of ameloblastoma cases are benign, the biological behaviour often suggests a more aggressive neoplasm[35,36,38]. Malignant ameloblastoma refers to a tumour that appears histologically benign, but demonstrates the ability to metastasize. Metastases most often involve the lymph nodes and lungs, although other sites may also be involved. Metastases develop following a mean interval of 11 years. Median survival after the development of metastasis is 2 years. However, metastatic disease may behave in an indolent manner, with long-term survival being described in the literature. Most deaths are related to aggressive local disease[35,39].

Malignant tumours

Ameloblastic carcinoma [35,40,41]

These tumours may be directly contiguous with an existing ameloblastoma (carcinoma ex ameloblastoma), or may arise independently (*de novo* ameloblastic carcinoma). Histologically, the tumour demonstrates areas of both ameloblastoma and squamous cell carcinoma. This tumour is locally aggressive, and has metastatic potential. These tumours are often managed in the same manner as an oral squamous cell carcinoma with primary surgery with/without post-operative radiation therapy.

Intraossesous carcinoma [35,38,42]

Primary intraosseous carcinoma represents a squamous cell carcinoma arising from foci of odontogenic epithelium (within the jaw). A precursor lesion such as an odontogenic cyst may be present in some cases. Subtypes of this carcinoma include cystic primary intraosseous carcinoma, carcinoma ex dentigerous cyst, carcinoma ex odontogenic keratocyst, and intraosseous mucoepidermoid carcinoma. The mean age of presentation is 52 years, and the tumour is more common in males. These tumours often present as a painful swelling in the posterior mandible. Paraesthesia occurs in ~16%. Approximately one-third of patients demonstrate cervical metastases at presentation. Treatment involves surgery followed by radiation therapy. The 5-year survival is ~38%.

Ghost cell odontogenic carcinoma [38,43–45]

Ghost cell odontogenic carcinoma represents a variant of ameloblastic carcinoma. This malignancy demonstrates features of ameloblastic carcinoma with ghost cell keratinization. Ghost cells are immunoreactive for amelogenin (a dental enamel protein). The mean age of presentation is 38 years, and the tumour occurs most often in males. These tumours may be more common in the Asian population. In general, the tumour presents in the maxilla. The biological behaviour of the tumour is quite variable. Locally destructive lesions may occur and involve the orbit and base of skull. Distant metastases are not common, and the behaviour of distant disease may be indolent. Primary treatment involves surgical resection and post-operative chemotherapy.

Clear cell odontogenic carcinoma [35,38,46–49]

Clear cell odontogenic carcinoma represents a low-grade carcinoma with ameloblastic features. Tumours are characterized by the presence of cells with clear cytoplasm, intermingled with islands of cells with eosinophilic cytoplasm. Squamous or ameloblastic differentiation may be noted. This tumour occurs predominantly in females in their 6th decade. This tumour often presents as a painful mass in the anterior mandible. This neoplasm may behave aggressively, including local destruction with dental pulp penetration and soft-tissue extension. Metastases to lymph nodes and lungs are also described. Optimal tumour control is with complete surgical resection. The role of neck dissection is unclear, but as ~20% of tumours have lymph node metastases, this form of surgical approach should be considered[48]. Post-operative radiation therapy should also be considered.

Haematological tumours

Plasma cell disorders

Plasma cell disorders involving the oral cavity are uncommon, but the ones found most commonly are solitary plasmacytoma of bone, extramedullary plasmacytoma, and multiple myeloma. Patients with these disorders present with non-specific complaints including swelling, ulceration, pain, numbness, bleeding, trismus, poorly fitting dentures, and macroglossia (due to amyloidosis). Diagnosis often requires a deep biopsy, as fine-needle aspiration may be non-diagnostic. Immunohistochemical staining demonstrates a monoclonal immunoglobulin (and thus a clonal population of plasma cells). A combination of the clinical picture and radiological imaging will guide the differential diagnosis[50].

Solitary plasmacytoma of bone

Solitary plasmacytoma of bone represents ~3% of plasma cell disorders. It is uncommon in the head and neck area. (The mandible is the most common site in the head and neck area). The average age of presentation is 50 years, and there is a male predominance.

Radiographic imaging demonstrates an expansile lytic lesion, often with endosteal scalloping and cortical thinning. Pathological fracture may also be evident. Magnetic resonance imaging (MRI) findings may include low-to-normal signal intensity on T1-weighted images, and high signal intensity on T2-weighted images. Osteogenic osteomalacia has also been described in association with solitary plasmacytoma of bone[50–52]. The spike of monoclonal protein in the blood or urine that is characteristic of multiple myeloma is absent, or is below the level required to make the diagnosis of multiple myeloma.

Treatment for solitary plasmacytoma of bone involves radical radiation therapy. Excellent local control is achieved with ~45 Gy. However, some clinicians suggest doses as high as 50–60 Gy (due to the propensity for local invasion). Surgery is reserved for patients who are unable to receive radiotherapy, or in whom local recurrence has occurred[51,53,54]. The median survival is ~11 years. The prognosis relates to the likelihood of evolution to multiple myeloma. A direct correlation exists between persistence of abnormal protein following radiation therapy and the development of multiple myeloma. Sixty-six percent of patients ultimately develop multiple myeloma[50,51,53,54].

Extramedullary plasmacytoma

Extramedullary plasmacytoma comprises ~3% of plasma cell disorders. The clonal proliferation of plasma cells arises in the soft tissues, and usually the submucosal lymphoid tissue. Approximately 80% occurs in the head and neck, often in the oral cavity or upper airway. Multiple sites of involvement can occur in a patient, and regional nodal involvement occurs in 15% of patients[51,55–57]. Extramedullary plasmacytoma affects a younger population than multiple myeloma[50].

A urine or serum monoclonal protein spike may be present, although the value is less than that required for a myeloma diagnosis.

Radiation therapy is the preferred therapeutic modality. Local control rates of ≥80% can be achieved with 40–50 Gy. Surgery is generally reserved for salvage treatment. The prognosis is excellent, with 10-year disease-specific rates as high as 90%. Myeloma develops in 8–30% of patients[50,51,56].

Multiple myeloma

Multiple myeloma represents a systemic plasma cell disorder. The median age of diagnosis is 68 years, and the disease is most common in men.

The criteria required for the diagnosis of multiple myeloma include presence of a monoclonal serum or urine protein, presence of monoclonal cells in the bone marrow or a plasmacytoma, and presence of end-organ damage such as increased serum calcium, lytic bone lesions, anaemia, or renal failure.

The treatment of multiple myeloma continues to evolve; traditional chemotherapies, new targeted therapies (e.g. bortezemib), thalidomide analogues, and haematopoietic stem cell transplantation all have a role in the treatment of this disease.

Lymphomas

A variety of lymphoid malignances can develop in the oral cavity. The majority are Non-Hodgkin's lymphomas, and are of B-cell origin. Low-grade, intermediate-grade, and high-grade lymphomas can all involve the oral cavity. Multiple classification systems remain in use, but commonly used ones are the Revised European and American Lymphoma (REAL) and World Health Organization (WHO) classifications of lymphoid neoplasms[58].

Lymphomas of the oral cavity can have a varied presentation, including intraoral mass, hypertrophy of Waldeyer's ring, cervical nodal mass, fatigue, and so-called 'B symptoms' (i.e. fever >38ºC, night sweats, and loss of >10% of total body weight over the previous 6 months).

An excisional or incisional biopsy is usually required to make the diagnosis (to allow for adequate immunohistochemical and flow cytometric studies). An accurate histological classification is crucial, since the treatment strategy is governed by the histological classification (and the stage of disease).

In general, these tumours are highly sensitive to chemotherapy and radiation therapy. The choice of treatment depends on the particular circumstances, and may involve either radiation therapy alone, chemotherapy alone, or a combination of these treatment modalities. The advent of monoclonal antibodies targeting proteins expressed on malignant B cells has significantly improved the outcome for some subgroups of lymphoma (e.g. rituximab).

Sarcomas

Sarcomas of the head and neck account for 2% of all head and neck tumours, and 5–10% of all sarcomas[59–62]. This section will focus on the most common primary malignant sarcomas in and around the oral cavity.

Bone tumours

Ewing sarcoma, osteosarcoma, and chondrosarcoma are the primary malignant bone sarcomas that occur in the head and neck region. Ewing sarcoma occurs more frequently in males, with a peak incidence of 10–20 years of age (with ~50% of all cases occurring in this age range)[63–65]. Approximately 3% occur in the skull and facial bones, and ~1% in the mandible[64,66]. Osteosarcoma also has a peak incidence between 10 and 20 years of age, with nearly 40% occurring in this age range. Between 5% and 9% occur in the skull and facial bones, and ~4% in the mandible[64,66]. Chondrosarcoma is rare below the age of 40, and increases in incidence with age[64]. It is the most common primary malignant bone tumour of the skull and facial bones[64,66,67].

The histological appearance of Ewing sarcoma is somewhat varied. The tumour cells are small, round, blue cells with scant cytoplasm. Nearly all tumours mark with CD99, and most mark for vimentin[68]. More mature tumours will also demonstrate some degree of neuronal differentiation with positive expression of NES and S-100[63]. One of the most important diagnostic features of Ewing sarcoma is the t(11;22)(q23;q12) translocation. This translocation is noted in >85% patients with Ewing sarcoma. The hallmark histological feature of osteosarcoma is the production of irregular osteoid by the tumour cells[69]. Most osteosarcomas are sporadic, although some are associated with rare cancer syndromes[70,71]. The histological appearance of chondrosarcomas is varied. The hallmark feature is the production of cartilage matrix[69].

These tumours usually present as a mass that can be painful, can interfere with function such as mastication, and/or erode through the mucosa. Symptoms may be present for weeks to months before they are brought to medical attention[63,72,73,75]. Furthermore 13–25% of patients with Ewing sarcoma and 10–20% of patients with osteosarcoma present with metastatic disease either to the lungs, other bones, or bone marrow (only Ewing sarcoma)[63,64]. Approximately 5% of patients with chondrosarcoma present with metastatic disease.

Primary surgical resection is important in all three tumour types, and is the only chance of cure for osteosarcoma and chondrosarcoma[63,72,73,75]. Radiation is a viable alternative for local control of Ewing sarcoma[76]. Osteosarcoma and chondrosarcoma are relatively radiation resistant[64]. However, in cases where complete surgical resection would cause excessive morbidity, radiation therapy with doses >60 Gy has been used[72,77,78]. Ewing sarcoma and osteosarcoma are both chemosensitive tumours. The current treatment strategies employ multi-agent chemotherapy regimens[63,64,73]. Chondrosarcomas are not chemosensitive.

At present, the long-term overall survival rate for Ewing sarcoma and osteosarcoma is ~50–60%[63,64,72,73]. The rates are nearly 70% for patients who present with local disease, but only 20% and 30% for patients with metastatic Ewing sarcoma and osteosarcoma, respectively[65,79]. The survival for chondrosarcoma is 75–90%. (Over 50% of patients with chondrosarcoma have localized disease.)

Soft-tissue sarcomas

Soft-tissue sarcomas have an estimated annual incidence of 3–4.5 per 100 000. The majority are in the extremities, with 1–2% located in the head and neck region[80–82]. The most common histology is rhabdomyosarcoma, which is more common in children than adults. The median age of diagnosis of head and neck soft-tissue sarcoma is 35–40 years when children are included, and 45–50 years when children are excluded[61,62,83–88].

The hallmark histological feature of rhabdomyosarcoma is rhabdomyoblasts forming cross-striations. Rhabdomyosarcoma marks for immature muscle-markers such as myosin, Myo-D, and myoglobin[89,90]. There are three histological subtypes: embryonal, alveolar, and pleomorphic, with embryonal being the most common subtype[91,92]. Embryonal rhabdomyosarcoma is usually associated with the loss of heterozygosity of chromosome 11p15[93]. Alveolar subtype, so named because it resembles the alveoli of the lungs, usually contains one of two translocations: t(2;13)(q35;q14), or t(1;13)(p36;q13).

The most common presentation is a painless mass. Depending on the location, and the grade of the tumour, the mass may have been present for a long time before coming to attention[85,88]. Tumour grading is important to determine the clinical nature of the tumour (as well as to help guide treatment). Low-grade tumours tend to be slow growing with low metastatic potential, whilst high-grade tumors are often more invasive and have an increased propensity for local recurrence and metastases[69,94]. Rhabdomyosaroma is considered a high-grade tumour.

The treatment of rhabdomyosarcoma is determined by the age, location, histology, and spread of the tumour[95]. The treatment involves resection, radiation therapy (in most circumstances), and chemotherapy. The survival is only ~35% for adults with head and neck rhabdomyosarcoma[61]. The overall survival for patients with soft-tissue sarcoma of the head and neck is 40–70%. The prognosis is generally dependent on two intertwined factors: the grade of the tumour and the resectability of the tumour. Complete resection with wide margins is the goal of primary treatment. However, this goal is often difficult to attain when tumours arise in the head and neck area[59,61,62,83–88,96–98].

Kaposi's sarcoma

Kaposi's sarcoma was an uncommon tumour until it was identified as a manifestation of acquired immune deficiency syndrome (AIDS). Kaposi's sarcoma is an AIDS-defining illness[99], and is still the most common human immunodeficiency virus (HIV)-associated tumour[100]. The incidence of Kaposi's sarcoma is inversely proportional to the use of antiretroviral therapy.

Kaposi's sarcoma in HIV patients is caused by an infection with human herpes virus 8 (Kaposi's sarcoma-associated herpes virus), with resultant oncogenic transformation of endothelial lymphatic cells[101,102]. The exact mechanism of oncogenesis is still being elucidated, but is felt to involve several pathways including vascular endothelial growth factor (VEGF), platelet-derived growth factor (PDGF), c-kit, phosphatidylinositol-3 kinase (PI3K), and Janus kinase (JAK/STAT).

Whilst Kaposi's sarcoma can affect most organs, the most common manifestations are cutaneous lesions. These lesions range from small red or purple papules to larger plaque-like lesions that can ulcerate. Approximately 20–30% will present with oral lesions commonly on the palate, buccal mucosa, and/or tongue (see Figure 20.6, see colour plate section). The lesions may be uncomfortable, and may interfere with oral functioning.

Diagnosis is confirmed by biopsy. The key histological feature is multiple, small, vascular channels with associated spindle cells that may be pleomorphic with varying numbers of mitotic figures[103]. If required, Kaposi's sarcoma-associated herpes virus can be identified within the lesion[104].

Treatment for Kaposi's sarcoma is dependent on the extent of disease. It is important for all patients to receive adequate antiviral therapy. For some patients, this may be adequate treatment of the Kaposi's sarcoma. Radiation therapy can lead to regression of tumours (and palliation of symptoms)[105,106]. In addition, intralesional chemotherapy, most often with vinblastine, has demonstrated efficacy[107]. Systemic cytotoxic chemotherapy is employed in patients with either aggressive or disseminated disease. The most common chemotherapy medications are liposomal doxorubicin and paclitaxel. Liposomal doxorubicin is the most efficacious chemotherapy regimen[108–111].

The AIDS clinical trial group categorizes patients with Kaposi's sarcoma into risk groups based on tumour extent, immune system function measured by the CD4 count, and presence of other AIDS-related illnesses[112]. Those with less extensive tumours, higher CD4 counts, and fewer systemic problems have a prognosis of 80–88%[113]. In developing countries, where antiretroviral therapy is not widely used, Kaposi's sarcoma is associated with a life expectancy of only 6 months[114,115].

References

1 Jemal A, Siegel R, Ward E, et al. (2008). Cancer statistics, 2008. *CA Cancer J Clin*, 58(2), 71–96.

2 Rice DH, Batsakis JG, McClatchey KD (1976). Postirradiation malignant salivary gland tumor. *Arch Otolaryngol*, 102(11), 699–701.

3 Katz AD, Preston-Martin S (1984). Salivary gland tumors and previous radiotherapy to the head and neck. Report of a clinical series. *Am J Surg*, 147(3), 345–8.

4 Ellis GL, Auclair PL (1996). *Tumors of the salivary glands. Atlas of Tumour Pathology*, 3rd series. Armed Forces Institute of Pathology, Washington DC.

5 Spiro RH, Huvos AG, Berk R, Strong EW (1978). Mucoepidermoid carcinoma of salivary gland origin. A clinicopathologic study of 367 cases. *Am J Surg*, 136(4), 461–8.

6 Stewart FW, Foote FW, Becker WF (1945). Muco-epidermoid tumors of salivary glands. *Ann Surg*, 122(5), 820–44.

7 Batsakis JG, Luna MA (1990). Histopathologic grading of salivary gland neoplasms: I. Mucoepidermoid carcinomas. *Ann Otol Rhinol Laryngol*, 99(10 Pt 1), 835–8.

8 Boahene DK, Olsen KD, Lewis JE, Pinheiro AD, Pankratz VS, Bagniewski SM (2004). Mucoepidermoid carcinoma of the parotid gland: the Mayo Clinic experience. *Arch Otolaryngol Head Neck Surg*, 130(7), 849–56.

9 Pires FR, de Almeida OP, de Araujo V, Kowalski LP (2004). Prognostic factors in head and neck mucoepidermoid carcinoma. *Arch Otolaryngol Head Neck Surg*, 130(2), 174–80.

10 Spiro RH, Huvos AG, Strong EW (1974). Adenoid cystic carcinoma of salivary origin. A clinicopathologic study of 242 cases. *Am J Surg*, 128(4), 512–20.

11 Batsakis JG, Luna MA, el-Naggar A (1990). Histopathologic grading of salivary gland neoplasms: III. Adenoid cystic carcinomas. *Ann Otol Rhinol Laryngol*, 99(12), 1007–9.

12 Sung MW, Kim KH, Kim JW, et al. (2003). Clinicopathologic predictors and impact of distant metastasis from adenoid cystic carcinoma of the head and neck. *Arch Otolaryngol Head Neck Surg*, 129(11), 1193–7.

13 Batsakis JG, Luna MA, el-Naggar AK (1990). Histopathologic grading of salivary gland neoplasms: II. Acinic cell carcinomas. *Ann Otol Rhinol Laryngol*, 99(11), 929–33.

14 Lewis JE, Olsen KD, Weiland LH (1991). Acinic cell carcinoma. Clinicopathologic review. *Cancer*, 67(1), 172–9.

15 Evans HL, Luna MA (2000). Polymorphous low-grade adenocarcinoma: a study of 40 cases with long-term follow up and an evaluation of the importance of papillary areas. *Am J Surg Pathol*, 24(10), 1319–28.

16 Cho KJ, el-Naggar AK, Mahanupab P, Luna MA, Batsakis JG (1995). Carcinoma ex-pleomorphic adenoma of the nasal cavity: a report of two cases. *J Laryngol Otol*, 109(7), 677–9.

17 Stephen J, Batsakis JG, Luna MA, von der Heyden U, Byers RM (1986). True malignant mixed tumors (carcinosarcoma) of salivary glands. *Oral Surg Oral Med Oral Pathol*, 61(6), 597–602.

18 Batsakis JG, el-Naggar AK, Luna MA (1992). "Adenocarcinoma, not otherwise specified": a diminishing group of salivary carcinomas. *Ann Otol Rhinol Laryngol*, 101(1), 102–4.

19 Waldron CA, el-Mofty SK, Gnepp DR (1988). Tumors of the intraoral minor salivary glands: A demographic and histologic study of 426 cases. *Oral Surg Oral Med Oral Pathol*, 66(3), 323–33.

20 Lopes MA, Santos GC, Kowalski LP (1998). Multivariate survival analysis of 128 cases of oral cavity minor salivary gland carcinomas. *Head Neck*, 20(8), 699–706.

21 Wang D, Li Y, He H, Liu L, Wu L, He Z (2007). Intraoral minor salivary gland tumors in a Chinese population: a retrospective study on 737 cases. *Oral Surg Oral Med Oral Pathol Oral Radiol Endod*, 104(1), 94–100.

22 Pires FR, Pringle GA, de Almeida OP, Chen SY (2007). Intra-oral minor salivary gland tumors: a clinicopathological study of 546 cases. *Oral Oncol*, 43(5), 463–70.

23 Pires FR, de Almeida OP, Pringle G, Chen SY (2008). Differences on clinicopathological profile from intraoral minor salivary gland tumors around the world. *Oral Surg Oral Med Oral Pathol Oral Radiol Endod*, 105(2), 136–8.

24 Terhaard CH, Lubsen H, Van der Tweel I, et al. (2004). Salivary gland carcinoma: independent prognostic factors for locoregional control, distant metastases, and overall survival: results of the Dutch head and neck oncology cooperative group. *Head Neck*, 26(8), 681–92.

25 Chen AM, Granchi PJ, Garcia J, Bucci MK, Fu KK, Eisele DW (2007). Local-regional recurrence after surgery without postoperative irradiation for carcinomas of the major salivary glands: implications for adjuvant therapy. *Int J Radiat Oncol Biol Phys*, 67(4), 982–7.

26 Terhaard CH (2007). Postoperative and primary radiotherapy for salivary gland carcinomas: indications, techniques, and results. *Int J Radiat Oncol Biol Phys*, 69(2 Suppl), S52–55.

27 Garden AS, Weber RS, Ang KK, Morrison WH, Matre J, Peters LJ (1994). Postoperative radiation therapy for malignant tumors of minor salivary glands. Outcome and patterns of failure. *Cancer*, 73(10), 2563–9.

28 Mendenhall WM, Morris CG, Amdur RJ, Werning JW, Villaret DB (2005). Radiotherapy alone or combined with surgery for salivary gland carcinoma. *Cancer*, 103(12), 2544–50.

29 Chen AM, Bucci MK, Quivey JM, Garcia J, Eisele DW, Fu KK (2006). Long-term outcome of patients treated by radiation therapy alone for salivary gland carcinomas. *Int J Radiat Oncol Biol Phys*, 66(4), 1044–50.

30 Laramore GE, Krall JM, Griffin TW, et al. (1993). Neutron versus photon irradiation for unresectable salivary gland tumors: final report of an RTOG-MRC randomized clinical trial. Radiation Therapy Oncology Group. Medical Research Council. *Int J Radiat Oncol Biol Phys*, 27(2), 235–40.

31 Chen AM, Garcia J, Granchi PJ, Johnson J, Eisele DW (2008). Late recurrence from salivary gland cancer: when does "cure" mean cure? *Cancer*, 112(2), 340–4.

32 Goldenberg D, Sciubba J, Koch W, Tufano RP (2004). Malignant odontogenic tumors: a 22-year experience. *Laryngoscope*, 114(10), 1770–4.

33 White DK. Odontogenic tumors (2004). *Oral Maxillofac Surg Clin North Am*, 16(3), ix–xi.

34 White DK, Lin YL (2004). Miscellaneous odontogenic tumors. *Oral Maxillofac Surg Clin North Am*, 16(3), 385–9.

35 Slootweg PJ (2002). Malignant odontogenic tumors: an overview. *Mund Kiefer Gesichtschir*, 6(5), 295–302.

36 Cohen DM, Bhattacharyya I (2004). Ameloblastic fibroma, ameloblastic fibro-odontoma, and odontoma. *Oral Maxillofac Surg Clin North Am*, 16(3), 375–84.

37 Kessler HP (2004). Intraosseous ameloblastoma. *Oral Maxillofac Surg Clin North Am*, 16(3), 309–22.

38 Slater LJ (2004). Odontogenic malignancies. *Oral Maxillofac Surg Clin North Am*, 16(3), 409–24.

39 Newman L, Howells GL, Coghlan KM, DiBiase A, Williams DM (1995). Malignant ameloblastoma revisited. *Br J Oral Maxillofac Surg*, 33(1), 47–50.

40 Elzay RP (1982). Primary intraosseous carcinoma of the jaws. Review and update of odontogenic carcinomas. *Oral Surg Oral Med Oral Pathol*, 54(3), 299–303.

41 Baden E, Doyle JL, Petriella V (1993). Malignant transformation of peripheral ameloblastoma. *Oral Surg Oral Med Oral Pathol*, 75(2), 214–19.

42 Suei Y, Tanimoto K, Taguchi A, Wada T (1995). Mucosal condition of the oral cavity and sites of origin of squamous cell carcinoma. *J Oral Maxillofac Surg*, 53(2), 144–7.

43 Folpe AL, Tsue T, Rogerson L, Weymuller E, Oda D, True LD (1998). Odontogenic ghost cell carcinoma: a case report with immunohistochemical and ultrastructural characterization. *J Oral Pathol Med*, 27(4), 185–9.

44 Lu Y, Mock D, Takata T, Jordan RC (1999). Odontogenic ghost cell carcinoma: report of four new cases and review of the literature. *J Oral Pathol Med*, 28(7), 323–9.

45 Jing W, Xuan M, Lin Y, et al. (2007). Odontogenic tumours: a retrospective study of 1642 cases in a Chinese population. *Int J Oral Maxillofac Surg*, 36(1), 20–5.

46 Brandwein M, Said-Al-Naief N, Gordon R, Urken M (2002). Clear cell odontogenic carcinoma: report of a case and analysis of the literature. *Arch Otolaryngol Head Neck Surg*, 128(9), 1089–95.

47 Ebert CS Jr, Dubin MG, Hart CF, Chalian AA, Shockley WW (2005). Clear cell odontogenic carcinoma: a comprehensive analysis of treatment strategies. *Head Neck*, 27(6), 536–42.

48 Braunshtein E, Vered M, Taicher S, Buchner A (2003). Clear cell odontogenic carcinoma and clear cell ameloblastoma: a single clinicopathologic entity? A new case and comparative analysis of the literature. *J Oral Maxillofac Surg*, 61(9), 1004–10.

49 Avninder S, Rakheja D, Bhatnagar A (2006). Clear cell odontogenic carcinoma: a diagnostic and therapeutic dilemma. *World J Surg Oncol*, 4, 91.

50 Lebowitz RA, Morris L (2003). Plasma cell dyscrasias and amyloidosis. *Otolaryngol Clin North Am*, 36(4), 747–64.

51 Pisano JJ, Coupland R, Chen SY, Miller AS (1997). Plasmacytoma of the oral cavity and jaws: a clinicopathologic study of 13 cases. *Oral Surg Oral Med Oral Pathol Oral Radiol Endod*, 83(2), 265–71.

52 Chua SC, O'Connor SR, Wong WL, Ganatra RH (2008). Solitary plasmacytoma of bone with oncogenic osteomalacia: recurrence of tumour confirmed by PET/CT. A case report with a review of the radiological literature. *Br J Radiol*, 81(964), e110–4.

53 Liebross RH, Ha CS, Cox JD, Weber D, Delasalle K, Alexanian R (1998). Solitary bone plasmacytoma: outcome and prognostic factors following radiotherapy. *Int J Radiat Oncol Biol Phys*, 41(5), 1063–7.

54 Ly JQ, Sandiego JW, Beall DP (2005). Plasmacytoma of the proximal humerus. *Clin Imaging*, 29(5), 367–9.

55 Liebross RH, Ha CS, Cox JD, Weber D, Delasalle K, Alexanian R (1999). Clinical course of solitary extramedullary plasmacytoma. *Radiother Oncol*, 52(3), 245–9.

56 Ozdemir R, Kayiran O, Oruc M, Karaaslan O, Kocer U, Ogun D (2005). Plasmacytoma of the hard palate. *J Craniofac Surg*, 16(1), 164–9.

57 Strojan P, Soba E, Lamovec J, Munda A (2002). Extramedullary plasmacytoma: clinical and histopathologic study. *Int J Radiat Oncol Biol Phys*, 53(3), 692–701.

58 Harris NL, Jaffe ES, Diebold J, Flandrin G, Muller-Hermelink HK, Vardiman J (2000). Lymphoma classification - from controversy to consensus: the R.E.A.L. and WHO classification of lymphoid neoplasms. *Ann Oncol*, 11(Suppl 1), 3–10.

59 Pellitteri PK, Ferlito A, Bradley PJ, Shaha AR, Rinaldo A (2003). Management of sarcomas of the head and neck in adults. *Oral Oncol*, 39(1), 2–12.

60 Brennan MF, Casper ES, Harrison LB, Shiu MH, Gaynor J, Hajdu SI (9991). The role of multimodality therapy in soft-tissue sarcoma. *Ann Surg*, 214(3), 328–36.

61 Penel N, Van Haverbeke C, Lartigau E, et al. (2004). Head and neck soft tissue sarcomas of adult: prognostic value of surgery in multimodal therapeutic approach. *Oral Oncol*, 40(9), 890–7.

62 Brockstein B (2004). Management of sarcomas of the head and neck. *Curr Oncol Rep*, 6(4), 321–7.

63 Bernstein M, Kovar H, Paulussen M, et al. (2006). Ewing's sarcoma family of tumors: current management. *Oncologist*, 11(5), 503–19.

64 Damron TA, Ward WG, Stewart A (2007). Osteosarcoma, chondrosarcoma, and Ewing's sarcoma: National Cancer Data Base Report. *Clin Orthop*, 459, 40–7.

65 Cotterill SJ, Ahrens S, Paulussen M, et al. (2000). Prognostic factors in Ewing's tumor of bone: analysis of 975 patients from the European Intergroup Cooperative Ewing's Sarcoma Study Group. *J Clin Oncol*, 18(17), 3108–14.

66 Bleyer A, Viny A, Barr R (2006). Cancer in 15- to 29-year-olds by primary site. *Oncologist*, 11(6), 590–601.

67 Bleyer A, O'Leary M, Barr R, Ries LA (2006). *Cancer epidemiology in older adolescents and young adults 15 to 29 years of age, including SEER incidence and survival: 1975–2000.* National Cancer Institute, Bethesda.

68 Lizard-Nacol S, Lizard G, Justrabo E, Turc-Carel C (1989). Immunologic characterization of Ewing's sarcoma using mesenchymal and neural markers. *Am J Pathol*, 135(5), 847–55.

69 Fletcher CD, Unni KK, Mertens F (2002). *Pathology and genetics of tumors of soft tissue and bone.* IARC Press, Lyon.

70 Fuchs B, Pritchard DJ (2002). Etiology of osteosarcoma. *Clin Orthop*, 397, 40–52.

71 Wang LL, Gannavarapu A, Kozinetz CA, et al. (2003). Association between osteosarcoma and deleterious mutations in the RECQL4 gene in Rothmund–Thomson syndrome. *J Natl Cancer Inst*, 95(9), 669–74.

72 Gelderblom H, Hogendoorn PC, Dijkstra SD, et al. (2008). The clinical approach towards chondrosarcoma. *Oncologist*, 13(3), 320–9.

73 Longhi A, Errani C, De Paolis M, Mercuri M, Bacci G (2006). Primary bone osteosarcoma in the pediatric age: state of the art. *Cancer Treat Rev*, 32(6), 423–36.

74 Jemal A, Siegel R, Ward E, et al. (2006). Cancer statistics, 2006. *CA Cancer J Clin*, 56(2), 106–30.

75 Meyers PA, Gorlick R (1997). Osteosarcoma. *Pediatr Clin North Am*, 44(4), 973–89.

76 Jenkin RD (1966). Ewing's sarcoma a study of treatment methods. *Clin Radiol*, 17(2), 97–106.

77 Krochak R, Harwood AR, Cummings BJ, Quirt IC (1983). Results of radical radiation for chondrosarcoma of bone. *Radiother Oncol*, 1(2), 109–15.

78 McNaney D, Lindberg RD, Ayala AG, Barkley HT Jr, Hussey DH (1982). Fifteen year radiotherapy experience with chondrosarcoma of bone. *Int J Radiat Oncol Biol Phys*, 8(2), 187–90.

79 Leavey PJ, Collier AB (2008). Ewing sarcoma: prognostic criteria, outcomes and future treatment. *Expert Rev Anticancer Ther*, 8(4), 617–24.

80 Landis SH, Murray T, Bolden S, Wingo PA (1999). Cancer statistics, 1999. *CA Cancer J Clin*, 49(1), 8–31.

81 Hartley AL, Blair V, Harris M, et al. (1992). Sarcomas in north west England: III. Survival. *Br J Cancer*, 66(4), 685–91.

82 Zahm SH, Fraumeni JF Jr (1997). The epidemiology of soft tissue sarcoma. *Semin Oncol*, 24(5), 504–14.

83 Dudhat SB, Mistry RC, Varughese T, Fakih AR, Chinoy RF (2000). Prognostic factors in head and neck soft tissue sarcomas. *Cancer*, 89(4), 868–72.

84 Greager JA, Patel MK, Briele HA, Walker MJ, Das Gupta TK(1985). Soft tissue sarcomas of the adult head and neck. *Cancer*, 56(4), 820–4.

85 Kraus DH, Dubner S, Harrison LB, et al. (1994). Prognostic factors for recurrence and survival in head and neck soft tissue sarcomas. *Cancer*, 74(2), 697–702.

86 Le Vay J, O'Sullivan B, Catton C, et al. (1994). An assessment of prognostic factors in soft-tissue sarcoma of the head and neck. *Arch Otolaryngol Head Neck Surg*, 120(9), 981–6.

87 Tran LM, Mark R, Meier R, Calcaterra TC, Parker RG (1992). Sarcomas of the head and neck. Prognostic factors and treatment strategies. *Cancer*, 70(1), 169–77.

88 Weber RS, Benjamin RS, Peters LJ, Ro JY, Achon O, Goepfert H (1986). Soft tissue sarcomas of the head and neck in adolescents and adults. *Am J Surg*, 152(4), 386–92.

89 Parham DM, Webber B, Holt H, Williams WK, Maurer H (1991). Immunohistochemical study of childhood rhabdomyosarcomas and related neoplasms. Results of an Intergroup Rhabdomyosarcoma study project. *Cancer*, 67(12), 3072–80.

90 Dias P, Parham DM, Shapiro DN, Webber BL, Houghton PJ (1990). Myogenic regulatory protein (MyoD1) expression in childhood solid tumors: diagnostic utility in rhabdomyosarcoma. *Am J Pathol*, 137(6), 1283–91.

91 Crist WM, Anderson JR, Meza JL, et al. (2001). Intergroup rhabdomyosarcoma study-IV: results for patients with nonmetastatic disease. *J Clin Oncol*, 19(12), 3091–102.

92 Wharam MD, Beltangady MS, Heyn RM, et al. (1987). Pediatric orofacial and laryngopharyngeal rhabdomyosarcoma. An Intergroup Rhabdomyosarcoma Study report. *Arch Otolaryngol Head Neck Surg*, 113(11), 1225–7.

93 Scrable HJ, Witte DP, Lampkin BC, Cavenee WK (1987). Chromosomal localization of the human rhabdomyosarcoma locus by mitotic recombination mapping. *Nature*, 329(6140), 645–7.

94 Carew JF, Singh B, Shaha AR (1999). Management of head and neck sarcomas. *Curr Opin Otolaryngol Head Neck Surg*, 7(2), 68–72.

95 Paulino AC, Okcu MF (2008). Rhabdomyosarcoma. *Curr Probl Cancer*, 32(1), 7–34.

96 Eeles RA, Fisher C, A'Hern RP, et al. (1993). Head and neck sarcomas: prognostic factors and implications for treatment. *Br J Cancer*, 68(1), 201–7.

97 Farhood AI, Hajdu SI, Shiu MH, Strong EW (1990). Soft tissue sarcomas of the head and neck in adults. *Am J Surg*, 160(4), 365–9.

98 Freedman AM, Reiman HM, Woods JE (1989). Soft-tissue sarcomas of the head and neck. *Am J Surg*, 158(4), 367–72.

99 Jessop S. HIV-associated Kaposi's sarcoma (2006). *Dermatol Clin*, 24(4), 509–20, vii.

100 Cheung MC, Pantanowitz L, Dezube BJ (2005). AIDS-related malignancies: emerging challenges in the era of highly active antiretroviral therapy. *Oncologist*, 10(6), 412–26.

101 Chang Y, Cesarman E, Pessin MS, et al. (1994). Identification of herpesvirus-like DNA sequences in AIDS-associated Kaposi's sarcoma. *Science*, 266(5192), 1865–9.

102 Gessain A, Duprez R (2005). Spindle cells and their role in Kaposi's sarcoma. *Int J Biochem Cell Biol*, 37(12), 2457–65.

103 Weedon D (2002). *Skin pathology*, 2nd edn. Churchill Livingstone, London.

104 Mendez JC, Procop GW, Espy MJ, Paya CV, Smith TF (1998). Detection and semiquantitative analysis of human herpesvirus 8 DNA in specimens from patients with Kaposi's sarcoma. *J Clin Microbiol*, 36(8), 2220–2.

105 Stelzer KJ, Griffin TW (1993). A randomized prospective trial of radiation therapy for AIDS-associated Kaposi's sarcoma. *Int J Radiat Oncol Biol Phys*, 27(5), 1057–61.

106 Swift PS (1996). The role of radiation therapy in the management of HIV-related Kaposi's sarcoma. *Hematol Oncol Clin North Am*, 10(5), 1069–80.

107 Ramirez-Amador V, Esquivel-Pedraza L, Lozada-Nur F, et al. (2002). Intralesional vinblastine vs. 3% sodium tetradecyl sulfate for the treatment of oral Kaposi's sarcoma. A double blind, randomized clinical trial. *Oral Oncol*, 38(5), 460–7.

108 Gill PS, Wernz J, Scadden DT, et al. (1996). Randomized phase III trial of liposomal daunorubicin versus doxorubicin, bleomycin, and vincristine in AIDS-related Kaposi's sarcoma. *J Clin Oncol*, 14(8), 2353–64.

109 Northfelt DW, Dezube BJ, Thommes JA, et al. (1998). Pegylated-liposomal doxorubicin versus doxorubicin, bleomycin, and vincristine in the treatment of AIDS-related Kaposi's sarcoma: results of a randomized phase III clinical trial. *J Clin Oncol*, 16(7), 2445–51.

110 Osoba D, Northfelt DW, Budd DW, Himmelberger D (2001). Effect of treatment on health-related quality of life in acquired immunodeficiency syndrome (AIDS)-related Kaposi's sarcoma: a randomized trial of pegylated-liposomal doxorubicin versus doxorubicin, bleomycin, and vincristine. *Cancer Invest*, 19(6), 573–80.

111 Stewart S, Jablonowski H, Goebel FD, et al. (1998). Randomized comparative trial of pegylated liposomal doxorubicin versus bleomycin and vincristine in the treatment of AIDS-related Kaposi's sarcoma. International Pegylated Liposomal Doxorubicin Study Group. *J Clin Oncol*, 16(2), 683–91.

112 Krown SE, Testa MA, Huang J (1997). AIDS-related Kaposi's sarcoma: prospective validation of the AIDS Clinical Trials Group staging classification. AIDS Clinical Trials Group Oncology Committee. *J Clin Oncol*, 15(9), 3085–92.

113 Nasti G, Talamini R, Antinori A, et al. (2003). AIDS-related Kaposi's Sarcoma: evaluation of potential new prognostic factors and assessment of the AIDS Clinical Trial Group Staging System in the Haart Era – the Italian Cooperative Group on AIDS and Tumors and the Italian Cohort of Patients Naive From Antiretrovirals. *J Clin Oncol*, 21(15), 2876–82.

114 Dal Maso L, Serraino D, Franceschi S (2001). Epidemiology of AIDS-related tumours in developed and developing countries. *Eur J Cancer*, 37(10), 1188–201.

115 Mwanda OW, Fu P, Collea R, Whalen C, Remick SC (2005). Kaposi's sarcoma in patients with and without human immunodeficiency virus infection, in a tertiary referral centre in Kenya. *Ann Trop Med Parasitol*, 99(1), 81–91.

Chapter 9

Overview of complications of oral surgery

Antonia Kolokythas and Michael Miloro

Introduction

Cancer of the oral cavity and oropharynx is among the top ten most common malignancies worldwide [1]. Over the last 30 years the philosophies of treatment of oral cancer has changed very little with regards to primary tumour extirpation (with the exception of marginal mandibular resection). However, there have been major changes in the approach to cervical lymph nodes at risk for metastases [2]. Thus, the radical neck dissection is now rarely performed in most centres[3]. In addition, the ability to offer a variety of reconstruction options has resulted in significant improvements in functional and aesthetic outcomes.

Nevertheless, the ablative process still results in the sacrifice of several functional and aesthetic organs during surgery for cancer of the oral cavity[3]. Early complications from ablative surgery for oral cancer are, for the most part, similar to those from other sites. However, long-term complications can be quite challenging for the oncological team and the patient, primarily due to the highly specialized tissues included in the surgical field. This chapter addresses some of the more common chronic complications associated with surgical treatment of oral cancer.

Complications associated with cancer resection

Treatment failure

The most significant negative outcome is failure to cure the disease. This failure may be due to local or regional recurrence, distant metastases, or presence of a second primary cancer. The vast majority of recurrences occur within the first 2–3 years following completion of treatment[1,3]. Local recurrences are mainly the result of failure to eradicate the primary cancer with surgery, and are often associated with failure to achieve 'negative margins'. In general, the head and neck surgeon attempts to remove the primary cancer with a 1–1.5-cm margin of healthy-looking tissue in order to try to achieve negative margins.

There is tremendous debate with regards to what precisely constitutes negative margins. A lack of dysplasia, carcinoma *in situ*, or invasive cancer within 5 mm of the resection margins of the pathological specimen is often considered to represent histopathologically negative margins. However, the validity of this interpretation has been challenged by various studies. The lack of universally accepted definitions, as well as clear distinction between mucosal and deep margins, has been identified as a major deficit when the status of the margins is examined[2,4–7].

To try to ensure adequate tumour resection, frozen tissue sections have been traditionally submitted for analysis during the surgical procedure. These have been proven to be valuable when found positive, as this then informs the need for additional tissue resection[8]. The diagnostic accuracy of frozen tissue specimens has been reported to be between 96% and 98%. 'Sampling error', inability to perform frozen sections to assess bone involvement, and difficulties with interpretation of histological changes in irradiated tissues are a few of the limitations of these procedures.

The benefit of removing the 'at risk' lymph nodes in the neck in advanced stage tumours has been clearly demonstrated (i.e. T3/T4 tumours). Controversy still exists as to whether one should watch or treat the neck nodes in early stage tumours with no clinical or radiographic evidence of nodal metastases (i.e. N0 tumours). This is an important issue, since metastases to the cervical lymph nodes have been shown to be a significant negative predictor of outcome (and is associated with tumour aggressiveness)[1,3,9,10].

A follow-up protocol is invariably proposed for all cancer patients; this recall includes frequent clinical examinations with radiographic surveillance, including computer tomography (CT) or magnetic resonance imaging (MRI), since these have been proven to be sensitive tests for assessing disease status. Most recently, positron emission tomography (PET), with or without CT and MRI, has been used for surveillance for local and regional tumour recurrence. The advantage of PET is that it may assist in the differentiation of post-surgical scarring from tumour recurrence[11,12].

In a non-irradiated field, local or regional failure may be treated with additional surgery alone, or in combination with radiation and chemotherapy[13,14]. One major clinical challenge is the case of local or regional failure following a full course of tumouricidal radiation treatment. It is best to treat these patients with additional surgery whenever feasible. If surgery is not possible, then additional radiation may be of use, but this is associated with serious complications and poor overall long-term therapeutic results[1,14,15].

Another major problem with the patients who fail surgery is the presence of distant metastases. This finding significantly decreases the chances of disease control, and impacts negatively on the life expectancy of the patient. Recent studies have demonstrated a significant increase in distant metastases, in spite of improved local and regional control, with current multimodality treatment[9]. New chemotherapeutic/biological therapeutic regimens may help to delay the progression of such advanced disease[16–18].

Speech and swallowing impairment

The harmonious coordination of the lips, tongue, buccal mucosa, and maxillomandibular complex is required for speech production (and more specifically articulation), and the initial phases of swallowing. Hence, surgical resection of malignancy within the vicinity of the oral cavity has a significant impact on speech and swallowing functions. As a general rule, ablative surgery that involves the most anterior portion of the oral tongue is associated with significantly altered speech, while resections that incorporate the posterior tongue affect swallowing function. As post-surgical time progresses, surgical site fibrosis further impairs speech and swallowing[19–21].

Unfortunately, the complexity of the function of the oral cavity structures cannot be restored to the pre-surgery status despite use of sensate free-tissue transfers (and various swallowing manoeuvres). Difficulties with articulation, and swallowing remain long-term problems for these patients, and adequate rehabilitation and support should be initiated early on. Consultations with speech and swallowing services are imperative in assisting the patient to try to regain their pre-treatment status, and to avoid recurrent aspiration and long-term dependence on enteral feeding tubes[1,3,22–24].

Masticatory insufficiency/trismus

The tongue, floor of mouth, maxilla, and mandible with the adjacent tissues are vital structures for mastication. Hence, masticatory function is adversely influenced by the surgical management of oral cancer. Mandibular or maxillary resection affects the grinding ability, either due to loss of stable stomatognathic system relationships, or due to loss of tooth-to-tooth contacts and diminished biting forces. In addition, loss of soft-tissue bulk and sensation causes difficulties with the patient's ability to manipulate the food bolus to the occlusal table, retrieve the bolus, and then consolidate it prior to deglutition. Composite reconstruction flaps can not only restore tissue bulk and facial aesthetics, but can also improve masticatory function[25,26].

Trismus is a common complaint following oral cancer surgery (see Chapter 11). Scar contraction and contraction of the muscles of mastication are the main reasons for inability of the patient to open the mouth. Common oral cancer procedures resulting in trismus include maxillary surgery involving the origin of the medial and lateral pterygoid muscles from the pterygoid plates, or mandibulectomy procedures involving any of the muscles of mastication (including the temporalis muscle insertion to the coronoid process, the masseter muscle insertion to the mandibular angle and ramus, and the pterygoid insertions to the medial ramus and condylar neck). Finally, disarticulation of the temporomandibular joint for tumour eradication will certainly lead to similar limited mouth opening. Exercise regimens and mouth opening assisting devices are prescribed to assist these patients. Unfortunately, if these steps are not incorporated early, and maintained long term, only limited improvement in trismus can be expected[1,27–30].

Nutritional considerations

The presence of trismus, difficulties with mastication, and difficulties with swallowing all contribute to limitations in food intake, and further compromise the nutritional status of patients. A significant number of these patients are forced to adopt dietary modifications that may lead to specific nutritional deficits. The usual problems are inadequate protein intake, and frequent episodes of dehydration. Indeed, some patients become dependent on enteral feeding tubes. Although feeding formulas are appropriately balanced, issues of intolerance, diarrhoea, dehydration, and electrolyte imbalance are very common. Nutritional education and support, along with close monitoring of nutritional intake, will assist in preventing long-term deficits and frequent hospital admissions[3,31]. It should be noted that patients may have a history of alcohol abuse, and so have pre-existing nutritional deficiencies.

Facial aesthetic considerations

Until recently, aesthetic considerations have not been a primary concern when tumour resection is planned. However, the change in patient demographics suffering from oral cancer, and concerns about the effects of long-term facial scarring, have forced surgeons to consider incision and flap design based upon facial aesthetic units. The stigmata of oral cancer surgery are no longer acceptable in the face and neck regions[32–37].

For surgical access to some of the tumours in the oral cavity, the lips may need to be divided, and incisions on the face may be required. The original lower lip-split procedure placed the incision at the middle of the lip and chin leading to severe scarring post-operatively. Since that time, various modifications have been described to this technique, with the main endpoint the achievement of an aesthetically acceptable result. Precise alignment and restoration of the vermilion border of the lip, alignment and interdigitation of the orbicularis oris muscle, and reorientation of the lip skin and oral mucosa are paramount to achieving excellent aesthetics (and lip competence and function)[34–36].

Incisions should try to follow natural skin creases, since those that do not have a higher incidence of dehiscence and unaesthetic scar formation. In addition, attempts should be made to handle tissue gently, to provide protection of the skin from iatrogenic trauma from traction or electrocautery, and to consider elevation of thick soft-tissue flaps with adequate blood supply in order to minimize the creation of unaesthetic scars[38].

Post-operative radiation may worsen soft-tissue scarring. Additionally, many oral cancer patients have a significant social history of tobacco use, and so the skin and soft- and hard-tissue vascularity may already be severely compromised. This may contribute to poor wound healing, wound dehiscence, and compromised flap viability (with resultant unaesthetic scarring).

Chronic fistulae

Any procedure that involves entering the mucosa of the upper aerodigestive tract via a neck incision may lead to formation of a fistulous tract due to salivary leakage into the neck wound. Fistulas often occur following oral oncologic surgery, and depend to a great deal on the type and stage of the tumour, the incision design, and the general physical and nutritional status of the patient.

Salivary fistulas can occur as early as 1 week, and as late as 3–4 weeks, post surgery. Patients may present with a low-grade fever of unknown origin, and other vague complaints indicating chronic inflammation. Usually, the skin flap under the area of dependant drainage becomes inflamed and indurated.

If a fistula is noted, then surgical exploration of the wound with an attempt to direct saliva away from vital structures such as the carotid vessels is indicated. The wound should be irrigated and packed, and the patient should be prescribed empiric antimicrobial therapy for oral and skin flora. If drainage persists for over 4 weeks, then excision of the fistulous tract with closure of the oral mucosa and the skin should be attempted[1,2,38,39]. Surgery may be combined with attempts to transiently decrease salivary flow with anti-cholinergic medications.

Wound breakdown and loose or contaminated hardware may be another reason for chronic fistulae. Usually, there is a nidus of bacteria that cannot be eliminated with antibiotics alone, and so local debridement with removal and/or replacement of existing hardware is indicated (and closure with local and regional flaps) [1].

Surgical airway complications

Surgical treatment of oral cancer, especially advanced stages, interferes with maintenance of air-way patency. This concern may require either prolonged intubation, or surgical securing of the airway with a tracheostomy. Surgical complications associated with tracheostomy are traditionally divided into peri-operative, immediate post-operative, and late post-operative complications based on the time of occurrence. Tracheal stenosis, tracheomalacia, tracheo-oesophageal fistula, and life-threatening bleeding are among the potential late post-surgical complications[38,40–42].

Tracheal stenosis

Tracheal stenosis is defined as an abnormal narrowing of the tracheal lumen, and occurs most commonly at the level of, or above, the stoma (and below the vocal cords). Two additional locations of potential stenosis include the site where the cuff and the tip the tracheostomy tube are located. Nearly all patients with a tracheostomy have some degree of trachea narrowing at the site of the stoma. About 3–12% of these patients develop a clinically significant stenosis that requires intervention.

Stenosis is believed to be the result of bacterial contamination of granulation tissue (which is the result of microtrauma around the stoma, the cuff, or the tip of the tracheal tube). The natural progression is maturation of this tissue to fibrous tissue that is covered with epithelium, and which results in narrowing of the airway. Multiple risks factors are associated with this complication (Table 9.1).

A high index of suspicion is the key to diagnosis. Difficulty clearing secretions and/or a persistent cough may be the initial presentation, but these symptoms may not occur until there

Table 9.1 Risks associated with tracheal stenosis

1. Sepsis
2. Stomal stenosis
3. Advanced Age
4. Male sex
5. Hypotension
6. Steroid Use
7. Ill fitting cannula
8. Oversized cannula
9. Excessive mobility
10. Excessive removal of tracheal cartilage
11. Prolonged use

is a 50–75% decrease in the tracheal lumen. The diagnosis is made by direct laryngoscopy or bronchoscopy. Excision of the granulation tissue, serial dilatations, stent placement, and surgical resection with anastomosis of the remaining tissue are some of the techniques employed to correct this problem (if the tracheal stenosis is symptomatic).

Tracheomalacia

Tracheomalacia is a weakening of the tracheal wall. Ischaemic injury leads to chondritis, and results in necrosis of the cartilage. This causes the airway to collapse during expiration, causing air trapping and difficulty with clearing of respiratory secretions. Treatment is based upon the severity of the condition, and may range from observation in mild cases to tracheal resection and reconstruction in the more severe cases.

Tracheo-oesophageal fistula

This is a rare complication (<1% patients who have had a tracheostomy), and is either due to direct trauma during the surgical procedure, or due to prolonged pressure from the cuff or the tip of the tube. Gastric distention (due to air leak into the stomach), persistent cuff leak, and food aspiration are some of the presentations of a tracheo-oesophageal fistula. Diagnosis is made with oesophagoscopy or a CT scan of the mediastinum. If the patient is a surgical candidate, repair via a thoracotomy approach may be attempted. Otherwise a stent can be used to manage the problem. In either scenario, the prognosis is generally not good.

Tracheo-innominate artery erosion

This is also a rare complication (<1% patients who have had a tracheostomy), and is either due to error in surgical technique by placing the tracheostomy too low in the neck, or erosion of the anterior wall of the trachea from the cuff or the tip of the tube. Mild bleeding around the tube can commonly be the first sign, and usually occurs 3–4 weeks following surgery. Massive bleeding, or haemoptysis, can alternatively be the first sign, and urgent surgical exploration may be indicated. The success of this repair is reported to be very low, and prevention remains the best treatment of this complication. (Erosion of the innominate artery is a complication with a nearly 100% mortality rate.)

Chronic aspiration and pneumonia

Tracheostomy interferes with swallowing, and places the patient at risk for aspiration. Indeed, silent aspiration is reported in >70% patients. In addition, chronically ventilated tracheostomy patients are found to be at highest risk for ventilator-associated pneumonitis and pneumonia.

Neurologic dysfunction

There are several nerves at risk for iatrogenic injury during extirpative surgery in the head and neck due to their anatomic proximity to the surgical field, especially when the surgery involves a nodal dissection.

Spinal accessory nerve (cranial nerve XI)

Transection of cranial nerve XI during radical surgery, or excessive manipulation during less radical procedures, as well as severing the anastomosis with the cervical plexus, may all result in the so-called 'shoulder syndrome'. This condition consists of pain, shoulder girdle deformity, and inability to abduct the upper extremity above 90 degrees (due to denervation of the trapezius muscle). Some debate exists in the literature regarding the actual incidence of developing shoulder syndrome even after preserving the spinal accessory nerve[43,44]. However, studies have clearly demonstrated that when the nerve trunk and its anastomosis with the cervical plexus are preserved, patients have better post-operative function with significantly less pain and deformity.

Careful dissection around the vicinity of the nerve, early identification based on known anatomical landmarks, and limited use of electrocautery may help to limit surgically induced neural trauma. Direct primary anastomosis of the iatrogenically severed nerve has also been described in the literature. There are no available techniques to restore the aesthetic component of 'shoulder syndrome', although immediate aggressive physical therapy can improve functional outcomes[1,2,38].

Phrenic nerve

Another neurologic complication that may be encountered during neck dissection is injury to the phrenic nerve. This causes paralysis to the ipsilateral diaphragm, since the phrenic nerve is the only motor innervation to this muscle. The diaphragm is responsible for 70% of the respiratory movement, and long-term pulmonary complications can originate from this type of injury. An attempt to limit the surgical dissection to a layer superficial to the pre-vertebral fascia, with identification of the nerve, may assist surgeons in preventing this complication[1,2,38].

Hypoglossal and lingual nerves

The hypoglossal nerve (cranial nerve XII) provides motor innervation to the ipsilateral tongue, and the lingual nerve (cranial nerve V3) provides sensation and gustatory innervation to the anterior two-thirds of the ipsilateral tongue (via the chorda tympani branch of the facial nerve). Both nerves may be injured during neck dissection, and excision of the tongue and floor of mouth may further endanger the lingual nerve.

Hypoglossal nerve dysfunction can present with dysarthria, accidental tongue biting, and deviation of the tongue to the ipsilateral side of injury. Patients may also experience increased difficulties with mastication and deglutition (see above). Atrophy of the muscles of the tongue can occur, and add to the functional difficulties experienced by these patients. In cases of bilateral hypoglossal nerve injury, upper airway obstruction can occur when the patient is placed in a supine position.

Ipsilateral loss of sensation to the tongue from lingual nerve injury can impact on speech, mastication, and swallowing, and leads to injury to the tongue during speech and mastication. A compromised ability to taste foods due to chorda tympani nerve injury may contribute to decreased food intake and malnutrition.

Rehabilitation for speech and swallowing is usually beneficial in these patients[38].

Vagus, recurrent laryngeal, and superior laryngeal nerves

Direct or indirect injury to the vagus nerve (cranial nerve X) or its branches, specifically the recurrent and superior laryngeal nerves, can occur during dissection around the carotid sheath.

Unilateral true vocal cord paralysis is the result of injury to the recurrent laryngeal nerve, and is generally well tolerated due to compensation from the intact contralateral vocal cord. However, mild-to-moderate hoarseness and diminished cough efforts are commonly experienced by patients. Upper airway obstruction may result in cases of bilateral nerve injury.

Injury to the branches of the superior laryngeal nerve may result in minor swallowing difficulties due to decreased sensation at the laryngeal inlet, or decreased tensor capability of the true vocal cord leading to early fatiguability and decreased ability to phonate high-pitched sounds.

Direct laryngoscopy alone, or in combination with motor speech evaluation, can assist in the diagnosis of these neurologic injuries.

Sympathetic trunk

Disruption of the sympathetic trunk nerve fibres may cause ipsilateral Horner's syndrome. This is usually due to a surgical dissection that extends too far medially behind the carotid sheath. Horner's syndrome involves blepharoptosis due to disruption of the innervation to Mueller's muscle, apparent enophthalmos, miosis (pupillary constriction), and anhidrosis (lack of perspiration) of the forehead skin ipsilateral to the injury. However, the clinical presentation can be somewhat variable.

Marginal mandibular branch of the facial nerve

The marginal mandibular branch of the facial nerve (cranial VII) is at risk during incision and elevation of the flaps for standard neck dissections, and access to the oral cavity for composite resections. Injury to this nerve causes alteration of the mobility of the corner of the mouth due to disruption of the innervation to the orbicularis oris and depressor angulae oris muscles. Inability to control the movement of the lower lip can interfere with liquid consumption, and gives the patient the appearance of having sustained an injury similar to a cerebrovascular accident.

Careful planning of incisions, and nerve identification early during flap elevation, is the best way of preventing inadvertent iatrogenic injury to this branch of the facial nerve. Some functionality is normally restored if the neurologic injury is due to traction and not severance, but it may take several months for such spontaneous recovery[1,2,38].

Complications associated with reconstruction and donor-site morbidity

Hardware failure

Mandibular osteotomies or resections require utilization of plates and screws to stabilize bone segments, span continuity defects, or secure bone flaps. Failure to adhere to basic reconstruction principles, fatigue of the metal due to over-manipulation, presence of extensive defects, and presence of unbalanced masticatory force distribution may all lead to hardware failure. The problems include fracture of the reconstruction plates, or loosening of the screws with mobility of the mandibular segments. The plates may become exposed, and secondarily infected. This leads further damage of the adjacent tissues and development of chronic fistulas.

Hardware exposure may occur even without fracture or mobility, if the overlying tissue is of inadequate thickness due to the resection, or atrophy occurs due to the effects of radiation. Careful incision planning, adequate soft-tissue coverage, and adherence to reconstruction principles is critical in order to avoid plate exposure.

In the cases of fractured or infected plates and screws, removal of the existing hardware is usually required. Preoperative preparation with hyperbaric oxygen treatments may be indicated in patients that have had adjuvant radiotherapy[1,45,46].

Donor-site problems

Composite tissue transfer from distant sites such as the fibula, radius, and iliac crest are considered the gold standard for reconstruction of defects of the oral cavity. Very acceptable aesthetic results and excellent functional outcomes can be achieved at the recipient sites. However, the donor sites are usually plagued by long scars and, occasionally, tissue mismatching and other bulk-related defects. Functional limitations such as limitation in range of motion and gait disturbances are some of the undesired long-term sequelae at the donor sites. Aggressive physical therapy is employed until near-normal function is regained, while scar revisions may be employed to address the aesthetic considerations. Similar problems may occur with other reconstruction techniques.

Quality of life

Quality of life is a critical outcome measure in head and neck cancer management, mainly due to the continued inability to improve survival (especially in cases of advanced disease).

Chronic pain, and difficulty with chewing, swallowing, and speech adversely impact on the quality of life. In general, studies have demonstrated that improved function post resection is achieved with utilization of free-tissue-composite flaps that correct bone-continuity defects, and can support dental implants as well as a future prosthesis. Both subjective perception of improved quality of life, and objectively measured improvement, have been demonstrated in multiple studies in the head and neck cancer literature[25,26,47,48].

Finally, facial disfigurement, inability to control secretions, speech impairment, and other functional impairments have a serious psychological impact on the oral cancer survivor. Indeed, this group has a high prevalence of clinical depression and other psychological/psychiatric problems.

References

1 Shah JP, Johnson NW, Batsakis JG (2002). *Oral Cancer*. Martin Dunitz, London.

2 Kim DD, Ord RA (2003). Complications in the treatment of head and neck cancer. *Oral Maxillofac Surg Clin North Am*, 15(2), 213–27.

3 Shah J (2001). *Cancer of the head and neck: a volume in the American Cancer Society Atlas of Clinical Oncology Series*. BC Decker, London.

4 Batsakis JG (1999). Surgical excision margins: a pathologist's perspective. *Adv Anat Pathol*, 6(3), 140–8.

5 Woolgar JA, Triantafyllou A (2005). A histopathological appraisal of surgical margins in oral and oropharyngeal cancer resection specimens. *Oral Oncol*, 41(10), 1034–43.

6 Looser KG, Shah JP, Strong EW (1978). The significance of "positive" margins in surgically resected epidermoid carcinomas. *Head Neck Surg*, 1(2), 107–11.

7 Batsakis JG (2003). Clinical pathology of oral cancer, in Shah JP, Johnson NW, Batsakis JG (eds) *Oral Cancer*, pp. 75–128. Martin Dunitz, London.

8 Byers RM, Bland KI, Borlase B, Luna M (1978). The prognostic and therapeutic value of frozen section determinations in the surgical treatment of squamous carcinoma of the head and neck. *Am J Surg*, 136(4), 525–8.

9 Genden EM, Ferlito A, Bradley PJ, Rinaldo A, Scully C (2003). Neck disease and distant metastases. *Oral Oncol*, 39(3), 207–12.

10 Calhoun KH, Fulmer P, Weiss R, Hokanson JA (1994). Distant metastases from head and neck squamous. *Laryngoscope*, 104(10), 1199–205.

11 Gregoire V, Bol A, Geets X, Lee J (2006). Is PET-based treatment planning the new standard in modern radiotherapy? The head and neck paradigm. *Semin Radiat Oncol*, 16(4), 232–8.

12 Schwartz DL, Rajendran J, Yueh B, et al. (2003). Staging of head and neck squamous cell cancer with extended-field FDG-PET. *Arch Otolaryngol Head Neck Surg*, 129(11), 1173–8.

13 Ord RA, Kolokythas A, Reynolds MA (2006). Surgical salvage for local and regional recurrence in oral cancer. *J Oral Maxillofac Surg*, 64(9),1409–14.

14 Pearlman NW. Treatment outcome in recurrent head and neck cancer. *Arch Surg*, 114(1), 39–42.

15 Krol BJ, Righi PD, Paydarfar JA, et al. (2000). Factors related to outcome of salvage therapy for isolated cervical recurrence of squamous cell carcinoma in the previously treated neck: A multi-institutional study. *Otolaryngol Head Neck Surg*, 123(4), 368–76.

16 Robert F, Ezekiel MP, Spencer SA, et al. (2001). Phase I study of anti–epidermal growth factor receptor antibody cetuximab in combination with radiation therapy in patients with advanced head and neck cancer. *J Clin Oncol*, 19(13), 3234–43.

17 Bonner JA, Harari PM, Giralt J, et al. (2006). Radiotherapy plus cetuximab for squamous- cell carcinoma of the head and neck. *N Engl J Med*, 354(6), 567–78.

18 Forastiere A, Koch W, Trotti A, Sidransky D (2001). Head and neck cancer. *N Engl J Med*, 345(26), 1890–900.

19 LaBlance GR, Kraus K, Steckol KF (1991). Rehabilitation of swallowing and communication following glossectomy. *Rehabil Nurs*, 16(5), 266–70.

20 Pauloski BR, Logemann JA, Colangelo LA, et al. (1998). Surgical variables affecting speech in treated patients with oral and oropharyngeal cancer. *Laryngoscope*, 108(6), 908–16.

21 Massengill R Jr, Maxwell S, Pickrell K (1970). An analysis of articulation following partial and total glossectomy. *J Speech Hear Disord*, 35(2), 170–3.

22 Rentschler GJ, Mann MB (1980). The effects of glossectomy on intelligibility of speech and oral perceptual discrimination. *J Oral Surg*, 38(5), 348–54.

23 Logemann, JA (1988). The role of the speech language pathologist in the management of dysphagia. *Otolaryngol Clin North Am*, 21(4), 783–8.

24 Pauloski BR, Logemann, JA, Rademaker AW, et al. (1993). Speech and swallowing function after anterior tongue and floor of mouth resection with distal flap reconstruction. *J Speech Hear Res*, 36(2), 267–76.

25 Vaughan ED (1982). An analysis of morbidity following major head and neck surgery with particular reference to mouth function. *J Maxillofac Surg*, 10(3), 129–34.

26 Vaughan ED, Bainton R, Martin IC (1992). Improvements in morbidity of mouth cancer using microvascular free flap reconstructions. *J Craniomaxillofac Surg*, 20(3), 132–4.

27 Ichimura K, Tanaka T (1993). Trismus in patients with malignant tumours in the head and neck. *J Laryngol Otol*, 107(11), 1017–20.

28 Dijkstra PU, Kalk WW, Roodenburg JL (2004). Trismus in head and neck oncology: a systematic review. *Oral Oncol*, 40(9), 879–89.

29 Dijkstra PU, Huisman PM, Roodenburg JL (2006). Criteria for trismus in head and neck oncology. *Int J Oral Maxillofac Surg*, 35(4), 337–42.

30 Buchbinder D, Currivan RB, Kaplan AJ, Urken ML (1993). Mobilization regimens for the prevention of jaw hypomobility in the radiated patient: a comparison of three techniques. *J Oral Maxillofac Surg*, 51(8), 863–7.

31 Hooley R, Levine H, Flores TC, Wheeler T, Steiger E (1983). Predicting postoperative head and neck complications using nutritional assessment: the prognostic nutritional index. *Arch Otolaryngol*, 109(2), 83–5.

32 Devine JC, Rogers SN, McNally D, Brown JS, Vaughan ED (2001). A comparison of aesthetic, functional and patient subjective outcomes following lip-split mandibulotomy and mandibular lingual releasing access procedures. *Int J Oral Maxillofac Surg*, 30(3), 199–204.

33 Cilento BW, Izzard M, Weymuller EA, Futran N (2007). Comparison of approaches for oral cavity cancer resection: lip-split versus visor flap. *Otolaryngol Head Neck Surg*, 137(3), 428–32.

34 Ramon Y, Hendler S, Oberman M (1984). A stepped technique for splitting the lower lip. *J Oral Maxillofac Surg*, 42(10), 689–91.

35 Hayter JP, Vaughan ED, Brown JS (1996). Aesthetic lip splits. *Br J Oral Maxillofac Surg*, 34(5), 432–5.

36 Thankappan KM, Sharan R, Iyer S Kuriakose MA (2009). Esthetic and anatomic basis of Modified lateral rhinotomy approach. *J Oral Maxillofac Surg*, 67(1), 231–4.

37 Kolokythas A, Fernandes RP, Ord R (2007). A non-lip-splitting double mandibular osteotomy technique applied for resection of tumors in the parapharyngeal and pterygomandibular spaces. *J Oral Maxillofac Surg*, 65(3), 566–9.

38 Cummings CW, Haughey BH, Thomas JR, et al. (2005). *Cummings otolaryngology: head and neck surgery*, 4th edn. Mosby, St Louis.

39 Friess CC, Fontaine DJ, Kornblut AD (1979). Complications of therapy of oral malignant disease. *Otolaryngol Clin North Am*, 12(1), 175–81.

40 Epstein SK (2005). Late Complications of tracheostomy. *Respir Care*, 50(4), 542–9.

41 Goldenberg D, Ari EG, Golz A, Danino J. Netzer A. Joachims HZ (2000). Tracheotomy complications: a retrospective study of 1130 cases. *Otolaryngol Head Neck Surg*, 123(4), 495–500.

42 Wood DE, Mathisen DJ, Late complications of tracheotomy (1991). *Clin Chest Med*, 12(3), 597–609.

43 Saunders JR Jr, Hirata RM, Jacques DA (1985). Considering the spinal accessory nerve in head and neck surgery. *Am J Surg*, 150(4), 491–4.

44 Cappiello J, Piazza C, Nicolai P (2007). The spinal accessory nerve in head and neck surgery. *Curr Opin Otolaryngol Head Neck Surg*, 15(2), 107–11.

45 Shibahara T, Noma H, Furuya Y, Takaki R (2002). Fracture of mandibular reconstruction plates used after tumor resection. *J Oral Maxillofac Surg*, 60(2), 182–5.

46 Neovius EB, Lind MG, Lind FG (1997). Hyperbaric oxygen therapy for wound complications after surgery in the irradiated head and neck: a review of the literature and a report of 15 consecutive patients. *Head Neck*, 19(4), 315–22.

47 Wilson KM, Rizk NM, Armstrong SL, Gluckman JL (1998). Effects of hemimandibulectomy on quality of life. Laryngoscope, 108(10), 1574–7.

48 Rogers SN, Lowe D, Fisher SE, Brown JS, Vaughan ED (2002). Health-related quality of life and clinical function after primary surgery for oral cancer. *Br J Oral Maxillofac Surg*, 40(1), 11–18.

Chapter 10

Overview of complications of radiotherapy (radiation therapy)

Kate Newbold and Kevin Harrington

Definition

Radiotherapy ('radiation therapy' or 'irradiation') is defined as 'the use of high-energy radiation from X-rays, gamma rays, neutrons, protons, and other sources to kill cancer cells and shrink tumors'[1].

Radiotherapy, often with concomitant chemotherapy, has a significant role in the 'curative' management of head and neck cancer. Primary chemo-radiation allows preservation of organ function, and is the treatment modality of choice for tumours arising in the oropharynx, nasopharynx, hypopharynx, and larynx. In oral cavity cancers, the best cure rates are obtained using surgical techniques with adjuvant or post-operative radiotherapy (with or without chemotherapy).

Radiotherapy also has an important role in the palliation of symptoms in patients with advanced/incurable head and neck cancer (e.g. shrinkage of tumour, prevention of ulceration, prevention of bleeding, pain control).

Differentiated thyroid cancers are treated with targeted radioisotope therapy (i.e. 'radioiodine': iodine 131). Medullary carcinoma of the thyroid is managed primarily by surgery and post-operative radiotherapy. Radiotherapy is also used in the management of other tumours arising in the head and neck region such as lymphoma, sarcoma, and tumours of the skin.

Radiobiology

Radiation can cause damage to any molecule in a cell, but damage to DNA is crucial in causing cell death. This damage occurs both directly, and indirectly through free radicals which are formed following the interaction of the radiation with intracellular water. Single- and double-strand DNA breaks can cause death of the cell (if such lesions are not appropriately repaired).

The '4Rs' of radiobiology were initially defined to explain the success or failure of localized radiotherapy[2]. Differential *Repair* of tumour and normal cells between treatment fractions, *Redistribution* of cells into more or less radiation-sensitive phases of the cell cycle, *Repopulation* of tumour cells between fractions, and *Re-oxygenation* of tumour cells during treatment were variously invoked to explain the net outcome of radiotherapy.

Later, the system was refined to include intrinsic *Radiosensitivity* in the '5Rs' of radiobiology[3]. With a few exceptions, this final addition to the quintet was an admission of our inability to explain at the mechanistic level the different radioresponsiveness of different tumour types (e.g. lymphoma – sensitive; glioblastoma – resistant)[4]. The 5Rs of radiobiology provides an invaluable framework within which to examine new therapeutic strategies from the point of view of both tumour and normal cells.

Each of the 'Rs' can be viewed as a double-edged sword, such that changes can occur in either direction to increase or decrease the net therapeutic effect. For example, if a tumour cell has acquired a defect in its DNA repair pathway, it is more likely than an adjacent normal cell to be killed by a dose of radiation[5–7]. However, the abnormal DNA repair pathway may allow the tumour cell to accumulate mutations in other genes that enable it to tolerate unrepaired DNA damage.

Similarly, the enhanced tumour cell division that occurs during a course of radiotherapy is generally viewed negatively as the driving force behind accelerated repopulation (see below), but it may also make a tumour cell more susceptible to radiation-induced death by causing it to enter mitosis with unrepaired DNA damage (so-called mitotic catastrophe)[4]. The 5Rs of radiobiology are reviewed briefly to highlight their importance to the radiation response.

Repair

Radiation (and/or chemotherapy) induces DNA damage in both normal and cancer cells. For every 1 Gy of radiation delivered, 1000 single-stranded and 40 double-stranded breaks will occur. Of these lesions, double-stranded breaks represent the greatest threat to the viability of a cell. In response to DNA damage, cells engage a number of repair mechanisms. The principal mechanisms involved in double-stranded breaks repair are (1) homologous recombination; and (2) non-homologous end-joining.

Homologous recombination is an extremely accurate form of DNA repair that operates in cells in S and G2 phases of the cell cycle (when a sister chromatid is present to act as a template for repair). In contrast, non-homologous end-joining is a 'quick and dirty' form of repair that operates throughout the entire cell cycle and is, therefore, the dominant process in response to radiation-induced DNA damage[8]. This form of repair does not require the presence of a template and, as a consequence, is error prone.

Normal tissues are more efficient at repairing damage than tumour cells and this difference is exploited in fractionated radiotherapy. Thus, the damage from each small fraction of radiotherapy is repaired better in the normal tissues and, over the course of many weeks, the differential cell kill between normal and tumour cells results in more complete tumour eradication with acceptable normal tissue toxicity.

Redistribution

Radiosensitivity varies as cells progress through the cell cycle. Although this phenomenon may be cell-line dependent, there is a general trend for cells to be most radiosensitive in the G2 and M phases of the cell cycle, and most resistant during the late S phase[9]. Thus, following a dose of radiation, there is a tendency towards synchronization of cells – with more cells in S phase surviving and progressing together round the cell cycle. This effect is compounded by the effect of radiation on cell cycle checkpoints (i.e. it causes arrest at the G1/S boundary and in G2). Another important consideration in delivering fractionated radiotherapy is the fact that cells in a radioresistant phase of the cell cycle on one day are likely to be in a more radiosensitive phase of the cell cycle on other days during treatment.

Repopulation

As cells within the tumour are lost during radiotherapy, the remaining cells continue to divide. Indeed, there are data to suggest that the rate of tumour cell division may increase as treatment progresses beyond 4 weeks[10]. This so-called accelerated repopulation of cells results in an effective 'dose-loss effect', as some of the radiation dose delivered is used in killing the cells that came in to being since the previous fraction of treatment.

Appreciation of the importance of this phenomenon has had a profound effect on the practice of radiation oncology. Accelerated fractionation regimens aim to deliver radiotherapy using abbreviated schedules to minimize the tumour's ability to repopulate, whilst growth factor-receptor blockers aim to slow down the rate of repopulation during treatment[4]. Another important therapeutic principle that stems directly from an understanding of repopulation is the desire to avoid unscheduled gaps in radiotherapy regimens (see below).

Reoxygenation

It has been known for over 50 years that the response of cells to radiation is strongly influenced by ambient oxygen levels, with hypoxic cells showing relative radiation resistance[11]. Once they grow beyond a certain size, tumours contain areas with varying levels of oxygenation, including hypoxic regions where cells are able to remain viable. Cells in these compartments are relatively radioresistant.

A consequence of using fractionated radiotherapy is the possibility for progressive reoxygenation of previously hypoxic tumour tissue. This can occur through radiation-induced reductions in tumour cell density, with corresponding increases in access to and availability of oxygen for the remaining cells.

Radiosensitivity

The most recently defined of the '5Rs' represents an increase in our knowledge of the molecular determinants of the radiation response. For example, there is emerging evidence that the Ras signal transduction pathway plays a role in determining the radiosensitivity of tumours[12]. Thus, overexpression of epidermal growth factor receptor (EGFR), activating mutations of Ras, and phosphorylation of Akt and phosphoinositide-3-kinase have all been associated with increased radiation resistance *in vitro* (and in the case of overexpression of EGFR, and phosphorylation of Akt, to radiation treatment failure in cancer patients)[12–15].

In contrast, Ras pathway inhibitors, such as the farnesyltransferase inhibitors, sensitize cells to radiation[16]. Similar results have also been obtained with the use of adenoviral vectors encoding an inactivating single-chain antibody against Ras[17].

Radiotherapy modalities

External beam radiotherapy

External beam radiotherapy uses X-rays from the high-energy end of the spectrum of electromagnetic radiation. All types of electromagnetic radiation can be considered as moving packets of energy called photons. These photons have sufficient energy that when they interact with matter, electrons are displaced from their orbit around the nucleus of the atoms in the irradiated tissue. The atom is left with a positive charge, and thus becomes an ion/'free radical', (hence the term 'ionizing radiation').

The displaced electrons in turn ionize other atoms, setting yet more electrons into motion. As the electrons interact they slow down, and lose energy more and more rapidly. The maximum rate of energy loss occurs just before they come to rest (the so-called 'Bragg peak'). The depth in the tissue that the Bragg peak occurs is dependent on the energy of the source photons, and this characteristic is utilized by the clinical oncologist (radiation oncologist) when determining what X-ray energy to prescribe.

External beam radiotherapy can be subdivided according to the X-ray energy:

◆ Superficial X-rays – superficial X-rays are of energy 50–150 kV, and in the head and neck region are used predominantly for surface lesions (e.g. skin cancers).

- Orthovoltage X-rays – orthovoltage X-ray machines produce energies of between 200 and 300 kV, which penetrate to a depth of approximately 3 cm (and are uncommonly used in the head and neck region).
- Megavoltage X-rays – megavoltage X-rays of energy 4–20 MV are produced by linear accelerators, whilst γ-rays with energy of around 1.2 MV are produced from the decay of a radioactive element such as cobalt-60.

Electron therapy

Linear accelerators also produce electron beams, which as particulate radiation have the advantage of a defined range within tissue, and a sharp cut-off where the energy is deposited. This property is particularly useful when treating superficial lesions that overlie critical structures.

Proton/neutron therapy

Unlike with X-rays, the absorbed dose of a proton beam increases very gradually with increasing depth and then suddenly rises to a peak at the end of a proton range. Protons have certain radiobiological advantages over conventional photon radiotherapy. The ionization caused by protons is greater than that caused by photons, and so they impart more damage on the target tissue (which is less likely to be repaired). Furthermore, there is also less dependence on the cells' position in the cell cycle, and a greater number of hypoxic cells are killed.

However, clinical data are somewhat limited, because clinical proton-beam facilities are only now being developed. Clinical studies suggest that there may be benefits to using protons for tumours characterized by poor radiosensitivity, and in critical locations such as for skull-base tumours (e.g. chordoma, chondrosarcoma), paranasal sinus carcinomas, and nasopharyngeal tumours[18,19]. Nevertheless, the role of proton therapy is still very much under investigation[20].

Neutrons have also been used to treat cancer, although the data on therapy with neutrons is very sparse. Some authors report that neutrons offer no advantages over X-rays[21].

Brachytherapy

Brachytherapy is the use of radioactive sources placed either within, or on the target site. The advantage of this type of treatment is that as a result of the 'inverse square law', there is a rapid fall off in dose at only a short distance from the source. Brachytherapy can be applied in several ways. Mould treatment places radioactive sources directly over a superficial tumour. Intracavitary treatment involves placing radioactive sources within a body cavity (most commonly used in gynaecological malignancies). The most common modality in the head and neck region is interstitial treatment, which involves placing radioactive needles or wire directly into the tumour[22].

Tumours that are appropriate for treatment with Iridium wires in the form of hairpins are superficial, small, and accessible tumours such as those on the lateral tongue, buccal mucosa, or anterior floor of mouth. Iridium 192 wire can also be placed within loops of plastic tubing which have been sutured into an operative bed before closure of the wound (a process called 'after-loading'). The latter technique has a role in treating recurrences at the site of previous radiotherapy, as re-irradiation with brachytherapy can minimize the dose to adjacent critical structures, which have most likely already received their tolerance dose of radiation[23].

Isotope therapy

Isotope therapy involves the systemic administration of a radioactive isotope, which is then concentrated in a specific tissue of the body (e.g. radioiodine treatment in thyroid cancer).

Total body irradiation

Total body irradiation (TBI) is a technique of delivering radiation to the whole body with the aim of eradicating malignant cells within sanctuary sites, and promoting engraftment of an allograft by its immunosuppressive effect. It is most commonly used, in conjunction with high dose chemotherapy, in patients with certain haematological malignancies.

Radiotherapy regimens

Standard regimens for external beam radiotherapy for squamous cell carcinoma, the most common cancer of the head and neck region, consist of 6–7 weeks of daily fractionation delivering doses of around 2 Gy to a total dose of 70 Gy (or equivalent). Patients are treated in the supine position, and immobilized with a thermoplastic mask/'shell' which covers the head, neck, and often the shoulders. Conformal planning is enabled by CT scanning the patient in this immobilization device, and a three-dimensional target is constructed by defining the target volume and volumes of organs at risk on axial image slices. The optimal beam arrangement is then determined so as to deliver the prescribed dose to the target, and to keep the critical organs within tolerance.

Altered fractionation regimens

Radiation regimens have been designed to improve clinical benefit by increasing dose intensity to targets, whilst attempting to minimize the toxicity. Hyperfractionated regimens involve giving multiple fractions per day with a smaller dose per fraction: this regimen invokes the radiobiological principle of repair (as discussed earlier). Accelerated regimens involve giving shorter courses of treatment with, for example, no breaks in treatment at the weekend: this regimen invokes the radiobiological principle of repopulation. The first evidence that hyperfractionation and acceleration improved locoregional control in head and neck was from the Radiation Therapy Oncology Group (RTOG) 90-03 study[24].

The Meta-Analysis of Radiotherapy in Carcinomas of Head and neck (MARCH) Collaborative Group reported on 15 trials (with 6515 patients) that compared hyperfractionated or accelerated radiotherapy with conventional regimens[25]. There was a significant survival benefit with altered fractionated radiotherapy, corresponding to an absolute benefit of 3.4% at 5 years. The benefit was significantly higher with hyperfractionated radiotherapy (8% at 5 years) than with accelerated radiotherapy (2% with no total dose reduction, and 1.7% with total dose reduction at 5 years). Unsurprisingly, prolonged overall treatment time, reduced overall radiation dose, and split-course radiotherapy does not improve tumour control[25].

Tissue-sparing techniques

There is much interest in preventing the severity of radiation-induced oral complications by increased conformity of the delivery of radiotherapy. This can be done with computed tomography (CT)-guided three-dimensional target definition and with intensity-modulated radiotherapy (IMRT). IMRT provides a tool to create concavities in the treatment volume, and hence spare tissues such as oral mucosa, salivary glands, or specific muscle groups (Figure 10.1, see colour plate section)[26].

The ability of IMRT to produce dose distributions that may allow preservation of salivary tissue has been the subject of several trials. Eisbruch et al. showed that IMRT can reduce the radiation dose to the contralateral parotid gland to 32% (compared with 93% for conventionally planned techniques)[27]. As a result, the spared parotid glands recovered 63% of their pre-treatment stimulated salivary flow rates at 1 year (compared with 3% for conventionally planned techniques)[27].

Radioprotectors

A number of strategies have been used to prevent/ameliorate the development of oral complications in patients receiving head and neck radiotherapy, including screening for pre-existing oral problems, maintenance of oral hygiene, stopping smoking, stopping drinking alcohol, as well as various specific interventions[1]. In addition, researchers have investigated the clinical utility of so-called 'radioprotectors'.

The thiols group of agents have been particularly investigated for their role as radioprotectors (e.g. amifostine). The mechanism of action of thiols is through the scavenging of radiation-induced free radicals (as discussed earlier). It is thought that there is preferential rapid uptake into normal tissues, with negligible or slow uptake into tumour tissues[28]. There is conflicting data on amifostine's ability to reduce oral side effects in patients receiving head and neck radiotherapy. However, amifostine is now approved by the Food and Drug Administration Agency (FDA) in the USA for the reduction of xerostomia following radiotherapy.

A phase III randomized controlled trial of 315 head and neck cancer patients showed a statistically significant reduction in the incidence of Grade 2 acute and late xerostomia, but no reduction in the incidence of Grade 3 acute mucositis, in patients treated with amifostine[29]. The amifostine arm also had improved patient symptom-benefit scores over the control arm[30]. Furthermore, there was no difference in antitumour efficacy between the two treatment arms, as measured by locoregional control and overall survival at 2 years[31]. However, 20% of the patients discontinued amifostine before the completion of radiotherapy, primarily due to related side effects (i.e. nausea, vomiting, and hypotension).

Other free-radical inhibitors undergoing investigation include N-acetylcysteine, manganese superoxide dismutase, and benzydamine[32].

Consequences of treatment gaps

It is well documented that breaks in radiotherapy, and prolongation of overall treatment time, reduce treatment efficacy due to rapid repopulation of squamous cell carcinomas during treatment[10,33]. Thus, Bese et al. reported that a 1-day break in treatment involving conventional fractionation (1.8–2.0 Gy per fraction, once a day) reduces local control rates by 1.4%, and requires compensating by either increasing the number of daily fractions (hyperfractionation), increasing the dose per fraction, or delivering an additional fraction[34].

Oral complications of radiotherapy

Radiotherapy applied to the head and neck region can cause a variety of local oral complications (see Table 10.1). A detailed discussion of these oral complications is beyond the scope of this chapter, and the reader is directed to other relevant chapters within the book (e.g. Chapter 11 – Trismus; Chapter 12 – Post-radiation osteonecrosis; Chapter 15 – Oral mucositis; Chapter 21 – Salivary gland dysfunction; Chapter 22 – Taste disturbance).

Radioiodine-induced salivary gland problems

Salivary glands have the ability to concentrate iodine, and are, therefore, at risk of radiation damage in patients treated with radioiodine for thyroid cancer. Soon after radioiodine, patients may experience acute salivary gland swelling and pain, which usually subsides over a period of

Table 10.1 Oral complications of head and neck radiotherapy [1].

Complication	Comment
Oral mucositis	Acute complication
Oral infections ♦ fungal ♦ bacterial	Acute/chronic complication
Taste disturbance	Acute/chronic complication
Salivary gland dysfunction	Acute/chronic complication
Osteonecrosis	Chronic complication
Soft tissue necrosis	Chronic complication
Soft tissue fibrosis	Chronic complication Trismus may result from fibrosis of muscles of mastication and/or temporomandibular joint
Dental/skeletal developmental problems	Chronic complication Occurs in paediatric patients
Induction of second malignancy	Chronic complication

a few days. Some patients will develop a slower onset of symptoms, and others may progress to a chronic radiation sialadenitis. The frequency of these complications is uncertain, but clinically significant problems occur in 11–30% of patients[56–58].

References

1 National Cancer Institute (2008). Oral complications of chemotherapy and head/neck radiation. Health Professional Version. Available from NCI website: http://www.cancer.gov/cancertopics/pdq/supportivecare/oralcomplications/healthprofessional

2 Withers HR (1975). The four R's of radiotherapy. *Adv Radiat Biol*, 5, 241–7.

3 Steel GG, McMillan TJ, Peacock JH (1989). The 5Rs of radiobiology. *Int J Radiat Biol*, 56(6), 1045–8.

4 Harrington K, Jankowska P, Hingorani M (2007). Molecular biology for the radiation oncologist: the 5Rs of radiobiology meet the hallmarks of cancer. *Clin Oncol (R Coll Radiol)*, 19(8), 561–71.

5 Banath JP, MacPhail SH, Olive PL (2004). Radiation sensitivity, H2AX phosphorylation, and kinetics of repair of DNA strand breaks in irradiated cervical cancer cell lines. *Cancer Res*, 64(19), 7144–9.

6 Berry SE, Garces C, Hwang HS, et al. (1999). The mismatch repair protein, hMLH1, mediates 5-substituted halogenated thymidine analogue cytotoxicity, DNA incorporation, and radiosensitization in human colon cancer cells. *Cancer Res*, 59(8), 1840–5.

7 Bishay K, Ory K, Lebeau J, Levalois C, Olivier MF, Chevillard S (2000). DNA damage-related gene expression as biomarkers to assess cellular response after gamma irradiation of a human lymphoblastoid cell line. *Oncogene*, 19(7), 916–23.

8 Helleday T, Petermann E, Lundin C, Hodgson B, Sharma RA (2008). DNA repair pathways as targets for cancer therapy. *Nat Rev Cancer*, 8(3), 193–204.

9 Sinclair WK, Morton RA (1965). X-ray and ultraviolet sensitivity of synchronized Chinese hamster cells at various stages of the cell cycle. *Biophys J*, 5, 1–25.

10 Withers HR, Maciejewski B, Taylor JM, Hliniak A (1988). Accelerated repopulation in head and neck cancer. *Front Radiat Ther Oncol*, 22, 105–10.

11 Wright EA, Howard-Flanders P (1957). The influence of oxygen on the radiosensitivity of mammalian tissues. *Acta Radiol*, 48(1), 26–32.

12 McKenna, WG, Muschel RJ, Gupta, AK, Hahn SM, Bernhard EJ (2003). The RAS signal transduction pathway and its role in radiation sensitivity. *Oncogene*, 22(37), 5866–75.

13 Gupta AK, McKenna WG, Weber CN, et al. (2002). Local recurrence in head and neck cancer: relationship to radiation resistance and signal transduction. *Clin Cancer Res*, 8(3), 885–92.

14 Gupta AK, Cerniglia GJ, Mick R, et al. (2003). Radiation sensitization of human cancer cells in vivo by inhibiting the activity of PI3K using LY294002. *Int J Radiat Oncol Biol Phys*, 56(3), 846–53.

15 Liang K, Ang KK, Milas L, Hunter N, Fan Z (2003). The epidermal growth factor receptor mediates radioresistance. *Int J Radiat Oncol Biol Phys*, 57(1), 246–54.

16 Bernhard EJ, Kao G, Cox AD, et al. (1996). The farnesyltransferase inhibitor FTI-277 radiosensitizes H-ras-transformed rat embryo fibroblasts. *Cancer Res*, 56(8), 1727–30.

17 Russell JS, Lang FF, Huet T, et al. (1999). Radiosensitization of human tumor cell lines induced by the adenovirus-mediated expression of an anti-Ras single-chain antibody fragment. *Cancer Res*, 59(8), 5239–44.

18 Tokuuye K, Akine Y, Kagei K, et al. (2004). Proton therapy for head and neck malignancies at Tsukuba. *Strahlenther Onkol*, 180(2), 96–101.

19 Slater JD, Yonemoto LT, Mantik DW, et al. (2005). Proton radiation for treatment of cancer of the oropharynx: early experience at Loma Linda University Medical Center using a concomitant boost technique. *Int J Radiat Oncol Biol Phys*, 62(2), 494–500.

20 Jereczek-Fossa BA, Krengli M, Orecchia R (2006). Particle beam radiotherapy for head and neck tumors: radiobiological basis and clinical experience. *Head Neck*, 28(8), 750–60.

21 Jones B (2008). The potential clinical advantages of charged particle radiotherapy using protons or light ions. *Clin Oncol (R Coll Radiol)*, 20(7), 555–63.

22 Dobbs J, Barrett A, Ash D (1999). *Practical radiotherapy planning*, 3rd edn. Hodder Arnold, London.

23 Hall CE, Harris R, A'Hern R, et al. (2003). Le Fort I osteotomy and low-dose rate Ir192 brachytherapy for treatment of recurrent nasopharyngeal tumours. *Radiother Oncol*, 66(1), 41–8.

24 Fu KK, Pajak TF, Trotti A, et al. (2000). A Radiation Therapy Oncology Group (RTOG) phase III randomized study to compare hyperfractionation and two variants of accelerated fractionation to standard fractionation radiotherapy for head and neck squamous cell carcinomas: first report of RTOG 9003. *Int J Radiat Oncol Biol Phys*, 48(1), 7–16.

25 Bourhis J, Overgaard J, Audry H, et al. (2006). Hyperfractionated or accelerated radiotherapy in head and neck cancer: a meta-analysis. *Lancet*, 368(9538), 843–54.

26 Guerrero Urbano MT, Nutting CM (2004). Clinical use of intensity-modulated radiotherapy: part 1. *Br J Radiol*, 77(914), 88–96.

27 Eisbruch A, Kim HM, Terrell JE, Marsh LH, Dawson LA, Ship JA (2001). Xerostomia and its predictors following parotid-sparing irradiation of head-and-neck cancer. *Int J Radiat Oncol Biol Phys*, 50(3), 695–704.

28 Capizzi RL (1999). The preclinical basis for broad-spectrum selective cytoprotection of normal tissues from cytotoxic therapies by amifostine. *Semin Oncol*, 26(2 Suppl 7), 3–21.

29 Brizel DM, Wasserman TH, Henke M, et al. (2000). Phase III randomized trial of amifostine as a radioprotector in head and neck cancer. *J Clin Oncol*, 18(19), 3339–45.

30 Wasserman T, Mackowiak JI, Brizel DM, et al. (2000). Effect of amifostine on patient assessed clinical benefit in irradiated head and neck cancer. *Int J Radiat Oncol Biol Phys*, 48(4), 1035–9.

31 Wasserman TH, Brizel DM, Henke M, et al. (2005). Influence of intravenous amifostine on xerostomia, tumor control, and survival after radiotherapy for head-and-neck cancer: 2-year follow-up of a prospective, randomized, phase III trial. *Int J Radiat Oncol Biol Phys*, 63(4), 985–90.

32 Epstein JB, Silverman S Jr, Paggiarino DA, et al. (2001). Benzydamine HCl for prophylaxis of radiation-induced oral mucositis: results from a multicenter, randomized, double-blind, placebo-controlled clinical trial. *Cancer*, 92(4), 875–85.

33 Koukourakis M, Hlouverakis G, Kosma L, et al. (1996). The impact of overall treatment time on the results of radiotherapy for nonsmall cell lung carcinoma. *Int J Radiat Oncol Biol Phys*, 34(2), 315–22.

34 Bese NS, Hendry J, Jeremic B (2007). Effects of prolongation of overall treatment time due to unplanned interruptions during radiotherapy of different tumor sites and practical methods for compensation. *Int J Radiat Oncol Biol Phys*, 68(3), 654–61.

Chapter 11

Trismus

Pieter Dijkstra and Jan Roodenburg

Definition

The word trismus comes from the Greek word 'trismos' meaning grating, grinding, or squeaking[1,2]. Originally, the term was used to refer to the inability to open the mouth as a result of tetanus. At present, the term is used to indicate severely restricted mouth opening of any aetiology[3].

Epidemiology

Trismus is frequently seen in head and neck cancer patients. The reported prevalence of trismus ranges from 0% to 100% in head and neck cancer patients[4–57]. This enormous range can be attributed to differences in research design (e.g. prospective assessment of patients, retrospective review of medical charts), differences in the assessment method (e.g. 'eyeballing' mouth opening, actual measurement of mouth opening), and differences in the criteria used to define trismus (see following sections). In addition, tumour site, tumour size, and treatment(s) utilized and sample variation may explain differences in the reported prevalence of trismus.

Table 11.1a shows data on the prevalence of trismus from studies of mixed groups of head and neck cancer[4–7]. Detailed information concerning site/type of tumour is provided in the studies of Ichimura and Tanaka[5], and Kent et al.[6]. However, the numbers of patients reported in the subgroups are small, resulting in very wide 95% confidence intervals. Tables 11.1b–d show the data on the prevalence of trismus from studies looking at specific groups of head and neck cancer[8–54]. Trismus has been reported to be present in 5–32% of the patients treated for maxillary sinus cancer (Table 11.1b)[8–13], 0–69% patients treated for oral/oropharyngeal cancer (Table 11.1c)[14–21], and 0–36% for patients treated for nasopharyngeal cancer (Table 11.1d)[22–30]. In patients who have been treated for large/unresectable tumours, the prevalence of trismus ranges from 3% to 26% [31–36] (Table 11.1e), whilst for patients treated for recurrent tumours the prevalence ranges from 2% to 61%. (Table 11.1f)[37–54]. Trismus has been reported to have been present in 9% (95% CI: 9; 28) to 20% (95% CI: 6; 51) patients treated for rhabdomyosarcoma in the head and neck area, but the sample sizes investigated were small (10–22)[55–57].

The data presented in the tables should be interpreted with caution, particularly as most of the studies were retrospective in design, and so the data available to the researchers was merely the data recorded in the medical charts. Additionally, in the majority of studies it is not clear whether trismus was present prior to cancer treatment, or developed during or following cancer treatment. Thus, cause–effect relationships cannot be inferred from these studies.

Table 11.1a Prevalence of trismus in studies involving mixed groups of head and neck patients

Study	Study design, participants, follow up	Treatment	Tumour location	Prevalence trismus % (95% CI*)
Olmi et al., 1990 [4]	Design not reported n = 53 Follow up ≥1 year	Radiotherapy (accelerated)	All head and neck tumours	6% (2; 15)
Ichimura and Tanaka, 1993 [5]	Retrospective study n = 212 Follow up not reported	Not reported	All head and neck tumours	10% (7; 15)
			Tongue	23% (11; 42)
			Floor of mouth	33% (6; 79)
			Buccal mucosa	50% (9; 91)
			Retromolar trigone	100% (34; 100)
			Hypopharynx /cervical oesophagus	6% (1; 28)
			Parotid gland	33% (6; 79)
			Nasal cavity	6% (1; 26)
			Nasopharynx	17% (5; 45)
			Maxillary sinus	57% (25; 84)
			Infratemporal fossa	100% (34; 100)
Kent et al., 2007 [6]	Retrospective study n = 40 Follow up ≥1 month	Surgery, radiotherapy, chemotherapy	All head and neck tumours	45% (31; 60)
			Tongue	35% (17; 59)
			Floor of mouth	50% (15; 85)
			Oropharynx	60% (23; 88)
			Tonsil	50% (24; 76)
			Hypopharynx	67% (21; 94)
			Salivary glands	33% (6; 79)
			Nasopharynx	50% (9; 91)
			Unknown	0% (0; 79)
Aref et al., 1997 [7]	Design not reported n = 21 Follow up ≥9 months	Neutron therapy	Salivary gland tumours	10% (3; 29)

*95% CI = 95% confidence interval

Aetiology

Trismus may be caused by either intra-articular or extra-articular problems[3,58]. In head and neck oncology, trismus may be the result of the tumour itself, or may be the result of the treatment for the tumour (i.e. surgery and/or radiotherapy).

Trismus may be the result of growth of the tumour into the temporomandibular joint (TMJ), or into the muscles involved in mouth closing (i.e. masseter, medial pterygoid, or temporalis muscles). Furthermore, tumours growing adjacent to these muscles may restrict their ability to stretch, and thereby reduce their ability to open the mouth. In a study of 212 head and neck cancer patients, 2% overall had trismus at the time of diagnosis, and another 1% overall had trismus at the time of recurrence[6]. In other studies, trismus was a presenting sign in 56% patients with malignant parapharyngeal space tumours[59], in 4–9% patients with nasopharyngeal tumours[60,61], and in 72% patients with advanced parotid gland tumours[33].

Surgery in the area of the TMJ and/or the masticatory muscles may lead to trismus. In the Ichimura and Tanaka study[5], 5% of patients with head and neck cancer developed trismus following surgery. Additionally, trismus may be the result of fractures of mandible due to failure of the materials used for reconstruction of the mandible[58].

Table 11.1b Prevalence of trismus in patients with maxillary sinus tumours

Study	Study design, participants, follow up	Tumour location	Treatment	Prevalence trismus % (95% CI)
Sakai et al., 1988 [8]	Survey n = 171 Follow up ≥10 years	Maxillary sinus	Surgery, radiotherapy, chemotherapy	32% (26; 39)
Jiang et al., 1991 [9]	Retrospective study n = 73 Follow up ≥9 months	Maxillary sinus	Surgery, radiotherapy	12% (7; 22)
Paulino et al., 1998 [10]	Retrospective study n = 48 Follow up ≥24 months	Maxillary sinus	Surgery, radiotherapy	6% (2; 17)
Nishino et al., 2000 [11]	Retrospective study n = 75 Follow up ≥4 months	Maxillary sinus	Surgery, radiotherapy, chemotherapy	5% (2; 13)
Ogawa et al., 2001 [12]	Retrospective study n = 41 Follow up ≥25 months	Maxillary sinus	Surgery, radiotherapy	5% (1; 16)
Özsaran et al., 2003 [13]	Retrospective study n = 79 Follow up ≥3 months	Maxillary sinus	Surgery, radiotherapy	5% (2; 12)

Similarly, radiotherapy in the area of the TMJ and/or masticatory muscles may lead to trismus; radiotherapy is associated with the development of tissue fibrosis. In the Ichimura and Tanaka study[5], 2% of patients with head and neck cancer developed trismus following radiotherapy. Mouth opening following radiotherapy decreases on average by 18% compared to mouth opening prior to radiotherapy[62]. In the first 9 months following radiotherapy, mouth opening decreases on average by 2.4 % per month[63]. In the second year, mouth opening decreases about 0.2% per month, and in the period from 24 to 48 months mouth opening decreases by 0.1% per month[63]. All in all, in the first 9 months following radiotherapy about two-thirds of the total reduction in mouth opening occurs[63]. The higher the dose delivered to the relevant tissues, the greater the decrease in mouth opening[62]. Additionally, trismus may be the result of fractures of mandible due to osteoradionecrosis[58].

It is important to remember that trismus in patients with cancer may develop independently of the tumour, or the treatment of the tumour. Common causes for trismus are internal derangement of the TMJ, osteoarthritis of the TMJ, dental infection, and alveolar infection.

Clinical features

Trismus is defined as severely restricted opening of the mouth. Intra-articular causes are associated with restricted horizontal movement of the mandible (towards the contralateral/unaffected side).

Table 11.1c Prevalence of trismus in patients with oral cavity/oropharynx tumours

Study	Study design, participants, follow up	Tumour location	Treatment	Prevalence trismus % (95% CI)
Thomas et al., 1988 [14]	Retrospective study n = 150 Follow up ≥3 months	Oropharynx	Radiotherapy – 4 fractions/week Radiotherapy – 5 fractions/week	21% (14; 30) 5% (2; 13)
Foote et al., 1990 [15]	Retrospective study n = 84 Follow up ≥2 years	Base of tongue	Radiotherapy	6% (3; 13)
Koka et al., 1990 [16]	Retrospective study n = 104 (Prior to treatment)	Oral cavity/ oropharynx	Hemi-mandibulectomy (for osteoradionecrosis)	17% (11; 26)
Pinheiro and Frame, 1994 [17]	Retrospective study n = 78 Follow up ≥1 month	Oral cavity	Laser treatment	1% (0; 7)
Ryu et al., 1995 [18]	Retrospective study n = 47 Follow up ≥3 months	Oral cavity/ oropharynx	Surgery, mandibular reconstruction, radiotherapy	2% (0; 11)
Bertrand et al., 2000 [19]	Retrospective study n = 64 Follow up ≥6 months	Oral cavity	Mandibular osteotomy, radiotherapy, chemotherapy	69% (57; 79)
Eisen et al., 2000 [20]	Retrospective study n = 30 Follow up ≥5 months	Oral cavity/ oropharnyx	Mandibulotomy, radiotherapy	0% (0; 11)
Karakoyun-Celik et al., 2005 [21]	Prospective study n = 40 Follow up ≥18 months	Base of tongue	Radiotherapy, brachytherapy, chemotherapy	5% (1; 17)

In contrast, extra-articular causes are generally not associated with restricted horizontal movement of the mandible. Most cases of oncology-related trismus are extra-articular in nature. The difference between passive and active opening of the mouth is usually small in oncology-related trismus (i.e. 1–2 mm).

Many different criteria for diagnosing trismus have been used in clinical practice:[64]

1. Dichotomous criteria:
   - <20 mm [28,47,49,53]
   - <25 mm [65]
   - <30 mm [26,61]
   - <35 mm [66]
   - <40 mm [32]

2. Categorical criteria:
   - Moderately restricted: 20–30 mm; severely restricted: <20 mm [8]
   - Light: >30 mm; moderate: 15–30 mm; severe: <15 mm [14]

Table 11.1d Prevalence of trismus in patients with nasopharynx tumours

Study	Study design, participants, follow up	Tumour location	Treatment	Prevalence trismus % (95% CI)
Qin et al., 1987 [22]	Retrospective study n = 1379 Follow up not reported	Nasopharynx	Radiotherapy	10% (8; 11)
Cmelaket et al., 1997 [23]	Prospective study n = 47 Follow up ≥1 month	Nasopharynx/skull base	Radiosurgery	2% (0; 11)
Choi et al., 1997 [24]	Retrospective study N = 21 Follow up ≥36 months	Nasopharynx/ paranasal sinuses	Chemotherapy, radiotherapy	0% (0; 15)
Zubizarreta et al., 2000 [25]	Design not reported n = 11 Follow up ≥23 months	Nasopharynx	Chemotherapy, radiotherapy	36% (15; 65)
Teo et al., 2000 [26]	Prospective study n = 159 Follow up ≥6 months	Nasopharynx	Radiotherapy - normal fractionation Radiotherapy - hyper-fractionation	9% (4; 17) 13% (7; 22)
Wolden et al., 2001 [27]	Retrospective study n = 68 Follow up ≥12 months	Nasopharynx	Radiotherapy, chemotherapy	4% (2; 12)
Jen et al., 2002 [28]	Prospective study n = 222 Follow up ≥8 months	Nasopharynx	Radiotherapy – 1 fraction/day Radiotherapy – 2 fractions/day	14% (9; 21) 17% (11; 26)
Fuchs et al., 2003 [29]	Retrospective study n = 101 Follow up not reported	Nasopharynx	Radiotherapy Radio-chemotherapy	9% (4; 20) 23% (13; 37)
Yeh et al., 2005 [30]	Retrospective study n = 849 Follow up ≥3 years	Nasopharynx	Radiotherapy	12% (10; 14)

3. Multidimensional categorical criteria

Grade 1: vertical mouth opening >40 mm and <25% difference in horizontal range of motion;
Grade 2: vertical mouth opening >30 mm and >25% difference in horizontal range of motion;
Grade 3: vertical mouth opening <25 mm and no horizontal movements[19].

Some of the categorical criteria lack scientific rigour. For instance, in the system of Thomas et al. a mouth opening of 32, 40, or 50 mm are all graded as lightly restricted[14]. Additionally, in the system used by Bertrand et al., it is impossible to classify a mouth opening of >31 mm with symmetrical horizontal movements of 1 mm[19].

The reasons for choosing specific cut-off points are seldom provided, and the cut-off points are probably based on the clinical judgement of the investigators. Recently, a mouth opening

Table 11.1e Prevalence of trismus in patients with advanced/unresectable tumours

Study	Study design, participants, follow up	Tumour location	Treatment	Prevalence trismus % (95% CI)
Nguyen et al., 1985 [31]	Design not reported n = 178 Follow up ≥2 yrs	Head and neck	Radiotherapy - 66 Gy Radiotherapy - 72 Gy	5% (2; 11) 9% (5; 16)
Nguyen et al., 1988 [32]	Design not reported n = 39 Follow up ≥2 years	Head and neck	Radiotherapy (hyperfractioned)	26% (15; 41)
Katsantonis et al., 1989 [33]	Design not reported n = 18 Follow up ≥1 years	Parotid gland	Stylo-hamular dissection, radiotherapy	17% (6; 39)
Chandrasekhar et al., 1990 [34]	Design not reported n = 29 Follow up ≥6 months	Head and neck	Surgery (parascapular flap reconstruction), radiotherapy	7% (2, 22)
Zidan et al., 1997 [35]	Design not reported n = 53 Follow up ≥3 years	Head and neck	Radiotherapy, chemotherapy	19% (11; 31)
MacKenzie et al., 1999 [36]	Prospective study n = 35 Follow up ≥12 months	Head and neck	Radiotherapy	3% (1; 15)

Table 11.1f Prevalence of trismus in patients with recurrent/new primary tumours

Study	Study design, participants, follow up	Tumour location	Treatment	Prevalence trismus % (95% CI)
MacNeese and Fletcher, 1981 [37]	Retrospective study n = 30 Follow up not reported	Nasopharynx	Re-irradiation	13% (5; 30)
Yan et al., 1983 [38]	Retrospective study n = 85 Follow up ≥5 years	Nasopharynx	Re-irradiation	29% (21; 40)
Langlois et al., 1985 [39]	Retrospective study n = 35 Follow up ≥2 years	Head and neck	Surgery, re-irradiation	6% (2; 19)
Emami et al., 1987 [40]	Retrospective study n = 99 Follow up ≥18 months	Head and neck	Surgery, re-irradiation	3% (1; 9)
Wang, 1987 [41]	Retrospective study n = 51 Follow up not reported	Nasopharynx	Re-irradiation	2% (0; 10)
Nagorsky and Sessions, 1987 [42]	Design not reported n = 28 Follow up ≥2 years	Oral cavity	Laser resection, radiotherapy	11% (4; 28)

Table 11.1f (continued)

Study	Study design, participants, follow up	Tumour location	Treatment	Prevalence trismus % (95% CI)
Pryzant et al., 1992 [43]	Retrospective study n = 53 Follow up ≥7 months	Nasopharynx	Re-irradiation	15% (8; 27)
Tercilla et al., 1993 [44]	Design not reported n = 10 Follow up ≥6 months	Head and neck	Re-irradiation	10% (2; 40)
Benchalal et al., 1995 [45]	Prospective study n = 17 Follow up ≥1 month	Head and neck	Surgery, chemotherapy, re-irradiation	12% (3; 34)
De Crevoisier et al., 1998 [46]	Retrospective study n = 169 Follow up ≥6 months	Head and neck	Re-irradiation Re-irradiation - 1 fraction/day & chemotherapy Re-irradiation - 2 fractions/day & chemotherapy	41% (25; 59) 23% (16; 31) 39% (25; 55)
Teo et al., 1998 [47]	Retrospective study n = 103 Follow up ≥2.5 months	Nasopharynx	Surgery, re-irradiation	61% (52; 70)
King et al., 2000 [48]	Retrospective study n = 31 Follow up ≥3 months	Nasopharynx	Surgery, re-irradiation	48% (32; 65)
Chang et al., 2000 [49]	Retrospective study n = 186 Follow up ≥12 months	Nasopharynx	Re-irradiation	5% (3; 9)
Nishioka et al., 2000 [50]	Design not reported n = 16 Follow up not reported	Nasopharynx	Re-irradiation	6% (1; 28)
Schaefer et al., 2000 [51]	Prospective study n = 26 Follow up ≥3 months	Head and neck	Re-irradiation, chemotherapy	4% (1; 19)
Dawson et al., 2001 [52]	Retrospective study n = 40 Follow up ≥5 months	Head and neck	Re-irradiation	20% (10; 35)
Low et al., 2006 [53]	Design not reported n= 36 Follow up ≥8 months	Nasopharynx	Stereotactic radio-surgery, radiotherapy	19% (10; 35)
Chen et al., 2007 [54]	Retrospective study n = 137 Follow up ≥1 month	Head and neck	Surgery, radiotherapy, chemotherapy	1% (0; 4)

of ≤35 mm has been proposed as a cut-off point for trismus on the basis of sensitivity/specificity analyses of two external criteria: (1) patients' experiences of limitation of mouth opening; and (2) mandibular function impairment assessed by means of the Mandibular Function Impairment Questionnaire (MFIQ)[67]. The MFIQ assesses perceived hindrance during 11 mandibular functions (i.e. speaking, taking a large bite, chewing hard food, chewing soft food, work and/or daily activities, drinking, laughing, chewing resistant food, yawning, and kissing) and perceived difficulty eating food with different consistencies (i.e. a hard cookie, meat, a raw carrot, French bread, peanuts/ almonds, and an apple)[68]. A more recent study has been confirmed this cut off point using other external criteria[69].

Trismus can have major consequences for food intake, communication, oral hygiene, dental care, and oncological follow-up. Patients with trismus may experience difficulties in eating [6,70]; limited mouth opening impedes intake of food, and leads to difficulties in chewing adequately. In extreme cases, patients cannot eat food of a normal consistency, and are forced to use mashed or liquidized food. Indeed, sometimes enteral tube feeding is required[71].

Patients with severely restricted mouth opening may experience difficulties in performing their oral hygiene, resulting in dental infections and other associated problems (see Chapter 6)[72]. In particular, they cannot reach the molar region, although sometimes a smaller tooth brush is helpful in reaching that region. In addition, some patients with trismus have difficulties inserting and removing their dentures.

From a medical point of view, restricted mouth opening may impede inspection of the oral cavity as needed for dental care, and particularly for oncological follow-up. In addition, intubation may be very difficult to perform, and made need to be performed transnasally[73,74].

The prognosis of trismus, if untreated, has not been extensively studied. However, it is clear that radiotherapy induces a progressive deterioration of mouth opening, which continues for some years following the end of treatment[62,63].

Investigations

Assessment of mouth opening should be performed in a standardized way using either a ruler, or sliding callipers with 1-mm gradations (Figure 11.1). (Measuring instruments should be made of materials that are easy to clean and sterilize.) 'Eye balling' mouth opening, or assessment of the number of fingers inserted between the teeth or alveolar ridges, lack precision and reliability. The measurements should be performed regularly, preferably prior to surgery, following surgery, prior to radiotherapy, following radiotherapy, and during follow-up.

Mouth opening should be measured in the following manner:

◆ The maximal inter-incisal distance (11–41)* in the case of a complete frontal (mandible and maxilla) dentition.

◆ The distance between the incisal edge of the 11 and the alveolar ridge of the mandible (location 41), in the case of an edentulous mandible and no denture.

◆ The distance between the incisal edge of the 41 and the alveolar ridge (location 11), in case of an edentulous maxilla and no denture.

◆ The distance between upper and lower dentures (11–41), in the case of edentulous mandible and maxilla and dentures present.

◆ The distance between upper and lower alveolar ridges (location 11–41) in the case of edentulous mandible and maxilla and dentures absent.

* = dental notation of teeth

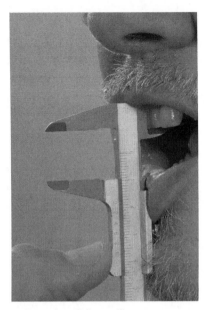

Fig. 11.1 Measuring mouth opening using sliding callipers.

If, during follow-up, the dentition changes in the region of the measurements, then this should be recorded in order to adequately compare mouth opening over time.

When a patient presents himself/herself with trismus following cancer treatment, it is important to determine whether the trismus is the result of the treatment, or is the first sign of a recurrence. In particular, if mouth opening decreases despite treatment (i.e. exercises), then a recurrence must be seriously considered. The use of imaging such as computed tomography (CT), magnetic resonance imaging (MRI), and positron emission tomography (PET) may be helpful in confirming/refuting a recurrence.

Management

The detection and management of trismus are the responsibility of all members of the multidisciplinary Head and Neck Oncology Team. The following discussion is based on the strategy employed in the Multidisciplinary Head and Neck Oncology Team of the University Medical Centre Groningen (The Netherlands), which is based on the available (limited) evidence, experience, and good clinical practice (Tables 11.2a–c).

Prevention

It is important to identify patients at risk of trismus (i.e. patients with tumour close to TMJ and masticatory muscles, patients scheduled to receive surgery and/or radiotherapy close to TMJ and masticatory muscles). The patient should be informed about the risk of developing trismus, the consequences of trismus, and the importance of ongoing exercising[76].

Exercise therapy features in various clinical recommendations, although the evidence for the effectiveness of exercise therapy is limited (Table 11.2a). Exercising should start as soon as possible following surgery, and should begin during radiotherapy. Exercising should be performed as often as possible (see below).

Table 11.2a Studies of exercise to prevent trismus

Study	Study design, participants, treatment, follow up	Mean change in mouth opening	Comment
Grandi et al., 2007 [75]	Randomized controlled trial n = 54 Exercise (during radiotherapy) Follow up not reported Group 1 – no exercise Group 2 – 6 exercise sessions*/day Group 3 – 3 exercise sessions**/day, and chewing gum for 15 min 3 times/day	 −4.9 mm (SD: 3.0) −3.8 mm (SD: 5.1) −1.4 mm (SD: 7.1)	* Exercise involved vertical and horizontal movements, repeated 10 times, with the end position held for 3 sec. ** Exercise as above, repeated 5 times, with the end position held for 3 sec. Changes in mouth opening were not significant between the groups.
Li et al., 2007 [76]	Cohort study n = not reported Exercise (during radiotherapy) Follow up 52 weeks after radiotherapy Group 1 – compliant with exercise instructions Group 2 – non-compliant with exercise instructions	 −5.8 mm (SD: 6.2) −24.2 mm (SD: 8.4)	Data based on English abstract (Chinese paper)
Cohen et al., 2005 [77]	Cohort study n = 11 (7 evaluable) Use of TheraBite® device (after surgery for oropharyngeal cancer) Follow up 12–48 weeks	+ 9.7 mm (SD: 8.1)	Effect size: 1.8 (mean $_{change}$/SD $_{pre-treatment}$) It is not clear whether these patients would have developed trismus.

In the case of tumour close to the coronoid process, it is recommended that a coronoidectomy is performed during tumour resection in order to try to prevent the development of trismus.

Treatment

Exercise therapy is the mainstay of the treatment of trismus, although again the evidence for the effectiveness of exercise therapy is limited (Table 11.2b). Exercise therapy should particularly involve a vertical range of motion exercises, but should also involve a horizontal range of motion exercises. Various strategies can improve exercise efficacy (e.g. stretching of mouth using thumb and index finger, wooden tongue blades, rubber plugs) (Figure 11.2–4). These strategies can also be used for goal setting for the patient (e.g. the number of tongue blades, the size of the plug). It is best to start with simple exercises, and to choose strategies that are acceptable to the patient. If the effects of these techniques are limited, then the use of a TheraBite® device should be considered [77,78] (Figure 11.5). Other stretching techniques such as using a dynamic bite openers, weights, and spring devices have not been systematically evaluated.

Table 11.2b Studies of exercise to treat trismus

Study	Study design, participants, treatment	Mean change in mouth opening	Effect size#	Comment
Buchbinder et al., 1993 [78]	Randomized controlled trial n = 21 Exercise (post radiotherapy; <5 yr) 10 exercise sessions/day over 10 weeks. Group 1 – forced manual opening Group 2 – wooden tongue blades Group 3 – TheraBite® device	+5.4 mm (SD: 4.4) +6.0 mm (SD: 2.6) +13.6 mm (SD: 6.6)	1.1 1.5 2.6	Mouth opening ≤30 mm at start of study. Changes in mouth opening with the TheraBite® device were significant (cf. other interventions). No long term follow-up.
Dijkstra et al., 2006 [79]	Historic cohort study n = 27 Exercise Various strategies used*	+5.5 mm (SD: 6.0)	0.7	* Strategies used were based on clinical findings, and included forced manual opening, use of wooden tongue blades, use of rubber plugs, use of dynamic bite openers, and use of the TheraBite® device. No long term follow-up.

Effect size = mean $_{change}$/SD $_{pre-treatment}$

It is important to measure mouth opening regularly to evaluate the degree of trismus, and also to encourage exercise adherence. The aim should be to strive for a mouth opening of >35 mm[67,69], and once this has been achieved then the exercise frequency may be reduced.

Other therapies that have been used to increase mouth opening following cancer treatment include pentoxifylline and microcurrent electrotherapy, although both of these therapies have only a limited effect on mouth opening (Table 11.2c)[65,80].

If conservative treatment fails, and the patient has a good prognosis, then it may be worth considering performing a coronoidectomy (Table 11.2c) [81,82]. It should be noted that radiation fibrosis is seldom limited to the temporalis region, and fibrosis of the other masticatory muscles and other subcutaneous tissues will not be corrected by coronoidectomy.

Note

In this chapter, a review of scientific papers concerning epidemiology, aetiology, clinical features, assessment, and management of trismus has been presented. The papers were identified in a literature search performed for a systematic review[67]. The search terms were 'trismus' or 'restricted mouth opening' combined with 'head and neck oncology'. The literature search was updated in December 2007. Papers describing less than 10 patients, expert review papers, clinical recommendations, and letters to the editor were not used for this chapter because of lack of scientific evidence. Case reports were only referred to as anecdotal illustrations.

Table 11.2c Studies of other treatments than exercise therapy for trismus

Study	Study design, participants, treatment	Mean change in mouth opening	Effect size*	Comment
Chua et al., 2001 [65]	Cohort study n = 20 (16 evaluable) Pentoxifylline 400 mg three times a day for 8 weeks and electrotherapy (post radiotherapy; ≥6 months)	+4.0 mm (SD: 6.3)	0.3	Mouth opening ≤25 mm at start of study. Follow-up 3 months.
Lennox et al., 2002 [80]	Cohort study n = 26 (23 evaluable) Microcurrent therapy –10 treatments in 5 days	+2.6 mm (SD: 2.4)	0.3	
Mardini et al., 2006 [81]	Cohort study n = 11 Coronoidectomy, scar release and free flap reconstruction (post surgery)	+15.8 mm (SD: 7.5)	3.5	Follow-up 22.7 months.
Bhrany et al., 2007 [82]	Cohort study n = 18 Coronoidectomy	+22.2 mm (SD: 3.5)	6.0	Mouth opening ≤20 mm at start of study. Follow-up 6 months.

* Effect size = mean $_{change}$/SD $_{pre-treatment}$

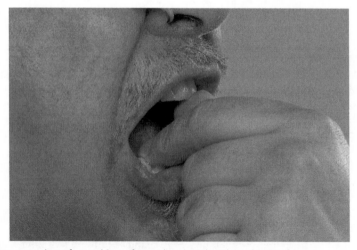

Fig. 11.2 Demonstration of stretching of mouth using thumb and index finger.

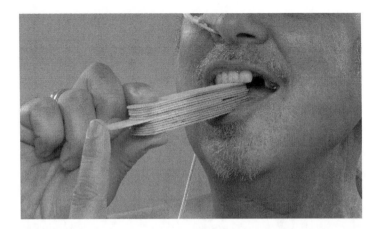

Instructions: "Insert as many tongue blades between your teeth as possible. Bite gently on the tongue blades for about 10 seconds. Relax and try to open the mouth a bit further". Any increase in mouth opening can be maintained by inserting a new tongue blade in the stack. Tongue blades should never be used as a wedge.

Fig. 11.3 Demonstration of use of wooden tongue blades.

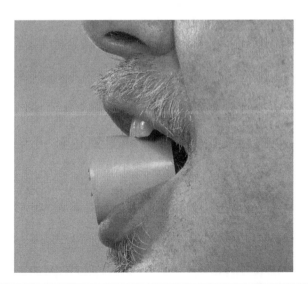

"Insert the largest possible plug between your teeth (gums). Bite gently on the plug for about 10 seconds. Relax and try to open the mouth a bit further". Any increase in mouth opening can be maintained by inserting the plug a bit further between the teeth (gums). Rubber plugs should never be used as a wedge.

Fig. 11.4 Demonstration of use of rubber plug.

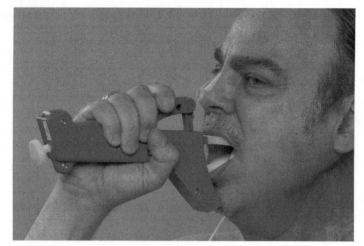

Fig. 11.5 Demonstration of use of the TheraBite® device. Printed with permission of the patient.

Acknowledgement

We would like to thank Mr Bert Tebbes for taking the photographs presented in this chapter, and Dr G Grandi for providing additional data needed for Table 11.2a.

References

1 Jablonski S (1982). *Illustrated dictionary of dentistry*. W.B. Saunders, Philadelphia.

2 Landau SI (1986). *International dictionary of medicine and biology*. Churchill Livingstone, New York.

3 Beekhuis GJ, Harrington EB (1965). Trismus. Etiology and management of inability to open the mouth. *Laryngoscope*, 75, 123–58.

4 Olmi P, Cellai E, Chiavacci A, Fallai C (1990). Accelerated fractionation in advanced head and neck cancer: results and analysis of late sequelae. *Radiother Oncol*, 17(3), 199–207.

5 Ichimura K, Tanaka T (1993). Trismus in patients with malignant tumours in the head and neck. *J Laryngol Otol*, 107(11), 1017–20.

6 Kent LM, Brennan MT, Noll JL, et al. (2008). Radiation-induced trismus in head and neck cancer patients. *Support Care Cancer*, 16(3), 305–9.

7 Aref A, Ben Josef E, Shamsa F, et al. (1997). Neutron radiotherapy for salivary gland tumors at Harper hospital. *J Brachytherapy Int*, 13(1), 17–22.

8 Sakai S, Kubo T, Mori N, et al. (1988). A study of the late effects of radiotherapy and operation on patients with maxillary cancer. A survey more than 10 years after initial treatment. *Cancer*, 62(10), 2114–17.

9 Jiang GL, Ang KK, Peters LJ, Wendt CD, Oswald MJ, Goepfert H (1991). Maxillary sinus carcinomas: natural history and results of postoperative radiotherapy. *Radiother Oncol*, 21(3), 193–200.

10 Paulino AC, Marks JE, Bricker P, Melian E, Reddy SP, Emami B (1998). Results of treatment of patients with maxillary sinus carcinoma. *Cancer*, 83(3), 457–65.

11 Nishino H, Miyata M, Morita M, Ishikawa K, Kanazawa T, Ichimura K (2000). Combined therapy with conservative surgery, radiotherapy, and regional chemotherapy for maxillary sinus carcinoma. *Cancer*, 89(9), 1925–32.

12 Ogawa K, Toita T, Kakinohana Y, et al. (2001). Postoperative radiotherapy for squamous cell carcinoma of the maxillary sinus: analysis of local control and late complications. *Oncol Rep*, 8(2), 315–19.

13 Ozsaran Z, Yalman D, Baltalarli B, Anacak Y, Esassolak M, Haydaroglu A (2003). Radiotherapy in maxillary sinus carcinomas: evaluation of 79 cases. *Rhinology*, 41(1), 44–8.

14 Thomas F, Ozanne F, Mamelle G, Wibault P, Eschwege F (1988). Radiotherapy alone for oropharyngeal carcinomas: the role of fraction size (2 Gy vs 2.5 Gy) on local control and early and late complications. *Int J Radiat Oncol Biol Phys*, 15(5), 1097–102.

15 Foote RL, Parsons JT, Mendenhall WM, Million RR, Cassisi NJ, Stringer SP (1990). Is interstitial implantation essential for successful radiotherapeutic treatment of base of tongue carcinoma? *Int J Radiat Oncol Biol Phys*, 18(6), 1293–8.

16 Koka VN, Deo R, Lusinchi A, Roland J, Schwaab G (1990). Osteoradionecrosis of the mandible: study of 104 cases treated by hemimandibulectomy. *J Laryngol Otol*, 104(4), 305–7.

17 Pinheiro AB, Frame JW (1994). An audit of CO_2 laser surgery in the mouth. *Braz Dent J*, 5(1), 15–25.

18 Ryu JK, Stern RL, Robinson MG, et al. (1995). Mandibular reconstruction using a titanium plate: the impact of radiation therapy on plate preservation. *Int J Radiat Oncol Biol Phys*, 32(3), 627–34.

19 Bertrand J, Luc B, Philippe M, Philippe P (2000). Anterior mandibular osteotomy for tumor extirpation: a critical evaluation. *Head Neck*, 22(4), 323–7.

20 Eisen MD, Weinstein GS, Chalian A, et al. (2000). Morbidity after midline mandibulotomy and radiation therapy. *Am J Otolaryngol*, 21(5), 312–7.

21 Karakoyun-Celik O, Norris CM, Jr., Tishler R, et al. (2005). Definitive radiotherapy with interstitial implant boost for squamous cell carcinoma of the tongue base. *Head Neck*, 27(5), 353–61.

22 Qin DX, Hu YH, Yan JH, et al. (1988). Analysis of 1379 patients with nasopharyngeal carcinoma treated by radiation. *Cancer*, 61(6), 1117–24.

23 Cmelak AJ, Cox RS, Adler JR, Fee WE, Jr., Goffinet DR (1997). Radiosurgery for skull base malignancies and nasopharyngeal carcinoma. *Int J Radiat Oncol Biol Phys*, 37(5), 997–1003.

24 Choi KN, Rotman M, Aziz H, et al. (1997). Concomitant infusion cisplatin and hyperfractionated radiotherapy for locally advanced nasopharyngeal and paranasal sinus tumors. *Int J Radiat Oncol Biol Phys*, 39(4), 823–9.

25 Zubizarreta PA, D'Antonio G, Raslawski E, et al. (2000). Nasopharyngeal carcinoma in childhood and adolescence: a single-institution experience with combined therapy. *Cancer*, 89(3), 690–5.

26 Teo PM, Leung SF, Chan AT, et al. (2000). Final report of a randomized trial on altered-fractionated radiotherapy in nasopharyngeal carcinoma prematurely terminated by significant increase in neurologic complications. *Int J Radiat Oncol Biol Phys*, 48(5), 1311–22.

27 Wolden SL, Zelefsky MJ, Hunt MA, et al. (2001). Failure of a 3D conformal boost to improve radiotherapy for nasopharyngeal carcinoma. *Int J Radiat Oncol Biol Phys*, 49(5), 1229–34.

28 Jen YM, Lin YS, Su WF, et al. (2002). Dose escalation using twice-daily radiotherapy for nasopharyngeal carcinoma: does heavier dosing result in a happier ending? *Int J Radiat Oncol Biol Phys*, 54(1), 14–22.

29 Fuchs S, Rodel C, Brunner T, et al. (2003). Patterns of failure following radiation with and without chemotherapy in patients with nasopharyngeal carcinoma. *Onkologie*, 26(1), 12–18.

30 Yeh SA, Tang Y, Lui CC, Huang YJ, Huang EY (2005). Treatment outcomes and late complications of 849 patients with nasopharyngeal carcinoma treated with radiotherapy alone. *Int J Radiat Oncol Biol Phys*, 62(3), 672–9.

31 Nguyen TD, Demange L, Froissart D, Panis X, Loirette M (1985). Rapid hyperfractionated radiotherapy. Clinical results in 178 advanced squamous cell carcinomas of the head and neck. *Cancer*, 56(1), 16–19.

32 Nguyen TD, Panis X, Froissart D, Legros M, Coninx P, Loirette M (1988). Analysis of late complications after rapid hyperfractionated radiotherapy in advanced head and neck cancers. *Int J Radiat Oncol Biol Phys*, 14(1), 23–5.

33 Katsantonis GP, Friedman WH, Rosenblum BN (1989). The surgical management of advanced malignancies of the parotid gland. *Otolaryngol Head Neck Surg*, 101(6), 633–40.

34 Chandrasekhar B, Lorant JA, Terz JJ (1990). Parascapular free flaps for head and neck reconstruction. *Am J Surg*, 160(4), 450–3.

35 Zidan J, Kuten A, Rosenblatt E, Robinson E (1997). Intensive chemotherapy using cisplatin and fluorouracil followed by radiotherapy in advanced head and neck cancer. *Oral Oncol*, 33(2), 129–35.

36 Mackenzie R, Balogh J, Choo R, Franssen E (1999). Accelerated radiotherapy with delayed concomitant boost in locally advanced squamous cell carcinoma of the head and neck. *Int J Radiat Oncol Biol Phys*, 45(3), 589–95.

37 McNeese MD, Fletcher GH (1981). Retreatment of recurrent nasopharyngeal carcinoma. *Radiology*, 138(1), 191–3.

38 Yan JH, Hu YH, Gu XZ (1983). Radiation therapy of recurrent nasopharyngeal carcinoma. Report on 219 patients. *Acta Radiol Oncol*, 22(1), 23–8.

39 Langlois D, Eschwege F, Kramar A, Richard JM (1985). Reirradiation of head and neck cancers. Presentation of 35 cases treated at the Gustave Roussy Institute. *Radiother Oncol*, 3(1), 27–33.

40 Emami B, Bignardi M, Spector GJ, Devineni VR, Hederman MA (1987). Reirradiation of recurrent head and neck cancers. *Laryngoscope*, 97(1), 85–8.

41 Wang CC (1987). Re-irradiation of recurrent nasopharyngeal carcinoma – treatment techniques and results. *Int J Radiat Oncol Biol Phys*, 13(7), 953–6.

42 Nagorsky MJ, Sessions DG (1987). Laser resection for early oral cavity cancer. Results and complications. *Ann Otol Rhinol Laryngol*, 96(5), 556–60.

43 Pryzant RM, Wendt CD, Delclos L, Peters LJ (1992). Re-treatment of nasopharyngeal carcinoma in 53 patients. *Int J Radiat Oncol Biol Phys*, 22(5), 941–7.

44 Tercilla OF, Schmidt-Ullrich R, Wazer DE (1993). Reirradiation of head and neck neoplasms using twice-a-day scheduling. *Strahlenther Onkol*, 169(5), 285–90.

45 Benchalal M, Bachaud JM, Francois P, et al. (1995). Hyperfractionation in the reirradiation of head and neck cancers. Result of a pilot study. *Radiother Oncol*, 36(3), 203–10.

46 De Crevoisier R, Bourhis J, Domenge C, et al. (1998). Full-dose reirradiation for unresectable head and neck carcinoma: experience at the Gustave-Roussy Institute in a series of 169 patients. *J Clin Oncol*, 16(11), 3556–62.

47 Teo PM, Kwan WH, Chan AT, Lee WY, King WW, Mok CO (1998). How successful is high-dose (> or = 60 Gy) reirradiation using mainly external beams in salvaging local failures of nasopharyngeal carcinoma? *Int J Radiat Oncol Biol Phys*, 40(4), 897–913.

48 King WW, Ku PK, Mok CO, Teo PM (2000). Nasopharyngectomy in the treatment of recurrent nasopharyngeal carcinoma: a twelve-year experience. *Head Neck*, 22(3), 215–22.

49 Chang JT, See LC, Liao CT, et al. (2000). Locally recurrent nasopharyngeal carcinoma. *Radiother Oncol*, 54(2), 135–42.

50 Nishioka T, Shirato H, Kagei K, Fukuda S, Hashimoto S, Ohmori K (2000). Three-dimensional small-volume irradiation for residual or recurrent nasopharyngeal carcinoma. *Int J Radiat Oncol Biol Phys*, 48(2), 495–500.

51 Schaefer U, Micke O, Schueller P, Willich N (2000). Recurrent head and neck cancer: retreatment of previously irradiated areas with combined chemotherapy and radiation therapy – results of a prospective study. *Radiology*, 216(2), 371–6.

52 Dawson LA, Myers LL, Bradford CR, et al. (2001). Conformal re-irradiation of recurrent and new primary head-and-neck cancer. *Int J Radiat Oncol Biol Phys*, 50(2), 377–85.

53 Low JS, Chua ET, Gao F, Wee JT (2006). Stereotactic radiosurgery plus intracavitary irradiation in the salvage of nasopharyngeal carcinoma. *Head Neck*, 28(4), 321–9.

54 Chen AM, Bucci MK, Singer MI, et al. (2007). Intraoperative radiation therapy for recurrent head-and-neck cancer: the UCSF experience. *Int J Radiat Oncol Biol Phys*, 67(1), 122–9.

55 Kaste SC, Hopkins KP, Bowman LC (1995). Dental abnormalities in long-term survivors of head and neck rhabdomyosarcoma. *Med Pediatr Oncol*, 25(2), 96–101.

56 Daya H, Chan HS, Sirkin W, Forte V (2000). Pediatric rhabdomyosarcoma of the head and neck: is there a place for surgical management? *Arch Otolaryngol Head Neck Surg*, 126(4), 468–72.

57 Estilo CL, Huryn JM, Kraus DH, et al. (2003). Effects of therapy on dentofacial development in long-term survivors of head and neck rhabdomyosarcoma: the Memorial Sloan Kettering Cancer Center experience. *J Pediatr Hematol Oncol*, 25(3), 215–22.

58 Tveteras K, Kristensen S (1986). The aetiology and pathogenesis of trismus. *Clin Otolaryngol Allied Sci*, 11(5), 383–7.

59 Miller FR, Wanamaker JR, Lavertu P, Wood BG (1996). Magnetic resonance imaging and the management of parapharyngeal space tumors. *Head Neck*, 18(1), 67–77.

60 Balm AJ, Plaat BE, Hart AA, Hilgers FJ, Keus RB (1997). [Nasopharyngeal carcinoma: epidemiology and treatment outcome]. *Ned Tijdschr Geneeskd*, 141(48), 2346–50.

61 Ozyar E, Cengiz M, Gurkaynak M, Atahan IL (2005). Trismus as a presenting symptom in nasopharyngeal carcinoma. *Radiother Oncol*, 77(1), 73–6.

62 Goldstein M, Maxymiw WG, Cummings BJ, Wood RE (1999). The effects of antitumor irradiation on mandibular opening and mobility: a prospective study of 58 patients. *Oral Surg Oral Med Oral Pathol Oral Radiol Endod*, 88(3), 365–73.

63 Wang CJ, Huang EY, Hsu HC, Chen HC, Fang FM, Hsiung CY (2005). The degree and time-course assessment of radiation-induced trismus occurring after radiotherapy for nasopharyngeal cancer. *Laryngoscope*, 115(8), 1458–60.

64 Dijkstra PU, Kalk WW, Roodenburg JL (2004). Trismus in head and neck oncology: a systematic review. *Oral Oncol*, 40(9), 879–89.

65 Chua DT, Lo C, Yuen J, Foo YC (2001). A pilot study of pentoxifylline in the treatment of radiation-induced trismus. *Am J Clin Oncol*, 24(4), 366–9.

66 Steelman R, Sokol J (1986). Quantification of trismus following irradiation of the temporomandibular joint. *Mo Dent J*, 66(6), 21–3.

67 Dijkstra PU, Huisman PM, Roodenburg JL (2006). Criteria for trismus in head and neck oncology. *Int J Oral Maxillofac Surg*, 35(4), 337–42.

68 Stegenga B, de Bont LG, de Leeuw R, Boering G (1993). Assessment of mandibular function impairment associated with temporomandibular joint osteoarthrosis and internal derangement. *J Orofac Pain*, 7(2), 183–95.

69 Scott B, Butterworth C, Lowe D, Rogers SN (2008). Factors associated with restricted mouth opening and its relationship to health-related quality of life in patients attending a Maxillofacial Oncology clinic. *Oral Oncol*, 44(5), 430–8.

70 Motta A, Louro RS, Medeiros PJ, Capelli J, Jr. (2007). Orthodontic and surgical treatment of a patient with an ankylosed temporomandibular joint. *Am J Orthod Dentofacial Orthop*, 131(6), 785–96.

71 Hujala K, Sipila J, Pulkkinen J, Grenman R (2004). Early percutaneous endoscopic gastrostomy nutrition in head and neck cancer patients. *Acta Otolaryngol*, 124(7), 847–50.

72 el-Sheikh MM, Medra AM (1997). Management of unilateral temporomandibular ankylosis associated with facial asymmetry. *J Craniomaxillofac Surg*, 25(3), 109–15.

73 Taller A, Horvath E, Ilias L, et al. (2001). Technical modifications for improving the success rate of PEG tube placement in patients with head and neck cancer. *Gastrointest Endosc*, 54(5), 633–6.

74 Lustberg A, Fleisher AS, Darwin PE (2001). Transnasal placement of percutaneous endoscopic gastrostomy with a pediatric endoscope in oropharyngeal obstruction. *Am J Gastroenterol*, 96(3), 936–7.

75 Grandi G, Silva ML, Streit C, Wagner JC (2007). A mobilization regimen to prevent mandibular hypomobility in irradiated patients: an analysis and comparison of two techniques. *Med Oral Patol Oral Cir Bucal*, 12(2), E105–9.

76 Li XH, Liao YP, Tang JT, Zhou JM, Wang GH (2007). [Effect of early rehabilitation training on radiation-induced trismus in nasopharyngeal carcinoma patients]. *Ai Zheng*, 26(9), 987–90.

77 Cohen EG, Deschler DG, Walsh K, Hayden RE (2005). Early use of a mechanical stretching device to improve mandibular mobility after composite resection: a pilot study. *Arch Phys Med Rehabil*, 86(7), 1416–19.

78 Buchbinder D, Currivan RB, Kaplan AJ, Urken ML (1993). Mobilization regimens for the prevention of jaw hypomobility in the radiated patient: a comparison of three techniques. *J Oral Maxillofac Surg*, 51(8), 863–7.

79 Dijkstra PU, Sterken MW, Pater R, Spijkervet FK, Roodenburg JL (2007). Exercise therapy for trismus in head and neck cancer. *Oral Oncol*, 43(4), 389–94.

80 Lennox AJ, Shafer JP, Hatcher M, Beil J, Funder SJ (2002). Pilot study of impedance-controlled microcurrent therapy for managing radiation-induced fibrosis in head-and-neck cancer patients. *Int J Radiation Oncol Biol Phys*, 54(1), 23–34.

81 Mardini S, Chang YM, Tsai CY, Coskunfirat OK, Wei FC (2006). Release and free flap reconstruction for trismus that develops after previous intraoral reconstruction. *Plast Reconstr Surg*, 118(1), 102–7.

82 Bhrany AD, Izzard M, Wood AJ, Futran ND (2007). Coronoidectomy for the treatment of trismus in head and neck cancer patients. *Laryngoscope*, 117(11), 1952–6.

Chapter 12

Post-radiation osteonecrosis (osteoradionecrosis) of the jaws

Fred Spijkervet and Arjan Vissink

Introduction

Radiotherapy plays an important role in the treatment of patients with head and neck cancer. At least 50% of these patients will receive radiotherapy, and approximately 50% of these patients will be long-term survivors. Radiotherapy is used either as a primary treatment (± chemotherapy), or as an adjunct treatment to surgery. Even with optimal fractionation schedules and optimal radiation techniques (e.g. intensity-modulated radiation therapy (IMRT)), unwanted radiation-induced changes will occur in the surrounding tissues[1]. Acute radiation tissue injuries are observed in most patients, and are seen during and shortly following the radiotherapy (e.g. oral mucositis). In contrast, late radiation tissue injuries are observed in a smaller number of patients, and develop months to years following the radiotherapy (e.g. soft-tissue necrosis). One such late radition tissue injury is post-radiation osteonecrosis (PRON), which is also known as osteoradionecrosis. The complications of radiotherapy are discussed in detail in Chapter 10.

Epidemiology

The incidence of PRON of the mandible varies from 2.6% to 22%, and is lower in more modern series (and is expected to decrease with increasing use of radiation techniques, such as IMRT)[2–6]. The incidence of osteonecrosis of the maxilla is much lower[4,7,8].

Aetiology

Gross changes in the matrix of bone develop relatively slowly after irradiation. The initial changes result from injury to the remodelling system, i.e. the osteocytes, osteoblasts, and osteoclasts. Osteoblasts tend to be more radiosensitive than osteoclasts (and so there may be a relative increase in lytic activity). The subsequent changes result from alterations of the vascular system[9,10]. Whether altered bone remodelling is the result of direct irradiation injury to the cells of the remodelling system, or the indirect result of irradiation-induced vascular injury, or a combination of both of these phenomena is still a matter of some debate.

Radiation injury to the fine vasculature of the bone (and surrounding tissues) first leads to hyperaemia, followed by endarteritis, thrombosis, and progressive occlusion and obliteration of the small vessels. This results in a further reduction of the number of cells and progressive fibrosis within the bone. With time, the marrow exhibits marked acellularity, hypo- or avascularity, and significant fatty degeneration and fibrosis. The endosteum atrophies with significant loss of active osteoblasts and osteoclasts. The periosteum demonstrates significant fibrosis, with a similar loss of remodelling elements[2,9–14].

In the early literature the pathogenesis of PRON was thought to be due to the triad of radiation, trauma, and infection[15–17]. In this model, the role of trauma was to act as a portal of entry for oral bacteria into the bone. Thus, PRON was considered to be primarily an infectious process. (The source of trauma may be anything, including tooth removal, denture irritation, sharp bony ridges, and hard/sharp food particles).

Subsequently, Marx suggested that PRON was a problem of wound healing rather than of infection (and in which micro-organisms are merely contaminants)[18,19]. Thus, the hypoxic–hypovascular– hypocellular tissues have reduced ability to replace normal cellular and collagen loss, which eventually results in tissue breakdown (i.e. cell death and collagen lysis exceed cell replication and collagen synthesis). Furthermore, the hypoxic–hypovascular–hypocellular tissues have reduced ability to heal relevant wounds, since the metabolic demands exceed the vascular supply[18,19]. It should be noted that PRON is as much a disease process of the covering soft tissues as of the underlying bone.

Some (35%) cases of PRON are apparently spontaneous in nature. Spontaneous PRON usually occurs within the first 2 years following radiotherapy[4,14,18,19], but it can occur at any later time following irradiation[3,4]. Spontaneous PRON is associated with increasing age, high radiation dose (>65 Gy), field of radiation (i.e. volume of bone in the field; proximity of bone to maximal dosing), hyperfractionation of radiation, use of implant sources close to bone, and combined interstitial and external beam irradiation[2,4,7,8,14,18–23]. Spontaneous PRON represents a greater outright cellular death from the radiotherapy.

Trauma-induced PRON usually occurs later than spontaneous PRON[4]. It is also related to high radiation dose. In dentulous patients, PRON is associated with tooth removal or other surgical procedures (e.g. periodontal procedures), ongoing periodontal or periapical infection, and poor oral hygiene[3,8,14,24,25]. In edentulous patients, trauma induced by prosthetic appliances is a predisposing factor, especially when related to certain mastication and parafunctional habits (e.g. teeth clenching/grinding)[26]. Inadequate healing time for pre-irradiation extractions is also known to predispose to PRON[2,8,14]. Other factors associated with PRON include higher body mass index and use of corticosteroids[23].

Clinical features

Patients with PRON present with an area of exposed (non-healing) bone within the treatment area sometime following completion of radiotherapy (Figure 12.1, see colour plate section). The mandible is more often involved than the maxilla. As discussed, the process may occur spontaneously, or more usually following a traumatic event (e.g. tooth removal). The lesion may cause (severe) pain, and there may be evidence of secondary infection. The process may progress to formation of a sequestrum, development of a pathological fracture (Figure 12.2), and/or development of a cutaneous fistula (Figure 12.3, see colour plate section)[2,3,6,8,18,19,27,28].

Investigation

The diagnosis of PRON is based on a combination of clinical features and radiological features. Plain X-rays show decreased bone density, and may show fractures. Computed tomography (CT) scans show bone abnormalities, such as focal lytic areas, cortical breaks, and loss of spongiosa trabeculation (Figure 12.2). Other imaging techniques (i.e. bone scanning, magnetic resonance imaging (MRI))will also show bone abnormalities.

Management

Prevention

The incidence of PRON should be reduced by the utilization of newer radiation techniques (e.g. IMRT).

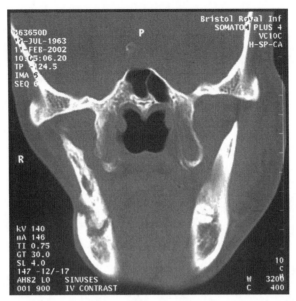

Fig. 12.2 CT scan showing osteoradionecrosis of right mandible [reproduced with permission from Davies A and Finlay I (2005), Oral Care in Advanced Disease. Oxford University Press, Oxford].

A vital step towards prevention of PRON is a thorough pre-treatment dental assessment (see Chapter 5). The aim of pre-treatment assessment is to identify factors that will increase the risk for PRON, and initiate measures to ameliorate/eliminate these factors before the radiotherapy begins[2,4,6,23,25,29–32]. The primary goal should be to reduce the potential for needing to perform high-risk procedures, such as extraction of teeth in the post-irradiation period[4,7,8,12,13, 23,25,29,30,32,33]. However, to maximize the impact of screening, adequate time for treatment and healing must be allowed[25,32].

It is now generally accepted that all teeth with a questionable prognosis must be extracted prior to radiotherapy[4,25,29–31]. The less motivated the patient is concerning dental care and hygiene, the more aggressive one should be in extracting teeth prior to radiotherapy[12,13,30,34–36]. The extractions should be performed as atraumatically as possible, and primary closure should be attempted[25,30]. Suggested healing intervals frequently range from 10 to 14 days[8,12,13,24,25, 30,36]. However, an interval of 14 days still poses a minor risk for the development of PRON[14]. The risk appears to be reduced to zero if there is a ≥21-day interval between extraction of teeth and initiation of radiation therapy.

Extraction of teeth during radiation therapy will result in an extremely high risk of PRON (and is strongly discouraged)[37]. Post-irradiation extractions have been shown to be the significant factor predisposing to PRON[4,7,8,24,25]. Indeed, Epstein et al. have identified a twofold increased risk of necrosis if teeth were extracted following radiotherapy compared with pre-irradiation-therapy dental extractions[27,28]. In general, post-irradiation extractions should be performed as atraumatically as possible, without radical alveolotomies, with smoothing of the alveolar ridge, and with primary wound closure not under tension[25,30]. Antibiotic coverage is also strongly recommended[8,30,32,38]. Antibiotic protocols include a 2-week course of a β-lactam antibiotic to be started 1 day prior to extraction (e.g. amoxicillin 500 mg tds). Clindamycin is a proven alterative in patients with β-lactam allergy (i.e. clindamycin 300 mg tds). A recent review by the Cochrane Collaboration suggested that hyperbaric oxygen treatment may be of benefit in preventing the development of PRON following tooth extraction in an irradiated field (see below)[39]. Hyperbaric oxygen therapy is the therapeutic administration of 100% oxygen at an environmental pressure greater than one atmosphere absolute, and usually of 2 atmospheres absolute. Hyperbaric oxygen therapy optimizes cellular levels of oxygen, and stimulates localized angiogenesis, thereby enhancing the healing potential of the irradiated tissues[40]. Hyperbaric oxygen treatment should be used both prior to and following dental surgery.

Treatment

The management of PRON remains difficult, due to the biological background of the radiation injury to the bone. Conservative management should be limited to early-onset PRON, and includes antibiotic treatment with limited curettage, debridement, and/or sequestrotomy (under local anaesthesia). The 'cure rate' of limited PRON with conservative therapy is 53%.

More extensive surgical therapies are indicated for advanced or refractory lesion[41]. The first step is debridement of all bone that is no longer vascularized. The removal of this dead bone eliminates any nidus for continued infection. Surgical techniques include extensive sequestrotomy combined with marginal or complete resection of affected parts of the mandible (and stabilization of the continuity defect). These interventions often need to be combined with soft-tissue reconstruction[42]. Indications for the different types of therapies have not been clearly defined. The 'cure rate' of surgical approaches in cases of failure of conservative therapy is 40%.

Antibiotic therapy is considered an adjuvant therapy (since PRON is a disease of hypovascularity and not necessarily of infection). Hyperbaric oxygen therapy is also considered an adjuvant therapy. A recent review by the Cochrane collaboration group concluded that there is some evidence that hyperbaric oxygen therapy improves the healing after hemi-mandibulectomy and reconstruction[39].

References

1　Vissink A, Burlage FR, Spijkervet FK, Jansma J, Coppes RP (2003). Prevention and treatment of the consequences of head and neck radiotherapy. *Crit Rev Oral Biol Med*, 14(3), 213–25.

2　Constantino PD, Friedman CD, Steinberg MJ (1995). Irradiated bone and its management. *Otolaryngol Clin North Am*, 28(5), 1021–38.

3　Epstein J, van der Meij E, McKenzie M, Wong F, Lepawsky M, Stevenson-Moore P (1997). Postradiation osteonecrosis of the mandible: a long-term follow-up study. *Oral Surg Oral Med Oral Pathol Oral Radiol Endod*, 83(6), 657–62.

4　Thorn JJ, Hansen SH, Specht L, Bastholt L (2000). Osteoradionecrosis of the jaws: clinical characteristics and relation to the field of irradiation. *J Oral Maxillofac Surg*, 58(10), 1088–93.

5　Annane D, Depondt J, Aubert P, et al. (2004). Hyperbaric oxygen therapy for radionecrosis of the jaw: a randomized, placebo-controlled, double-blind trial from the ORN96 Study Group. *J Clin Oncol*, 22(24), 4893–900.

6　Sciubba JJ, Goldenberg D (2006). *Oral complications of radiotherapy. Lancet Oncol*, 7(2), 175–83.

7　Curi MM, Dib LL (1997). Osteoradionecrosis of the jaws: a retrospective study of the background factors and treatment in 104 cases. *J Oral Maxillofac Surg*, 55(6), 540–4.

8　Tong AC, Leung AC, Cheng JC, Sham J (1999). Incidence of complicated healing and osteoradionecrosis following tooth extraction in patients receiving radiotherapy for treatment of nasopharyngeal carcinoma. *Aust Dent J*, 44(3), 187–94.

9　Assael LA (2004). New foundations in understanding osteonecrosis of the jaws. *J Oral Maxillofac Surg*, 62(2), 125–6.

10　Al-Nawas B, Duschner H, Grotz KA (2004). Early cellular alterations in bone after radiation therapy and its relation to osteoradionecrosis. *J Oral Maxillofac Surg*, 62(8), 1045.

11 Silverman S Jr, Chierici G (1965). Radiation therapy of oral carcinoma. I. Effects on oral tissues and management of the periodontium. *J Periodontol*, 36(6), 478–84.

12 Beumer J, Curtis T, Harrison RE (1979). Radiation therapy of the oral cavity: sequelae and management, part 1. *Head Neck Surg*, 1(4), 301–12.

13 Beumer J, Curtis T, Harrison RE (1979). Radiation therapy of the oral cavity: sequelae and management, part 2. *Head Neck Surg*, 1(5), 392–408.

14 Marx RE, Johnson RP (1987). Studies in the radiobiology of osteoradionecrosis and their clinical significance. *Oral Surg Oral Med Oral Pathol*, 64(4), 379–90.

15 Watson WJ, Scarborough JE (1938). Osteoradionecrosis in intraoral cancer. *Am J Roentgenol*, 40, 524–34.

16 Meyer I (1958). Osteoradionecrosis of the jaws. *PDM*, 26, 1–51.

17 Meyer I. (1970). Infectious diseases of the jaws. *J Oral Surg*, 28(1), 17–26.

18 Marx RE (1983). Osteoradionecrosis: a new concept of its pathophysiology. *J Oral Maxillofac Surg*, 41(5), 283–8.

19 Marx RE (1983). A new concept in the treatment of osteoradionecrosis. *J Oral Maxillofac Surg*, 41(6), 351–7.

20 Murray CG, Herson J, Daly TE, Zimmerman S (1980). Radiation necrosis of the mandible: a 10-year study. Part I. Factors influencing the onset of necrosis. *Int J Radiat Oncol Biol Phys*, 6(5), 543–8.

21 Kluth EV, Jain PR, Stuchell RN, Frich JC Jr (1988). A study of factors contributing to the development of osteoradionecrosis of the jaws. *J Prosthet Dent*, 59(2), 194–201.

22 Glanzmann C, Gratz KW (1995). Radionecrosis of the mandibula: a retrospective analysis of the incidence and risk factors. *Radiother Oncol*, 36(2), 94–100.

23 Goldwaser BR, Chuang SK, Kaban LB, August M (2007). Risk factor assessment for the development of osteoradionecrosis. *J Oral Maxillofac Surg*, 65(11), 2311–16.

24 Murray CG, Daly TE, Zimmerman SO (1980). The relationship between dental disease and radiation necrosis of the mandible. *Oral Surg Oral Med Oral Pathol*, 49(2), 99–104.

25 Koga DH, Salvajoli JV, Alves FA (2008). Dental extractions and radiotherapy in head and neck oncology: review of the literature. *Oral Dis*, 14(1), 40–4.

26 Marunick MT, Leveque F (1989). Osteoradionecrosis related to mastication and parafunction. *Oral Surg Oral Med Oral Pathol*, 68(5), 582–5.

27 Epstein JB, Wong FL, Stevenson-Moore P (1987). Osteoradionecrosis: clinical experience and a proposal for classification. *J Oral Maxillofac Surg*, 45(2), 104–10.

28 Epstein JB, Rea G, Wong FL, Spinelli J, Stevenson-Moore P (1987). Osteonecrosis: Study of the relationship of dental extractions in patients receiving radiotherapy. *Head Neck Surg*, 10(1), 48–54.

29 Stevenson-Moore P (1990). Oral complications of cancer therapies. Essential aspects of a pretreatment oral examination. *NCI Monogr*, 9, 33–6.

30 Jansma J, Vissink A, Spijkervet FK, et al. (1992). Protocol for the prevention and treatment of oral sequelae resulting from head and neck radiation therapy. *Cancer*, 70(8), 2171–80.

31 Schiodt M, Hermund NU (2002). Management of oral disease prior to radiation therapy. *Support Care Cancer*, 10(1), 40–3.

32 Koga DH, Salvajoli JV, Kowalski LP, Nishimoto IN, Alves FA (2008). Dental extractions related to head and neck radiotherapy: ten-year experience of a single institution. *Oral Surg Oral Med Oral Pathol Oral Radiol Endod*, 105(5), e1–6.

33 Beumer J, Brady FA (1978). Dental management of the irradiated patient. *Int J Oral Surg*, 7(3), 208–20.

34 Horiot JC, Maingon P, Barillot I (1994). Radiotherapy for head and neck cancers including chemoradiotherapy. *Curr Opin Oncol*, 6(3), 272–6.

35 Toljanic JA, Heshmati RH, Bedard JF (2002). Dental follow-up compliance in a population of irradiated head and neck cancer patients. *Oral Surg Oral Med Oral Pathol Endod*, 93(1), 35–8.

36 Cramer CK, Epstein JB, Sheps SB, Schechter MT, Busser JR (2002). Modified Delphi survey for decision analysis for prophylaxis of post-radiation osteonecrosis. *Oral Oncol*, 38(6), 574–83.

37 Friedman RB (1990). Osteoradionecrosis: causes and prevention. *NCI Monogr*, 9, 145–9.

38 Maxymiw WG, Wood RE, Liu FF (1991). Postradiation dental extractions without hyperbaric oxygen. *Oral Surg Oral Med Oral Pathol*, 72(3), 270–4.

39 Bennett MH, Feldmeier J, Hampson N, Smee R, Milross C (2008). Hyperbaric oxygen therapy for late radiation tissue injury. *Cochrane Database Syst Rev*, 3, CD005005.

40 Myers RA, Marx RE (1990). Use of hyperbaric oxygen in postradiation head and neck surgery. *NCI Monogr*, 9, 151–7.

41 Pitak-Arnnop P, Sader R, Dhanuthai K, et al. (2008). Management of osteoradionecrosis of the jaws: an analysis of evidence. *Eur J Surg Oncol*, 34(10), 1123–34.

42 Notani K, Yamazaki Y, Kitada H, et al. (2003). Management of mandibular osteoradionecrosis corresponding to the severity of osteoradionecrosis and the method of radiotherapy. *Head Neck*, 25(3), 181–6.

Chapter 13

Overview of complications of systemic chemotherapy

Douglas Peterson and Rajesh Lalla

Introduction

Chemotherapy has long been a mainstay of cancer management. The primary goals of treatment vary, depending on stage of the disease and overall patient status. These goals can range from intention-to-cure, through prolongation of life, to provision of comfort (i.e. palliation). There have been major advances in the chemotherapeutic management of malignant disease over the past decade[1]. These advances have included introduction of more targeted treatments, together with significant improvements in supportive oncology[2]. However, despite important progress, normal tissues continue to be at risk for either reversible or irreversible injury secondary to the chemotherapy. This chapter will provide an overview of the most frequent and clinically significant oral complications encountered with chemotherapy (Table 13.1)[3].

Epidemiology

Estimates for the collective incidence of oral complications secondary to chemotherapy are[1]: (1) 10% with adjuvant chemotherapy; (2) 40% with primary chemotherapy; and (3) 80% with myeloablative conditioning regimens utilized in haematopoietic stem cell transplantation. The frequency of oral tissue involvement is governed by class, mechanism of action, dose, and frequency of the chemotherapeutic agents utilized.

Aetiology

Oral toxicities secondary to chemotherapy can arise as a result of a direct injurious effect on oral tissues, as well as from chemotherapy-induced systemic compromise (i.e. indirect effects). The interactions that result in oral complications of cancer chemotherapy can be highly complex. For example, systemic chemotherapy can predispose to oral candidosis through oral mucosal damage, salivary gland dysfunction, and/or systemic immunosuppression.

High-dose chemotherapy is frequently being incorporated into the management of head and neck squamous cell carcinoma[4]. Regimens can include 2–3 cycles of induction chemotherapy, followed by 6–7 weeks of head and neck radiation with concurrent weekly chemotherapy. The collective injury to oral tissue is influenced by the dose and type of the chemotherapeutic component as well as the dose and type of the radiotherapy component.

The development of oral complications is governed by the pre-existing oral status. Indeed, management of coexistent oral/dental pathology pre-chemotherapy, and oral hygiene measures during chemotherapy, can be highly effective in preventing or minimizing the acute oral toxicities associated with this type of treatment. These interventions are discussed in detail in Chapter 5.

Table 13.1 Oral complications of chemotherapy [3].

Oral complication	Direct risk factor	Indirect risk factor
Oral mucositis	Mucosal toxicity Physical/chemical trauma	Decreased local/systemic immunity Oral infection
Oral viral infection		Decreased systemic immunity
Oral fungal infection	Inadequate oral/denture hygiene Mucosal breakdown	Decreased systemic immunity Salivary gland dysfunction Altered oral flora (e.g. antibiotics, steroids)
Oral bacterial infection	Inadequate oral hygiene Mucosal breakdown Acquired pathogens	Decreased systemic immunity Salivary gland dysfunction
Taste dysfunction	Taste receptor toxicity Neuropathy (see below)	Salivary gland dysfunction
Xerostomia	Salivary gland toxicity	Anticholinergic drugs
Neuropathy	Vinca alkaloids Platinum-based agents Taxanes Other specific drugs	Anaemia Dental hypersensitivity Temporomanadibular dysfunction/ myofascial pain
Dental/craniofacial growth and development problems (paediatric patients)	Tissue toxicity	Stage of dental/skeletal maturation
Gastrointestinal mucositis – causing secondary changes in oral status (e.g. poor oral hygiene, taste dysfunction)	Mucosal toxicity	Nausea and vomiting
Haemorrhage	Oral mucositis Oral infection (e.g. periodontal disease, herpes simplex virus) Physical trauma	Thrombocytopenia Decreased clotting factors (e.g. disseminated intravascular coagulation)

Clinical features

Most oral sequelae occur in association with the acute phase of treatment (Table 13.1)[3]. Long-term effects are not usually encountered, except for specific toxicities such as impaired dental and craniofacial development in children.

Oral toxicities can result in considerable patient morbidity, as well as impact on the family and caregivers[5]. Oral complications can also cause additional sequelae including dehydration and nutritional compromise. In addition, patients experiencing profound myelosuppression are at risk of developing systemic infection secondary to oral infection (which may be associated with mortality as well as morbidity).

Severe oral toxicities may result in the patient taking a temporary break from cancer treatment, or even withdrawing altogether from further cancer treatment (e.g. severe oral mucositis)[6]. Moreover, severe toxicities may necessitate a dose reduction in future chemotherapy cycles[6]. Such a course of action may result in a decreased tumour response, and so a decreased chance of long-term survival.

Oral mucositis

Clinically significant oral mucositis occurs in up to 14% of patients receiving conventional chemotherapy for solid tumours, and 27–52% of patients receiving high-dose chemotherapy prior to haematopoietic stem cell transplantation[7,8]. Certain drugs and regimens are more likely to cause oral mucositis than others[7]. The pain and associated sequelae are sufficiently severe in ~50% of these patients, so as to require medical intervention including opioid analgesics, hospitalization, and/or modification of the chemotherapeutic regimen[9–11].

Oral mucositis is discussed in detail in Chapter 15.

Salivary gland dysfunction

The predominance of research suggests that chemotherapy does not directly cause clinically significant compromise in salivary gland function[3]. However, several types of medication utilized in the supportive care of chemotherapy patients exert a direct anti-cholinergic effect on the major and minor salivary glands (e.g. anti-emetic drugs, analgesic drugs). As a result, chemotherapy patients may develop salivary gland dysfunction.

Salivary gland dysfunction is discussed, in detail, in Chapter 21.

Oral infection

Acute oral infection can arise for three principal reasons in the chemotherapy patient:

1. Chemotherapy can cause acute oral mucosal injury – the disrupted tissue architecture is more susceptible to colonization/infection.

2. Chemotherapy can compromise oral mucosal immune defence mechanisms – this renders oral tissues more susceptible to infection, caused by either opportunistic or newly acquired organisms. (The risk is increased when there is co-existent salivary gland dysfunction.)

3. Pre-existent latent or low-grade clinical infection can undergo acute flares during periods of myelosuppression (e.g. chronic periodontal disease, latent herpes simplex virus 1 infection)[3].

Oral infections are discussed in detail in Chapters 17–20.

Haemorrhage

Clinically significant thrombocytopaenia may occur in patients treated with certain chemo-therapeutic regimens. Spontaneous oral haemorrhage can occur when the platelet count is $<25\ 000/mm^3$, and is more likely in the setting of pre-existent periodontal disease (i.e. gingivitis, periodontitis). Severe ulcerative oral mucositis can also result in oral mucosal haemorrhage. In general, although oral haemorrhage can be disconcerting to the patient and family, it is typically not a major concern in the overall context of patient management.

Oral haemorrhage is discussed in more detail in Chapter 25.

Neurotoxicity

Some chemotherapeutic agents are directly neurotoxic, including the vinca alkaloids (e.g. vincris-tine, vinblastine). These drugs can, in some instances, produce a throbbing pain that mimics irreversible pulpal disease secondary to dental caries. If the pain is a result of chemotherapy-induced neuropathy, the symptom typically resolves 7–10 days following discontinuation of the chemotherapy[3].

In relatively rare cases, patients may develop dental hypersensitivity to thermal stimuli in the weeks or months following discontinuation of the chemotherapy. It is important to rule out dental disease before implicating chemotherapy as the cause of the problem. Patients may experience symptomatic relief in these instances from the topical application of fluorides and/or a desensitizing dentrifice.

Nutritional compromise

Patients undergoing chemotherapeutic management can experience nutritional compromise for several reasons. Nausea and vomiting can occur secondary to chemotherapy regimens. In addition, several other chemotherapy-related complications can adversely impact on nutritional intake, including oral mucositis, salivary gland dysfunction, and taste disturbance.

Given the importance and complexity of this complication, it is extremely important that a dietician is involved in the management of affected patients. This integration should be comprehensive, beginning with development of the treatment plan, and followed by ongoing monitoring of the patient's ability to comply with any nutritional interventions.

Taste disturbance

Chemotherapy has been demonstrated as having an important effect on taste in patients receiving chemotherapy for various malignancies[12]. Abnormalities in taste can occur secondary to direct injury to the taste buds, damage to the nerves innervating the taste cells, and decrease in saliva secretion. In addition, conditioned food aversions may develop in association with the chemotherapy regimen. Fortunately, normal taste sensation usually returns in the first few months following cessation of the chemotherapy.

Tasted disturbance is discussed in detail in Chapter 22.

Skeletal/dental malformation in children

High-dose chemotherapy can adversely impact craniofacial development and growth in children, as a result of direct effects on the tissues and disturbances modulated via growth hormone. In children younger than 12 years of age, the effects include altered timing of dental eruption and alterations in tooth maturation. Morphological changes include diminished size of the crowns of teeth, as well as shortened and/or conical shape root structures[3].

Compromised wound healing

High-dose chemotherapy can result in delayed soft and hard tissue healing, and/or altered structural formation. The risk of compromised wound healing can be increased by selected co-morbidities (e.g. diabetes mellitus).

Guidelines regarding dental extractions prior to chemotherapy are based on a limited number of retrospective trials conducted in the 1980s[13,14]. The guidelines include: (1) performing extractions at least 10 days prior to the absolute neutrophil count becoming $<500/mm^3$; (2) minimizing trauma to the tissues, and obtaining primary closure with multiple interrupted sutures (whenever possible); (3) platelet support if the platelet count is $<40\,000/mm^3$; and (4) antibiotic prophylaxis if the white blood cell count is $<2000/mm^3$ (and/or neutrophil count is $<1000/mm^3$).

Halitosis

The genesis of halitosis in chemotherapy patients may be multifactorial. Key causes include: (1) pre-existing oral tumour; (2) pre-existing oral infection; (3) compromised oral hygiene; and (4) altered diet. In many patients, the cause of halitosis is related to accumulation of food and other debris on the dorsum of the tongue. Halitosis in such patients can be treated effectively by the use of a tongue scraper or gentle toothbrushing of the tongue, as well as the use of non-medicated oral rinses several times per day.

Halitosis is discussed, in detail, in Chapter 23.

References

1 Chabner BA, Longo DL (2006). *Cancer chemotherapy and biotherapy: principles and practice*, 4th edn. Lippincott Williams & Wilkins, Philadelphia.

2 Duffy MJ, Crown J (2008). A personalized approach to cancer treatment: how biomarkers can help. *Clin Chem*, 54(11), 1770–9.

3 National Cancer Institute website: http://www.cancer.gov/cancertopics/pdq/supportivecare/oralcomplications/HealthProfessional

4 Haddad RI, Shin DM (2008). Recent advances in head and neck cancer. *N Engl J Med*, 359(11), 1143–54.

5 Honea N, Brant J, Beck SL (2007). Treatment-related symptom clusters. *Semin Oncol Nurs*, 23(2), 142–51.

6 Trotti A, Bellm LA, Epstein JB, et al. (2003). Mucositis incidence, severity and associated outcomes in patients with head and neck cancer receiving radiotherapy with or without chemotherapy: a systematic literature review. *Radiother Oncol*, 66(3), 253–62.

7 Jones JA, Avritscher EB, Cooksley CD, Michelet M, Bekele BN, Elting LS (2006). Epidemiology of treatment-associated mucosal injury after treatment with newer regimens for lymphoma, breast, lung, or colorectal cancer. *Support Care Cancer*, 14(6), 505–15.

8 Sonis ST, Elting LS, Keefe D, et al. (2004). Perspectives on cancer therapy-induced mucosal injury: pathogenesis, measurement, epidemiology, and consequences for patients. *Cancer*, 100(9 Suppl), 1995–2025.

9 Keefe DM, Schubert MM, Elting LS, et al. (2007). Updated clinical practice guidelines for the prevention and treatment of mucositis. *Cancer*, 109(5), 820–31.

10 Lalla RV, Sonis ST, Peterson DE (2008). Management of oral mucositis in patients who have cancer. *Dent Clin North Am*, 52(1), 61–77.

11 Sonis ST, Oster G, Fuchs H, et al. (2001). Oral mucositis and the clinical and economic outcomes of hematopoietic stem-cell transplantation. *J Clin Oncol*, 19(8), 2201–5.

12 Steinbach S, Hummel T, Bohner C, et al. (2009). Qualitative and quantitative assessment of taste and smell changes in patients undergoing chemotherapy for breast cancer or gynecologic malignancies. *J Clin Oncol*, 27(11), 1899–905.

13 Williford SK, Salisbury PL, Peacock JE, et al. (1989). The safety of dental extractions in patients with hematologic malignancies. *J Clin Oncol*, 7(6), 798–802.

14 Overholser CD, Peterson DE, Bergman SA, Williams LT (1982). Dental extractions in patients with acute nonlymphocytic leukemia. *J Oral Maxillofac Surg*, 40(5), 296–8.

Chapter 14

Oral complications of haematopoietic stem cell transplantation

Sharon Elad, Judith Raber-Durlacher, and
Michael Y. Shapira

Introduction

Haematopoietic stem cell transplantation (HSCT) is widely applied as a potentially curative treatment for selected malignancies (e.g. leukaemia, lymphoma, multiple myeloma), and selected other diseases associated with damage to, or deficiency of, the bone marrow constituents (e.g. aplastic anaemia, severe combined immunodeficiency)[1]. HSCT can reconstitute the haematopoietic system when damaged by high dose chemo-radiotherapy, because haematopoietic stem cells possess the capacity for self-renewal, and for differentiating into all of the blood cell lineages.

In the past, haematopoietic stem cells were exclusively derived from the bone marrow, which involves aspiration of bone marrow from the posterior iliac crest while the donor is placed under sedation or anaesthesia (due to the discomfort of the procedure). Peripheral blood is now the preferred source for harvesting of stem cells in adults, and umbilical cord blood is an accepted alternative source of stem cells for paediatric transplantation. Autologous HSCT (in which stem cells are derived from the patient) is mainly used to treat chemosensitive malignancies. Its anti-cancer effect is entirely derived from the high dose 'conditioning regimen'; it involves the risk of infusing contaminated bone marrow back into the patient. Allogeneic HSCT (in which the stem cells are derived from a donor) is often the preferred treatment option, particularly in patients with acute leukaemia. Its anti-cancer effect depends on both the conditioning regimen, and an accompanying graft versus tumour/leukaemia effect (GVT/GVL effect), i.e. the donor immune cells mounting a response against the host malignant cells.

In the late 1990s, a better understanding of the GVL effect led to the development of less intensive conditioning regimens. These new regimens are primarily immunosuppressive (rather than primarily myeloablative), so as to facilitate engraftment of the transplanted donor cells. The approach is sometimes complemented by the infusion of donor lymphocytes (to enhance the GVL effect). These reduced-intensity conditioning (RIC) transplants are associated with less early morbidity and mortality as compared to standard conditioning transplants. Hence, RIC transplants can be conducted in patients previously ineligible for HSCT, because of their age and/or underlying medical condition[2]. However, RIC transplants may be associated with significant late complications, such as acute-like chronic graft-versus-host disease and a higher risk of relapse.

Oral complications

Oral complications significantly contribute to transplant-related morbidity and, in some cases, transplant-related mortality. The most common oral complications are shown in Table 14.1.

Table 14.1 Oral complications of haematopoietic stem cell transplantation

Category	Tissue	Oral complication
Tissue-specific complications	Oral mucosa	Oral mucositis
		Mucosal GVHD
		Anaemia-related atrophy
		Neutropenic ulcer
		Pyogenic granuloma
	Salivary glands	Xerostomia/salivary gland hypofunction
		GVHD
		Sialadenitis
	Musculoskeletal tissues	Trismus
		Restricted movement of tongue
		Bisphosphonate-related osteonecrosis
	Nervous tissues	Taste disturbance
		Neuropathy
		Tooth sensitivity
	Dental/periodontal tissues	Dental caries
		Periodontal disease
		Gingival hyperplasia
Non-tissue specific complications	Infection	Bacterial
		Fungal
		Viral
	Haemorrhage	
	Secondary malignancies	Post-transplant lymphoproliferative disease
		Squamous cell carcinoma
	Developmental abnormalities	Dental abnormalities
		Skeletal abnormalities

Oral mucosa

Oral Mucositis

Oral mucositis is a major complication of HSCT, particularly following myeloablative conditioning[3]. It is highly distressing to patients, and associated with significant local and systemic complications[4,5]. In a large prospective study, oral mucositis was experienced by 99% of patients undergoing myeloablative conditioning, and was most frequently grades III or IV on the World Health Organization mucositis scale[6]. It should be noted that there is little information available on the incidence and severity of oral mucositis following RIC regimens, although the incidence and severity of oral mucositis is reported to be lower in this situation[7].

Oral mucositis begins approximately 5–10 days following myeloablative conditioning therapy, and resolves within 2–3 weeks in over 90% patients. Some studies have shown that the resolution of oral mucositis coincides with recovery of the white cell count[8], although other studies have not confirmed the phenomenon of simultaneous recovery[6]. Its clinical presentation is very similar to that induced by other high-dose chemotherapeutic regimens (see Chapter 15). The most severe grade of oral mucositis has been shown to be significantly associated with the number of days of parenteral opioid therapy, the number of days of total parenteral nutrition, the incidence of significant infection, the number of days with fever, the overall time in hospital, and the total inpatient charges[9].

The management of oral mucositis starts with a pretreatment oral assessment aimed at reducing pre-existent oral infection and trauma-inducing factors (see Chapter 5)[10]. Education on the importance of performing good oral hygiene should be undertaken at this time, and should be reinforced during the HSCT procedure[11,12]. Chlorhexidine has not proved to be effective for the prevention of oral mucositis, although it may be indicated for the reduction of dental plaque[13,14]. Some centres also employ antifungal prophylaxis[15].

Human recombinant keratinocyte-growth factor (palifermin) has been approved as a prophylactic treatment for oral mucositis in patients undergoing HSCT[16–18]. There is evidence that low-level-laser therapy may be similarly beneficial for reducing the incidence of oral mucositis, although low-level-laser therapy requires expensive equipment and specialized training[19]. In addition, cryotherapy is recommended for prophylaxis in patients receiving melphalan in the conditioning regimen[18,19]. A variety of additional agents have been suggested for the prevention/treatment of oral mucositis, such as amifostine, calcium phosphate and iseganan[20–22]. However, the evidence to support these agents is somewhat limited, and so none have become standard treatments within HSCT.

The discomfort of oral mucositis may be reduced with regular oral hygiene, and the use of topical anaesthetics, topical analgesics, or coating agents. However, systemic analgesics are frequently needed[5], and the recommended modality is patient-controlled analgesia using morphine (or a similar 'opioid for moderate-to-severe pain')[22]. In published studies, opioids for moderate-to-severe pain were prescribed in 47–66% of patients, for a median of 6 days following myeloablative HSCT[4,6].

Oral mucositis is discussed in detail in Chapter 15.

Oral Graft-Versus-Host Disease (GVHD)

GVHD is an alloimmune inflammatory process, which results from the donor cells response against the host tissues. It occurs as 'acute' GVHD (aGVHD) in 50–70%, and 'chronic' GVHD (cGVHD) in 30–50%, of allogeneic transplant patients (and 40–80% of long-term survivors)[23].

Originally, GVHD was classified according to time of onset of clinical presentation; GVHD presenting <100 days following stem cell infusion was considered aGVHD, and >100 days following stem cell infusion was considered cGVHD. At present, GVHD is usually classified according to the type of clinical presentation[24]. Thus, cGVHD can occur as early as 50 days following transplantation[25], and aGVHD may occur much later than 100 days in patients transplanted using RIC regimens.

aGVHD is divided into three pathological stages: (1) the conditioning regimen results in mucosal injury leading to expression of allo-antigens; (2) host antigen-presenting cells present these allo-antigens to donor T cells, which results in their activation, proliferation, and the production of pro-inflammatory cytokines; and (3) multiple effector cells and cytokines then produce tissue damage. The translocation of bacterial cell wall products such as lipopolysacccharide through damaged gastrointestinal tract mucosa may further upregulate cytokine and chemokine production (and so contribute to tissue damage)[26]. The pathophysiology of cGVHD remains relatively poorly understood[27]. It is now recognized that cGVHD is not a temporal extension of aGVHD, but rather a distinct clinical entity. cGVHD evolves as a consequence of dysregulated alloreactive reactions between donor-derived immune cells and host cell populations, which combine the features of autoimmunity and immunodeficiency, and which lead to chronic inflammation and fibrosis of target organs.

Oral involvement may be seen in 35–60 % of patients who develop aGvHD, and in up to 80% of patients affected by cGvHD. Oral involvement is often indicative of the presence of systemic disease [28], although the oral cavity may be the only site of GVHD. Recently it has been reported that the incidence of oral aGVHD may be less following RIC transplantation compared to traditional myeloablative HSCT (at least in the first 3 months post-transplant)[29].

Common areas of involvement include the tongue, buccal mucosa, and labial mucosa. In aGVHD, oral lesions are often hyperkeratotic, erythematous, ulcerative, and desquamative (Figure 14.1, see colour plate section). The extent and severity of these oral lesions can become disabling. The presentation of cGVHD is similar, although lichenoid lesions may be more prominant in cGVHD, and mucocoeles may be present in cGVHD (Figure 14.2, see colour plate section)[28,30]. Scleroderma-like stiffness of the oral soft tissues can limit the mouth opening[31]. Painful mucosal lesions may represent a significant impediment to nutritional intake and performing oral hygiene. Additionally, cGVHD may be associated with progressive salivary gland dysfunction (see below). GVHD is a risk factor for the development of secondary solid cancers (see below)[32].

Histopathologic evaluation may be complementary to clinical evaluation[33]. The histopathologic features of aGVHD and cGVHD are similar (although there have been no large studies on the histopathology of oral aGVHD) [34]. Histopathologically, oral GVHD is best characterized as lichen planus-like, or lichenoid manifestations. Lesions may demonstrate varying degrees of epithelial atrophy and perivascular inflammation. Disruption of the basement membrane zone by inflammatory cells is often noted [30]. Additionally, an inflammatory infiltrate caused by superimposed infection may be present, possibly with histopathologic evidence of microscopic colonies or infiltrate.

Prophylaxis of GVHD is more successful than treatment, and first-line preventive pharmacological treatments include various immunosuppressive and immune-modulating drugs, such as steroids, cyclosporine, tacrolimus, methotrexate, and mycophenolate mofetil (Table 14.2).

The management of oral GVHD consists of appropriate systemic therapy, combined with proper oral hygiene and use of topical agents (Table 14.2). Systemic therapy will initially include systemic steroids and, when unsuccessful, may be followed by other immunosuppressives and immunomodulators, such as azathioprine, mycophenolate mofetil, thalidomide, and others (often in combination) [35]. The treatment of oral GVHD also needs to address pain management, prevention of limitation of mouth opening, prevention of dental and periodontal disease, and nutritional intake.

Topical therapy is preferred when the oral mucosa is the only site not responding to high doses of systemic corticosteroids, or when GVHD is only manifested in the oral mucosa [36]. In general, topical steroid preparations are the mainstay of local treatment for GVHD (e.g. budesonide).[37,38] Additional approaches to the local management of oral GVHD include topical anti-inflammatory and immunosuppressive agents such as azathioprine[39,40], cyclosporine [41], tacrolimus [42], and oral psoralen plus ultraviolet A (PUVA) therapy[43,44]. There are anecdotal reports of success with other local modalities including ultraviolet B (UVB) and CO_2 laser [45,46].

Other oral mucosal problems

Anaemia-related mucosal changes may occur in patients undergoing cancer treatment. Anaemia is characterized by oral epithelial atrophy (with loss of normal keratinization) [47]. Hence, the tongue may become smooth due to atrophy of the filiform and fungiform papillae. Oral mucosal sensitivity may occur in this situation.

Table 14.2 Management of oral mucosal graft versus host disease (GVHD)

Prevention	Systemic agents	Ciclosporin (cyclosporin)
		Methotrexate
		Tacrolimus
		Mycophenolate mofetil
		Graft manipulation (T-cell depletion)
		Anti-thymocyte globulin
Treatment	Topical/local agents	Steroids
		Azathioprine
		Ciclosporin (cyclosporin)
		Tacrolimus
		Phototherapy (PUVA/UVB)
	Systemic agents	Steroids
		Tacrolimus
		Sirolimus
		Mycophenolate mofetil
		Phototherapy (PUVA/extra-corporeal plasmaphotopheresis)
		Hydroxychloroquine
		Clofazimine
		Thalidomide
		Pentostatin
		Methotrexate
		Rituximab
		Daclizumab
		Alefacept
		Etanercept
Palliation	Topical/local agents	Anaesthetics
		Analgesics
		Antiseptics
		CO_2 laser

Patients undergoing HSCT usually become neutropaenic, and may subsequently develop 'neutropaenic' ulcers (see Chapter 4). These ulcers are usually well defined, often very painful, and usually heal with the recovery of the blood count. Standard measures can be used to relieve pain and prevent secondary infection.

Pyogenic granuloma has also been reported to occur in HSCT patients [31]. It is thought that its development is related to continuous mucosal inflammation associated with GVHD. Treatment involves excisional biopsy, and elimination of any local trauma.

Salivary glands

Salivary gland dysfunction is a common complication following HSCT. Indeed, both xerostomia (subjective dryness of the mouth) and hyposalivation (objective reduction in saliva flow) are observed in HSCT patients. Salivary gland dysfunction is a multifactorial condition in HSCT patients. The most common causes are the conditioning regimen, cGVHD, and chronic adminis-tration of various medications. In addition, altered oral intake may result in dehydration.

Salivary secretion is substantially reduced during the conditioning stage of HSCT [48]. An increase in saliva flow rate typically begins a few days following HSCT. Patients conditioned with chemotherapy, or chemotherapy and total lymph node irradiation, display early and complete recovery of saliva secretion (i.e. 2–5 months following engraftment). However, recovery is delayed and incomplete when total body irradiation (TBI) is added to the conditioning regimen.

The histological changes found in salivary glands as a result of cancer chemotherapy, include ductal dilation, cyst formation, acinar degeneration, and infiltration of inflammatory cells [49]. These effects are enhanced when TBI is included in the conditioning regimen. Ionizing radiation can cause permanent damage to salivary glands, which is manifested as acinar cell destruction with subsequent atrophy and fibrosis of the glands, and changes to the vasculature and connective tissue [48,50].

Salivary gland dysfunction affects 90% of aGVHD patients, and 60% of cGVHD patients [51]. A direct correlation is observed between the degree of hyposalivation and the severity of GVHD [51]. GVHD also results in various salivary biochemical and immunological composi-tional alterations [52–54]. For example, patients with GVHD have significantly higher salivary concentrations of electrolytes, albumin, total protein, and epidermal growth factor, and possibly lower salivary concentrations of immunoglobulin A (IgA; as compared with controls) [52,55]. These alterations may result in compromised saliva function.

GVHD-induced salivary gland dysfunction results from injury caused by donor lymphocytes reacting against ductal and acinar tissue [56]. GVHD-induced salivary gland dysfunction histologically resembles Sjögren's syndrome. Lymphocytic infiltration of salivary ducts results in epithelial necrosis; the end-result is obstruction and eventual acinar damage and fibrosis [57]. Cytokines (e.g. interleukin 2, interleukin 6, interferon gamma, tissue necrosis factor), adhesion molecules, and heat-shock proteins have been suggested to play a role in this process [57,58].

As hyposalivation progresses, inspection of the oral cavity may disclose dryness of the oral mucosa, dryness of the lips, absence of a 'pool' of saliva in the floor of the mouth, cobblestone appearance/fissuring of the oral mucosa (especially of the tongue), and cracking of the lips [59]. The most typical manifestation of minor salivary gland involvement is multiple mucocoeles, with the labial and soft-palate mucosae being the most frequently involved sites (Figure 14.2). Mucocoeles often produce a disturbed sensation in the mouth [31]. In rare cases, mucocoeles may evolve into a large mucocoele or ranule. The clinical features of salivary gland dysfunction are discussed, in detail, in Chapter 21.

Salivary gland dysfunction may be palliated with saliva stimulants or saliva substitutes. Systemic sialogogues may be effective in selected patients with GVHD (i.e. pilocarpine, cevimel-line) [30,60]. Topical fluorides are indicated in dentate patients in order to prevent rampant dental caries. Calcium phosphorous solutions may also be needed to maintain mineralization of teeth [61]. The management of salivary gland dysfunction is also discussed in detail in Chapter 21.

Musculoskeletal tissues

cGVHD commonly involves the skin and underlying fascia, and the clinical presentation may resemble sclerodema. Perioral fibrosis may decrease oral opening, limit tongue movement, and so interfere with oral function [31].

TBI administered during the conditioning regimen may contribute to fibrosis (and so limitation of mouth opening). However, the effect of radiotherapy used in myeloablative HSCT (typical dose: 1200 Gy) is not as pronounced as that used to treat head and neck cancers (typical dose: 4500–7000 Gy). The effect of TBI is most pronounced when administered at a young age [62]. Trismus is discussed, in detail, in Chapter 11.

Bisphosphonates are used in HSCT patients for treatment of the underlying disease, and steroid-induced osteoporosis. Hence, bisphosphonate-related osteonecrosis of the jaw may develop post-HSCT. Bisphosphonate-related osteonecrosis of the jaw is discussed in detail in Chapter 16.

Nervous tissues

Taste disturbance often occurs with chemotherapy and radiotherapy. A controlled pilot study assessed taste perception following HSCT [63]: immediately following transplantation, there was significant hypogeusia (decreased ability to taste) for all four taste modalities compared to measurements prior to HSCT (and compared to measurements in healthy controls). Although some normalization of taste thresholds was found after 3–6 months, most subjects still experienced some disturbance of taste. The most frequently recorded change was an elevated threshold for salt. Taste acuity had recovered in ~80% patients by 1 year following transplantation. Other reasons for taste disturbance include anaemia, nutritional deficiency, and drugs. Taste disturbance is discussed in detail in Chapter 22.

Most neuropathies involving the oral and perioral tissues are chemotherapy induced [5,64]. An asymmetric neuropathy should alert the clinician to possible recurrence of the malignant disease.

Dental and periodontal tissues

Dental caries may be a problem for HSCT patients with salivary gland dysfunction (see above) Thus, an active preventive approach is indicated in this group of patients (i.e. meticulous oral hygiene, use of a topical fluoride). A recent study reported that the risk of developing dental caries (or periodontal attachment loss) after transplantation is associated with human leucocyte antigen (HLA type) [65].

Data are scarce on the risk of periodontal disease post HSCT. Pattni et al. did not find periodontal health to be decreased when patients were followed up post allogeneic HSCT [66]. However, this study involved patients with relatively good periodontal health prior to HSCT, and the follow-up time was relatively short (i.e. 6 months).

There is anecdotic evidence that periodontal infection may trigger GVHD, and that oral GVHD improves when periodontal treatment is provided [28].

Infection

HSCT-associated myeloablation is associated with an increased risk for both oral infections and systemic infections of oral origin [67]. Indeed, oral bacterial, fungal, and viral infections are all common in HSCT patients. It should be noted that infected periodontal pockets act as a niche for a wide variety of microorganisms that may translocate into the bloodstream, and so induce systemic infectious complications [68].

The shift to RIC protocols will not necessarily decrease the incidence of oral infections. Thus, a recent study reported that the prevalence of oral opportunistic infections in patients receiving RIC HSCT was no different when compared to that in patients receiving myeloablative HSCT (despite a shorter duration of neutropaenia) [29]. In other words, RIC causes sufficient immune suppression to allow opportunistic pathogens to produce clinical disease.

Oral infections are discussed in detail in Chapters 17–20.

Haemorrhage

Oral haemorrhage may be due to a number of factors; the main factors are the cancer itself, thrombocytopaenia due to chemotherapy, and coagulopathy due to liver dysfunction (associated with the conditioning regimen, the supportive care regimen, or GVHD) [31].

Oral haemorrhage is discussed in detail in Chapter 25.

Secondary malignancies

Solid tumours

The oral cavity is one of the most prevalent sites for solid cancers following HSCT. The risk of a new oral cancer is increased 70-fold in 10-yr survivors of HSCT [69,70]. The vast majority of cases are oral squamous cell carcinomas [71], although salivary gland tumours are seen as well [32].

The risk for any solid cancer following HSCT, including oral cancer, is higher for recipients who are younger at the time of transplantation than for those who were older, and for patients treated with higher doses of total body irradiation. Furthermore, specific risk factors for oral cancer have been identified, including cGVHD [32,71], and GVHD treatment[72]. Additional risk factors have been suggested to contribute to the development of post-transplant neoplasms, including genetic predisposition, male sex, viral infection, and antigenic stimulation by viral or donor–recipient histocompatibility differences[71].

The increased cancer risk over time after transplantation necessitates lifelong surveillance of HSCT patients. HSCT patients should avoid carcinogenic exposure, such as tobacco smoking and excess alcohol consumption.

Post-transplantation lymphoproliferative disorder

Post-transplantation lymphoproliferative disorder (PTLD) has been defined as 'a lymphoid proliferation or lymphoma that develops as a consequence of immunosuppression in a recipient of a solid organ or bone marrow allograft'[73]. PTLD is the most common malignancy in the first year following allogeneic HSCT. PTLD is associated with compromised immune function and Epstein–Barr virus infection[69,70].

The manifestations of PTLD include compression of anatomical structures by a malignant mass, lymphoma-related 'B' symptoms (i.e. fever, sweats, weight loss), or an illness mimicking a viral infection[74,75]. Oral involvement of PTLD is rare, and is usually reported following solid organ transplantation[75]. PTLD may manifest as a crater-like defect of the gingiva, or an ulcerated dark-red mass post HSCT[76,77].

Treatment involves anti-viral medication and reduction of immunosuppression (which may lead to complete resolution). Other treatments include chemotherapy, radiotherapy, interferon, interleukin-6, intravenous IgG, anti-B-cell antibodies, and cellular immunotherapy[75]. Surgery may be considered when the lesion is accessible.

Developmental abnormalities

Dental growth abnormalities may develop in paediatric HSCT recipients. The conditioning regimen, and cancer therapy prior to transplantation, can damage the tooth buds resulting in enamel hypoplasia and disturbances in root formation[78]. Alterations to the size and shape of the teeth, and delayed eruption of the teeth are commonplace[31,79].

Skeletal growth abnormalities may also develop in paediatric HSCT recipients. Modifications in growth of the craniofacial complex are commonplace[31]. However, in many cases, the problem is symmetrical in nature, and so is not necessarily obvious on inspection[80].

References

1 Copelan EA (2006). Hematopoietic stem-cell transplantation. *N Engl J Med*, 354(17), 1813–26.

2 Shapira MY, Tsirigotis P, Resnick IB, Or R, Abdul-Hai A, Slavin S (2007). Allogeneic hematopoietic stem cell transplantation in the elderly. *Crit Rev Oncol Hematol*, 64(1), 49–63.

3 Epstein JB, Schubert MM (1999). Oral mucositis in myelosuppressive cancer therapy. *Oral Surg Oral Med Oral Pathol Oral Radiol Endod*, 88(3), 273–6.

4 Bellm LA, Epstein JB, Rose-Ped A, Martin P, Fuchs HJ (2000). Patient reports of complications of bone marrow transplantation. *Support Care Cancer*, 8(1), 33–9.

5 Epstein JB, Elad S, Eliav E, Jurevic R, Benoliel R (2007). Orofacial pain in cancer: part II -clinical perspectives and management. *J Dent Res*, 86(6), 506–18.

6 Wardley AM, Jayson GC, Swindell R, et al. (2000). Prospective evaluation of oral mucositis in patients receiving myeloablative conditioning regimens and haemopoietic progenitor rescue. *Br J Haematol*, 110(2), 292–9.

7 Takahashi K, Soga Y, Murayama Y, et al (2010). Oral mucositis in patients receiving reduced-intensity regimens for allogeneic hematopoietic cell transplantation: comparison with conventional regimen. *Support Care Cancer*, 18(1), 115–9.

8 Woo SB, Sonis ST, Monopoli MM, Sonis AL (1993). A longitudinal study of oral ulcerative mucositis in bone marrow transplant recipients. *Cancer*, 72(5), 1612–7.

9 Vera-Llonch M, Oster G, Ford CM, Lu J, Sonis S (2007). Oral mucositis and outcomes of allogeneic hematopoietic stem-cell transplantation in patients with hematologic malignancies. *Support Care Cancer*, 15(5), 491–6.

10 Elad S, Epstein JB, Meyerowitz C, Peterson DE, Schubert M (2005). Oral and dental management for cancer patients, in Buchsel PC, Yarbro CH (eds) *Oncology Nursing in the Ambulatory Setting: Issues and Models of Care,* 2nd edn. Jones and Bartlett Publishers, Sudbury.

11 Borowski B, Benhamou E, Pico JL, Laplanche A, Margainaud JP, Hayat M (1994). Prevention of oral mucositis in patients treated with high-dose chemotherapy and bone marrow transplantation: a randomised controlled trial comparing two protocols of dental care. *Eur J Cancer B Oral Oncol*, 30B(2), 93–7.

12 McGuire DB, Correa ME, Johnson J, Wienandts P (2006). The role of basic oral care and good clinical practice principles in the management of oral mucositis. *Support Care Cancer*, 14(6), 541–7.

13 Barasch A, Elad S, Altman A, Damato K, Epstein J (2006). Antimicrobials, mucosal coating agents, anesthetics, analgesics, and nutritional supplements for alimentary tract mucositis. *Support Care Cancer*, 14(6), 528–32.

14 Addy M, Moran JM (1997). Clinical indications for the use of chemical adjuncts to plaque control: chlorhexidine formulations. *Periodontol 2000*, 15, 52–4.

15 Elad S, Wexler A, Garfunkel AA, Shapira MY, Bitan M, Or R (2006). Oral candidiasis prevention in transplantation patients: a comparative study. *Clin Transplant*, 20(3), 318–24.

16 Spielberger R, Stiff P, Bensinger W, et al. (2004). Palifermin for oral mucositis after intensive therapy for hematologic cancers. *N Engl J Med*, 351(25), 2590–8.

17 von Bultzingslowen I, Brennan MT, Spijkervet FK, et al. (2006). Growth factors and cytokines in the prevention and treatment of oral and gastrointestinal mucositis. *Support Care Cancer*, 14(6), 519–27.

18 Keefe DM, Schubert MM, Elting LS, et al. (2007). Updated clinical practice guidelines for the prevention and treatment of mucositis. *Cancer*, 109(5), 820–31.

19 Migliorati CA, Oberle-Edwards L, Schubert M (2006). The role of alternative and natural agents, cryotherapy, and/or laser for management of alimentary mucositis. *Support Care Cancer*, 14(6), 533–40.

20 Worthington HV, Clarkson JE, Eden OB (2007). Interventions for preventing oral mucositis for patients with cancer receiving treatment. *Cochrane Database Syst Rev* 2007(4): CD000978.

21 Clarkson JE, Worthington HV, Eden OB (2007). Interventions for treating oral mucositis for patients with cancer receiving treatment. *Cochrane Database Syst Rev* 2007(2): CD001973.

22 Rubenstein EB, Peterson DE, Schubert M, et al. (2004). Clinical practice guidelines for the prevention and treatment of cancer therapy-induced oral and gastrointestinal mucositis. *Cancer*, 100(9 Suppl), 2026–46.

23 Sullivan KA (2004). Graft-vs-host disease, in Thomas ED, Blume KG, Forma SJ (eds) *Hematopoietic Stem Cell Transplantation*, pp. 635–64. Blackwell Science, Maiden.

24 Filipovich AH, Weisdorf D, Pavletic S, et al. (2005). National Institutes of Health consensus development project on criteria for clinical trials in chronic graft-versus-host disease: I. Diagnosis and staging working group report. *Biol Blood Marrow Transplant*, 11(12), 945–56.

25 Deeg HJ, Antin JH (2006). The clinical spectrum of acute graft-versus-host disease. *Semin Hematol*, 43(1), 24–31.

26 Ferrara JL, Reddy P (2006). Pathophysiology of graft-versus-host disease. *Semin Hematol*, 43(1), 3–10.

27 Vogelsang GB, Lee L, Bensen-Kennedy DM (2003). Pathogenesis and treatment of graft-versus-host disease after bone marrow transplant. *Annu Rev Med*, 54, 29–52.

28 Schubert MM, Correa ME (2008). Oral graft-versus-host disease. *Dent Clin North Am*, 52(1), 79–109.

29 Elad S, Shapira MY, McNeal S, et al. (2008). Oral effects of nonmyeloablative stem cell transplantation: a prospective observational study. *Quintessence Int*, 39(8), 673–8.

30 Woo SB, Lee SJ, Schubert MM (1997). Graft-vs.-host disease. *Crit Rev Oral Biol Med*, 8(2), 201–16.

31 Schubert MM, Peterson DE, Lloid ME (2004). Oral complications, in Thomas ED, Blume KG, Forma SJ (eds) *Hematopoietic Stem Cell Transplantation*, pp. 911–28. Blackwell Science, Malden.

32 Curtis RE, Rowlings PA, Deeg HJ, et al. (1997). Solid cancers after bone marrow transplantation. *N Engl J Med*, 336(13), 897–904.

33 Vendrell Rankin K, Jones D, Redding SW (2003). *Oral health in cancer therapy: a guide for Health Care Professionals*, 2nd edn. Dental Oncology Education Program, San Antonio.

34 Shulman HM, Kleiner D, Lee SJ, et al. (2006). Histopathologic diagnosis of chronic graft-versus-host disease: National Institutes of Health Consensus Development Project on Criteria for Clinical Trials in Chronic Graft-versus-Host Disease: II. Pathology Working Group Report. *Biol Blood Marrow Transplant*, 12(1), 31–47.

35 Imanguli MM, Pavletic SZ, Guadagnini JP, Brahim JS, Atkinson JC (2006). Chronic graft versus host disease of oral mucosa: review of available therapies. Oral Surg Oral Med Oral *Pathol Oral Radiol Endod*, 101(2), 175–83.

36 Couriel D, Carpenter PA, Cutler C, et al. (2006). Ancillary therapy and supportive care of chronic graft-versus-host disease: national institutes of health consensus development project on criteria for clinical trials in chronic Graft-versus-host disease: V. Ancillary Therapy and Supportive Care Working Group Report. *Biol Blood Marrow Transplant*, 12(4), 375–96.

37 Elad S, Or R, Garfunkel AA, Shapira MY (2003). Budesonide: a novel treatment for oral chronic graft versus host disease. *Oral Surg Oral Med Oral Pathol Oral Radiol Endod*, 95(3), 308–11.

38 Sari I, Altuntas F, Kocyigit I, et al. (2007). The effect of budesonide mouthwash on oral chronic graft versus host disease. *Am J Hematol*, 82(5), 349–56.

39 Epstein JB, Nantel S, Sheoltch SM (2000). Topical azathioprine in the combined treatment of chronic oral graft-versus-host disease. *Bone Marrow Transplant*, 25(6), 683–7.

40 Epstein JB, Gorsky M, Epstein MS, Nantel S (2001). Topical azathioprine in the treatment of immune-mediated chronic oral inflammatory conditions: a series of cases. *Oral Surg Oral Med Oral Pathol Oral Radiol Endod*, 91(1), 56–61.

41 Epstein JB, Truelove EL (1996). Topical cyclosporine in a bioadhesive for treatment of oral lichenoid mucosal reactions: an open label clinical trial. *Oral Surg Oral Med Oral Pathol Oral Radiol Endod*, 82(5), 532–6.

42 Eckardt A, Starke O, Stadler M, Reuter C, Hertenstein B (2004). Severe oral chronic graft-versus-host disease following allogeneic bone marrow transplantation: highly effective treatment with topical tacrolimus. *Oral Oncol*, 40(8), 811–14.

43 Redding SW, Callander NS, Haveman CW, Leonard DL (1998). Treatment of oral chronic graft-versus-host disease with PUVA therapy: case report and literature review. *Oral Surg Oral Med Oral Pathol Oral Radiol Endod*, 86(2), 183–7.

44 Wolff D, Anders V, Corio R, et al. (2004). Oral PUVA and topical steroids for treatment of oral manifestations of chronic graft-vs.-host disease. *Photodermatol Photoimmunol Photomed*, 20(4), 184–90.

45 Elad S, Garfunkel AA, Enk CD, Galili D, Or R (1999). Ultraviolet B irradiation: a new therapeutic concept for the management of oral manifestations of graft-versus-host disease. *Oral Surg Oral Med Oral Pathol Oral Radiol Endod*, 88(4), 444–50.

46 Elad S, Or R, Shapira MY, et al. (2003). CO2 laser in oral graft-versus-host disease: a pilot study. *Bone Marrow Transplant*, 32(10), 1031–4.

47 DeRossi SS, Garfunkel AA, Greenberg MS (2003). *Hematologic diseases*, 10th edn. BC Decker Inc, Hamilton.

48 Chaushu G, Itzkovitz-Chaushu S, Yefenof E, Slavin S, Or R, Garfunkel AA (1995). A longitudinal follow-up of salivary secretion in bone marrow transplant patients. *Oral Surg Oral Med Oral Pathol Oral Radiol Endod*, 79(2), 164–9.

49 Lockhart PB, Sonis ST (1981). Alterations in the oral mucosa caused by chemotherapeutic agents. A histologic study. *J Dermatol Surg Oncol*, 7(12), 1019–25.

50 Schubert MM, Izutsu KT (1987). Iatrogenic causes of salivary gland dysfunction. *J Dent Res*, 66 (Spec Iss), 680–8.

51 Nagler R, Marmary Y, Krausz Y, Chisin R, Markitziu A, Nagler A (1996). Major salivary gland dysfunction in human acute and chronic graft-versus-host disease (GVHD). *Bone Marrow Transplant*, 17(2), 219–24.

52 Izutsu KT, Menard TW, Schubert MM, et al. (1985). Graft versus host disease-related secretory immunoglobulin A deficiency in bone marrow transplant recipients. Findings in labial saliva. *Lab Invest*, 52(3), 292–7.

53 Hiroki A, Nakamura S, Shinohara M, Oka M (1994). Significance of oral examination in chronic graft-versus-host disease. *J Oral Pathol Med*, 23(5), 209–15.

54 Nagler RM, Laufer D, Nagler A (1996). Parotid gland dysfunction in an animal model of chronic graft-vs-host disease. *Arch Otolaryngol Head Neck Surg*, 122(10), 1057–60.

55 Nagler RM, Nagler A (2001). The effect of pilocarpine on salivary constituents in patients with chronic graft-versus-host disease. *Arch Oral Biol*, 46(8), 689–95.

56 Alborghetti MR, Correa ME, Adam RL, et al. (2005). Late effects of chronic graft-vs.-host disease in minor salivary glands. *J Oral Pathol Med*, 34(8), 486–93.

57 Nagler RM, Nagler A (2004). The molecular basis of salivary gland involvement in graft-vs.-host disease. *J Dent Res*, 83(2), 98–103.

58 Izutsu KT, Sullivan KM, Schubert MM, et al. (1983). Disordered salivary immunoglobulin secretion and sodium transport in human chronic graft-versus-host disease. *Transplantation*, 35(5), 441–6.

59 Guggenheimer J, Moore PA (2003). Xerostomia: etiology, recognition and treatment. *J Am Dent Assoc*, 134(1), 61–9.

60 Singhal S, Mehta J, Rattenbury H, Treleaven J, Powles R (1995). Oral pilocarpine hydrochloride for the treatment of refractory xerostomia associated with chronic graft-versus-host disease. *Blood*, 85(4), 1147–8.

61 Atkinson JC, Grisius M, Massey W (2005). Salivary hypofunction and xerostomia: diagnosis and treatment. *Dent Clin North Am*, 49(2), 309–26.

62 Dahllof G, Krekmanova L, Kopp S, Borgstrom B, Forsberg CM, Ringden O (1994). Craniomandibular dysfunction in children treated with total-body irradiation and bone marrow transplantation. *Acta Odontol Scand*, 52(2), 99–105.

63 Mattsson T, Arvidson K, Heimdahl A, Ljungman P, Dahllof G, Ringden O (1992). Alterations in taste acuity associated with allogeneic bone marrow transplantation. *J Oral Pathol* Med, 21(1), 33–7.

64 Benoliel R, Epstein J, Eliav E, Jurevic R, Elad S (2007). Orofacial pain in cancer: part I -mechanisms. *J Dent Res*, 86(6), 491–505.

65 Dobr T, Passweg J, Weber C, et al. (2007). Oral health risks associated with HLA-types of patients undergoing hematopoietic stem cell transplantation. *Eur J Haematol*, 78(6), 495–9.

66 Pattni R, Walsh LJ, Marshall RI, Cullinan MP, Seymour GJ, Bartold PM (2000). Changes in the periodontal status of patients undergoing bone marrow transplantation. *J Periodontol*, 71(3), 394–402.

67 Donnelly JP, Muus P, Horrevorts AM, Sauerwein RW, De Pauw BE (1993). Failure of clindamycin to influence the course of severe oromucositis associated with streptococcal bacteraemia in allogeneic bone marrow transplant recipients. *Scand J Infect Dis*, 25(1), 43–50.

68 Raber-Durlacher JE, Epstein JB, Raber J, et al. (2002). Periodontal infection in cancer patients treated with high-dose chemotherapy. *Support Care Cancer*, 10(6), 466–73.

69 Witherspoon RP, Fisher LD, Schoch G, et al. (1989). Secondary cancers after bone marrow transplantation for leukemia or aplastic anemia. *N Engl J Med*, 321(12), 784–9.

70 Bhatia S, Ramsay NK, Steinbuch M, et al. (1996). Malignant neoplasms following bone marrow transplantation. *Blood*, 87(9), 3633–9.

71 Demarosi F, Lodi G, Carrassi A, Soligo D, Sardella A (2005). Oral malignancies following HSCT: graft versus host disease and other risk factors. *Oral Oncol*, 41(9), 865–77.

72 Deeg HJ, Socie G, Schoch G, et al. (1996). Malignancies after marrow transplantation for aplastic anemia and fanconi anemia: a joint Seattle and Paris analysis of results in 700 patients. *Blood*, 87(1), 386–92.

73 Harris NL, Swerdlow SH, Frizzera G, Knowles DM (2001). *World Health Organization Classification of Tumours: Pathology & Genetics. Tumours of Haematopoietic and Lymphoid Tissues.* IARC press, Lyon.

74 Micallef IN, Chhanabhai M, Gascoyne RD, et al. (1998). Lymphoproliferative disorders following allogeneic bone marrow transplantation: the Vancouver experience. *Bone Marrow Transplant*, 22(10), 981–7.

75 Loren AW, Porter DL, Stadtmauer EA, Tsai DE (2003). Post-transplant lymphoproliferative disorder: a review. *Bone Marrow Transplant*, 31(3), 145–55.

76 Elad S, Meyerowitz C, Shapira MY, Glick M, Bitan M, Amir G (2008). Oral posttransplantation lymphoproliferative disorder: an uncommon site for an uncommon disorder. *Oral Surg Oral Med Oral Pathol Oral Radiol Endod*, 105(1), 59–64.

77 Raut A, Huryn J, Pollack A, Zlotolow I (2000). Unusual gingival presentation of post-transplantation lymphoproliferative disorder: a case report and review of the literature. Oral Surg *Oral Med Oral Pathol Oral Radiol Endod*, 90(4), 436–41.

78 Nasman M, Bjork O, Soderhall S, Ringden O, Dahllof G (1994). Disturbances in the oral cavity in pediatric long-term survivors after different forms of antineoplastic therapy. *Pediatr Dent*, 16(3), 217–23.

79 Vaughan MD, Rowland CC, Tong X, et al. (2005). Dental abnormalities after pediatric bone marrow transplantation. *Bone Marrow Transplant*, 36(8), 725–9.

80 National Cancer Institute (2008). Oral complications of chemotherapy and head/neck radiation. Health Professional Version. Available from NCI website: http://www.cancer.gov/cancertopics/pdq/supportivecare/oralcomplications/healthprofessional

Chapter 15

Oral mucositis

Stephen Sonis and Nathaniel Treister

Introduction

Mucositis is one of the most common, debilitating, and disruptive toxicities of chemotherapy and radiation therapy (radiotherapy) used for the treatment of malignant disease. Whilst mucositis may occur in virtually any segment of the gastrointestinal tract, it has been best documented and studied in its oral manifestation.

Epidemiology

Oral mucositis will affect approximately 450 000 patients, this year, in the United States [1]. One can only speculate on its worldwide incidence.

It is highly likely that the incidence of mucositis has been under-reported. This has occurred for a number of reasons, but one of the most significant is the fact that most incidence figures are based on the reporting of mucositis as an adverse event (toxicity) in studies evaluating the efficacy of a cancer treatment. Similar to other toxicities, when mucositis is not the focus of the investigation, the rigour with which it is pursued is somewhat diluted. A comparison of similar patient cohorts in which mucositis is the focus of the study, or where it is simply reported as an adverse event, illustrates this point clearly as the difference in rate is markedly higher in focused studies.

Incidence data based on large databases is often derived from International Classification of Diseases (ICD-9) codes. This not only depends on accurate coding, but also assumes that the individual making the diagnosis is correct. Mucositis was only assigned an ICD-9 code recently, and previously it was often assigned to categories such as candidiasis, viral infection, or non-specific stomatitis. Thus, a recent study in patients with colorectal cancer demonstrated that the incidence of mucositis is markedly higher than was previously thought [2]. Additional prospective studies in which diagnostic criteria are clearly established are necessary to accurately quantify the frequency with which the condition occurs.

Aetiology

The incidence and risk of mucositis is not the same for all cancer patients [1]. A number of factors govern its frequency, including the location and type of cancer, treatment choice, and factors associated with the patient including age, gender, and genetics (Table 15.1).

Patients receiving radiation treatment which includes sites within the oral cavity or oropharynx uniformly develop mucositis. While the frequency is less, mucositis is a common event in patients receiving treatment for cancers of the salivary glands, nasopharynx, hypopharynx, and larynx. In fact, the frequency of patient-reported mouth pain is no different in patients being treated for cancers of the hypopharynx or larynx than those being irradiated for cancers of the mouth or oropharynx [3].

Table 15.1 The risk of oral mucositis among newly diagnosed cancer patients

Risk of oral mucositis	Cancer treatment	Cancer patients
Significant risk (>50% patients will develop oral mucositis)	Patients receiving radiotherapy to head and neck area; some conditioning regimens for HSCT*; induction chemotherapy for acute leukaemia	8% newly diagnosed cancer patients (~112,000 patients in United States)
Some risk (<50% patients will develop oral mucositis)	Many chemotherapy regimens	49% newly diagnosed cancer patients (~651,000 patients in United States)
Little or no risk	Patients receiving surgery; patients receiving radiotherapy to non- head and neck areas; some chemotherapy regimens (non-stomatotoxic; low dose)	43% newly diagnosed cancer patients (~571,000 patients in United States)

* HSCT – haematopoietic stem cell transplant

Mucositis is commonly reported as a consequence of conditioning regimens administered prior to haematopoietic stem cell transplantation. However, the frequency with which mucositis occurs in this setting varies widely, and is largely dependent on the stomatotoxicity of the conditioning regimen used. In general, the incidence and severity of oral mucositis is increased amongst patients receiving total body irradiation. For example, in an intervention study in which palifermin was studied as a therapy for mucositis, virtually every patient in the placebo group developed World Health Organization (WHO) grade 3 or 4 mucositis in response to a conditioning regimen consisting of cyclophosphamide and total body irradiation (TBI) [4]. In contrast, in the absence of TBI, severe mucositis incidence can be as low as 27%[1]. The choice of chemotherapy used is also a driver of mucositis risk. Thus, the risk of mucositis amongst multiple myeloma patients who receive high-dose melphalan (200mg/m^2) is in excess of 50% [5].

The reported frequency of ulcerative mucositis in the largest groups of cancer patients – those being treated with cycled chemotherapy for solid cancers of the breast, colon, and rectum – is a function of the drugs used, the treatment schedule, and the cycle of treatment. While patients treated with the most popular chemotherapy courses for these diseases (AC+T for breast cancer and FOLFOX for colorectal cancer) have a risk of ulcerative mucositis in cycle 1 of about 20% or less, the risk goes up significantly in subsequent cycles amongst developers of ulceration during the first cycle [6]. Thus, a patient who develops mucositis in cycle 1 is approximately 4 times more likely to develop mucositis in cycle 2 than their non-mucositis counterpart. In general, mucositis risk increases with chemotherapy dose and duration of administration. Hence, infusion of 5-fluorouracil (5-FU) over a number of days for the treatment of colorectal cancer is far more likely to cause mucositis than a more acute infusion. This observation has, in fact, led to modifications in 5-FU dosing regimens.

The impact of a patient's age on mucositis risk is unclear as data are inconsistent, and hard to evaluate as childhood cancers and treatments are not equivalent to those received by adults. Nonetheless, it appears that children receiving haematopoietic stem cell transplant-conditioning regimens that include TBI are at slightly lower risk (42%) of developing mucositis compared to adults who receive TBI (64%)[7]. Women treated with 5-FU are at higher risk of developing oral mucositis than are their male counterparts.[8] Although the reason for this observation is unclear, it is consistent with an increased risk of females to other 5-FU-associated toxicities [9]. It may be that the most important risk factors are genetically related (Table 15.2). Other potential risk factors include nutritional status, salivary function, and concomitant systemic disease.

Table 15.2 The hypothetical role of genetics in oral mucositis

Observations suggesting genetic basis for toxicity	Potential genetic determinants of toxicity
◆ High inter-patient variability in response to many forms of chemotherapy	◆ Drug metabolism
	◆ Direct cell response to drug
◆ Toxicity in the first cycle is often followed by toxicity in subsequent cycles despite dose de-escalation	◆ Bystander biological targets of drug
◆ Metabolic and mechanistic determinants of toxicity are genetically controlled	

Pathophysiology

Mucositis is the consequence of a complex series of biological events that ultimately induce damage or apoptosis to the basal stem cells of the epithelium[10]. This seminal concept of mucositis development contrasts sharply with the historic concept that mucositis developed as a result of direct cell injury by radiation or chemotherapy.

Mucositis develops through a series of overlapping/integrated events that have been packaged, for the sake of convenience, into five phases or steps (Figure 15.1, see colour plate section)[11]. The first phase ('initiation') occurs immediately following tissue exposure to radiation or chemotherapy, and is characterized by two events: (1) DNA strand breaks within cells of the epithelium; and (2) the generation of reactive oxygen species. The DNA strand breaks result in immediate injury and death of the affected cells, while the reactive oxygen species serve as important initiators and mediators of downstream biological events. Importantly, it is injury to cells of the submucosa, which ultimately plays the biggest role in regimen-related mucositis.

It is during the second phase ('primary damage response') when the consequences of the initiation phase activate a host of biological mediators and controllers. DNA strand breaks trigger transduction pathways that lead to the activation of several transcription factors, including p53 and nuclear factor kappa-B (NF-κB). NF-κB serves as a controller for the expression of a broad range of genes, which subsequently results in the release of a series of mediators, including pro-inflammatory cytokines and both pro- and anti-apoptotic cellular changes. Other pathways are also activated during this phase including the ceramide pathway – through the activation of sphingomyelinase and ceramide synthase – which results in tissue injury. Breakup of fibronectin in the connective tissue of the submucosa leads to the production of a series of damaging matrix metalloproteinase enzymes. These changes are seen in the cells and tissues of the submucosa causing injury below the epithelium, but also damaging the epithelium. It is important to note that these changes occur very soon after radiation or chemotherapy is administered and that, despite the physiological *mêlée* that is occurring beneath the epithelium, the mucosa appears clinically healthy during this phase.

During the signal amplification phase (phase III) pro-inflammatory cytokines provide positive feedback to augment and accelerate the process of injury. As a consequence of the continued biological barrage that targets the cells and tissues of the submucosa and mucosa, the epithelium breaks down and ulceration occurs. The ulceration phase of mucositis (phase IV) is the most symptomatic stage. Once ulceration occurs, it is not unusual for the surface to become secondarily colonized by bacteria. Bacterial cell wall products enter the submucosa, and stimulate the accumulating population of macrophages to secrete additional amounts of pro-inflammatory cytokines.

In the majority of cases, mucositis healing occurs spontaneously. During the healing stage (phase V), signals from the connective tissue to the bordering epithelium stimulate migration, proliferation, and differentiation of cells to result in a healed mucosa that is devoid of scarring.

Clinical features

Whether induced by chemotherapy or radiation, mucositis generally develops in a predictable sequence that presents as erythema, atrophy, ulceration, and healing [12]. For patients receiving radiation therapy to treat tumours of the head and neck, the initial clinical signs of mucositis occur with cumulative radiation doses as low as 10 Gy, and consist of mucosal erythema, superficial sloughing, and discomfort. Although the mucosa is intact at this stage, it is not uncommon for patients to complain of mucosal burning analogous to pain associated with a food or chemical burn. By cumulative radiation doses of 20 Gy–30 Gy (usually occurring between the second and 3rd week of treatment in a typical radiation schedule), the intact mucosa starts to break down and ulceration occurs (Figure 15.2, see colour plate section)[13]. No site in the mouth is immune to the effects of radiation-induced injury, but the most reported areas for lesions are the buccal and lingual mucosae, floor of the mouth, and soft palate. At this stage, mucositis appears as a penetrating ulcerative lesion with uneven borders. A pseudomembrane consisting of necrotic tissue laden with bacteria often covers the ulceration. This phase is characterized by severe pain often requiring opioid analgesia and resulting in patient's inability to eat normally. This severe phase of mucositis typically persists for up to 3 weeks following the completion of the radiation course.

Ulcerative mucositis induced by chemotherapy tends to have a more acute course and begins within days of drug infusion [14]. Initial changes in the oral mucosa are noted within 5 days of chemotherapy administration. Painful ulceration is usually apparent by day 7. Lesions can involve any area of the movable oral mucosa; the more heavily keratinized areas such as the hard palate, dorsal tongue, and gingiva are spared. This site distribution is important and, often, helpful in differentiating mucositis from lesions of infectious origin such as candidiasis or viral infections. As with radiation-induced mucositis, mucosal injury caused by chemotherapy is extremely painful and requires opioids for reasonable control. The ulcerative phase lasts for about a week to 10 days and, in most cases, goes on to heal spontaneously by 3 weeks of its origin.

Mucositis often causes intolerable pain. Indeed, amongst patients who receive myeloablative chemotherapy regimens or radiation to the head and neck, mucositis is often recalled as the worst side effect of treatment [15]. The pain associated with mucositis often results in patients not being able to tolerate any foods by mouth, whether in liquid or solid form. Consequently, it is a driver of alternative nutritional supplement use. For patients being treated for cancers of the head and neck, mucositis is so predictable and of such severity that many institutions place gastrostomy tubes prophylactically so that patients can be tube fed once mucositis develops[16]. Aside from being a driver of non-oral feeding, mucositis is a common reason why patients seek unscheduled medical care, either in the form of office visits or visits to the emergency room (and may result in patients being hospitalized). For patients hospitalized for their care and, in particular, patients receiving haematopoietic stem cell transplants, mucositis extends hospital stays. As a result, the cost for patients who develop mucositis is higher than for patients who avoid the condition.

Aside from its symptomatic costs, mucositis contributes to patient morbidity and mortality. The mouth is richly colonized by a range of microorganisms including bacteria, fungi, and viruses. In the healthy individual, these organisms are maintained in the mouth by the intact epithelial barrier of the mucosa, and controlled by the interaction of salivary, humoral, and cellular immune systems. Amongst patients receiving myeloablative therapy, the bone marrow's ability to replenish white cells is reduced or eliminated. Consequently, patients no longer have the ability to effectively deal with potentially infective agents[17]. The nadir of patients' white blood count usually coincides with the breakdown of the oral mucosa. The damaged mucosa becomes a portal of systemic entry for oral bacteria that can then enter the bloodstream. In fact, the mouth is the most identifiable site for bacteraemias in granulocytopaenic cancer patients [18].

A number of grading/scoring systems have been developed for oral mucositis[19], and Box 15.1, shows some of those used more commonly in clinical practice [20].

Management

In an effort to optimize treatment, the Mucositis Study Section of the Multinational Association of Supportive Care in Cancer has published clinical practice guidelines for the prevention and treatment of mucositis (Box 15.2) [5]. The guidelines are evidence-based and follow the format described for other forms of oncological treatment. The recommendations demonstrate the relative paucity of mucositis interventions that are clinically available. Importantly, the guidelines do speak to a variety of treatments that have arisen as a function of 'folklore' rather than rigorous clinical studies. The National Comprehensive Cancer Network also created a taskforce, which recently published their report on the prevention and treatment of mucositis [21]. Not surprisingly, the conclusions of both panels were similar in nature.

There seems to be consensus that mucositis management should involve a defined preventative oral care regimen that includes aggressive oral hygiene procedures (brushing, flossing, and use of bland rinses). These measures are not to prevent mucositis *per se*, but to ensure that the oral

---

Box 15.1 Selected mucositis grading/scoring systems

World Health Organization:

Grade 0 No signs or symptoms
Grade 1 Mild soreness or painless ulcers with oedema or erythema
Grade 2 Pain, erythema, ulcers, ability to eat solids
Grade 3 Pain, erythema, ulcers, requires soft or liquid diet
Grade 4 Alimentation not possible

National Cancer Institute Common Terminology Criteria for Adverse Events (CTCAE) version 3: Mucositis (clinical exam):

Grade 1 Erythema of the mucosa
Grade 2 Patchy ulcerations or pseudomembranes
Grade 3 Confluent ulcerations or pseudomenbranes; bleeding with minor trauma
Grade 4 Tissue necrosis; significant spontaneous bleeding; life-threatening consequences
Grade 5 Death

National Cancer Institute Common Terminology Criteria for Adverse Events (CTCAE) version 3: Mucositis (functional/symptomatic):

Grade 1 Minimal symptoms, normal diet
Grade 2 Symptomatic but can eat and swallow modified diet
Grade 3 Symptomatic and unable to adequately aliment or hydrate orally
Grade 4 Symptoms associated with life-threatening consequences
Grade 5 Death

Box 15.2 Summary of the MASCC clinical practice guidelines on the management of oral mucositis [5].

Basic oral care and good clinical practices

♦ The panel suggests multidisciplinary development and evaluation of oral care protocols, and patient and staff education in the use of such protocols to reduce the severity of oral mucositis from chemotherapy and/or radiation therapy. As part of the protocols, the panel suggests the use of a soft toothbrush that is replaced on a regular basis. Elements of good clinical practice should include the use of validated tools to regularly assess oral pain and oral cavity health. The inclusion of dental professionals is vital throughout the treatment and follow-up phases.

♦ The panel recommends patient-controlled analgesia with morphine as the treatment of choice for oral mucositis pain in patients undergoing HSCT. Regular oral pain assessment using validated instruments for self-reporting is essential.

Radiotherapy: prevention

♦ The panel recommends the use of midline radiation blocks and 3-dimensional radiation treatment to reduce mucosal injury.

♦ The panel recommends benzydamine for prevention of radiation-induced mucositis in patients with head and neck cancer receiving moderate-dose radiation therapy.

♦ The panel recommends that chlorhexidine not be used to prevent oral mucositis in patients with solid tumours of the head and neck who are undergoing radiotherapy.

♦ The panel recommends that antimicrobial lozenges not be used for the prevention of radiation-induced oral mucositis.

Radiotherapy: treatment

♦ The panel recommends that sucralfate not be used for the treatment of radiation-induced oral mucositis.

Standard-dose chemotherapy: prevention

♦ The panel recommends that patients receiving bolus 5-FU chemotherapy undergo 30min of oral cryotherapy to prevent oral mucositis.

♦ The panel suggests the use of 20–30min of oral cryotherapy to decrease mucositis in patients treated with bolus doses of edatrexate.

♦ The panel recommends that acyclovir and its analogues not be used routinely to prevent mucositis.

Standard-dose chemotherapy: treatment

♦ The panel recommends that chlorhexidine not be used to treat established oral mucositis.

High-dose chemotherapy with or without total body irradiation plus HCST: prevention

♦ In patients with hematologic malignancies who are receiving high-dose chemotherapy and total body irradiation with autologous stem cell transplantation, the panel recommends the use of keratinocyte growth factor-1 (palifermin) in a dose of 60 µg/kg per day for 3 days prior to conditioning treatment and for 3 days post transplantation for the prevention of oral mucositis.

♦ The panel suggests the use of cryotherapy to prevent oral mucositis in patients receiving high-dose melphalan.

♦ The panel doses not recommend the use of pentoxifylline to prevent mucositis in patients undergoing HSCT.

♦ The panel suggests that GM-CSF mouthwashes not be used for the prevention of oral mucositis in patients undergoing HSCT.

♦ The panel suggests the use of LLLT to reduce the incidence of oral mucositis and its associated pain in patients receiving high-dose chemotherapy or chemoradiotherapy before HSCT if the treatment centre is able to support the necessary technology and training.

HSCT = haematopoietic stem cell transplantation
5-FU = 5 fluorouracil
GM-CSF = granulocyte macrophage colony stimulating factor
LLLT = low-level laser therapy

---

cavity is maintained as clean and healthy as possible in the event that ulceration does occur. Oral hygiene is discussed in detail in Chapter 5.

Palifermin is a keratinocyte growth factor (KGF1) that is approved in the United States for the prevention of mucositis in patients with haematological malignancies who are receiving stomatotoxic conditioning regimens followed by a haematopoietic stem cell transplantation. Palifermin is given in a six-dose regimen, with three doses being given prior to the start of conditioning, and three more doses administered starting on the day of stem cell infusion. Palifermin, which is administered intravenously, successfully reduces the incidence and duration of severe mucositis [4]. This is most likely due to a combination of modulation of some of the mediators of mucositis, as well as direct stimulation of basal keratinocytes resulting in tissue regeneration [22].

Cryotherapy, in the form of ice chips, has been shown to favourably alter the incidence of severe oral mucositis associated with high dose melphalan infusion (and represents a safe and very cost-effective intervention). Patients should be instructed to hold ice chips in the mouth starting about 30 min prior to the infusion, during the infusion, and then for several hours afterwards [23]. Localized vasoconstriction physically prevents the chemotherapy from reaching the oral tissues. This is, therefore, only useful during short infusions with agents that are rapidly cleared from the body (e.g. bolus 5FU, bolus edatrexate)[5].

Mucositis is painful. Symptom control is a major goal of treatment, and remains the mainstay of mucositis management. For less severe mucositis, topical agents including bland rinses, or those containing topical anaesthetics (such as viscous xylocaine), or diphenhydramine may be helpful. However, more aggressive pain management is often required. The use of systemic analgesics of increasing strengths at adequate dosing levels should be prescribed. The WHO pain/ analgesic ladder is an excellent guide (see Chapter 24). In general, regular dosing of analgesics is more efficacious than waiting until the pain level requires intervention. For patients receiving opioid analgesics, attention should be paid to the prevention of constipation.

Mucositis is not an infectious disease. Consequently, antibiotics, antifungals, and antivirals are not recommended as mucositis interventions. However, especially in the myelosuppressed patient, simultaneous infections may occur and the clinician must be vigilant for their development.

The lack of an easily available, cost-effective, efficacious treatment for mucositis has been a source of frustration for healthcare providers and patients. A number of agents, approved as medical devices, have been marketed as mucositis treatments. Unlike pharmaceuticals or biologicals, the threshold for device approval is generally not rigorous. Consequently, efficacy data derived from multi-centre, randomized, placebo-controlled double-blind studies is, for the most part, non-existent for these products. While it is possible that patients might benefit from their use, it is impossible to recommend their application (at significant cost) based on the available anecdotal data.

References

1   Sonis ST, Elting LS, Keefe D, et al. (2004). Perspectives on cancer therapy-induced mucosal injury: pathogenesis, measurement, epidemiology, and consequences for patients. *Cancer*, 100(9 Suppl), 1995–2025.

2   Grunberg S, Hesketh P, Randolph-Jackson P, et al. (2007). Risk and quality of life impact of mucosal injury among colorectal cancer patients receiving FOLFOX chemotherapy [abstract P-50]. *Supportive Care Cancer* 15(6), 704.

3   Elting LS, Keefe DM, Sonis ST, et al. (2008). Patient-reported measurements of oral mucositis in head and neck cancer patients treated with radiotherapy with or without chemotherapy: demonstration of increased frequency, severity, resistance to palliation and on quality of life. *Cancer*, 113, 2704–2713.

4   Spielberger R, Stiff P, Bensinger W, et al. (2004). Palifermin for oral mucositis after intensive therapy for hematologic cancers. *N Engl J Med*, 351(25), 2590–8.

5   Keefe DM, Schubert MM, Elting LS, et al. (2007). Updated clinical practice guidelines for the prevention and treatment of mucositis. *Cancer*, 109(5), 820–31.

6   Sonis ST. Personal communication.

7   Tomlinson D, Judd P, Hendershot E, et al. (2007). Measurement of oral mucositis in children: a review of the literature. *Support Care Cancer*, 15, 1251–1258.

8   Chansky K, Benedetti J, Macdonald JS (2005). Differences in toxicity between men and women treated with 5-fluorouracil therapy for colorectal carcinoma. *Cancer*, 103(6), 1165–71.

9   Sloan JA, Goldberg RM, Sargent DJ, et al. (2002). Women experience greater toxicity with fluorouracil-based chemotherapy for colorectal cancer. *J Clin Oncol*, 20(6), 1491–8.

10 Sonis ST (2007). Pathobiology of oral mucositis: novel insights and opportunities. *J Support Oncol*, 5(9 Suppl 4), 3–11.

11 Sonis ST (2004). The pathobiology of mucositis. *Nat Rev Cancer*, 4(4), 277–84.

12 Scully C, Epstein J, Sonis S (2003). Oral mucositis: a challenging complication of radiotherapy, chemotherapy, and radiochemotherapy: part 1, pathogenesis and prophylaxis of mucositis. *Head Neck*, 25(12), 1057–70.

13 Bentzen SM, Saunders MI, Dische S, Bond SJ (2001). Radiotherapy-related early morbidity in head and neck cancer: quantitative clinical radiobiology as deduced from the CHART trial. *Radiother Oncol*, 60(2), 123–35.

14 Woo SB, Sonis ST, Monopoli MM, Sonis AL (1993). A longitudinal study of oral ulcerative mucositis in bone marrow transplant recipients. *Cancer*, 72(5) 1612–7.

15 Bellm LA, Epstein JB, Rose-Ped A, Martin P, Fuchs HJ (2008). Patient reports of complications of bone marrow transplantation. *Support Care Cancer*, 8(1), 33–9.

16 Vera-Llonch M, Oster G, Hagiwara M, Sonis S (2006). Oral mucositis in patients undergoing radiation treatment for head and neck carcinoma. *Cancer*, 106(2), 329–36.

17 Ruescher TJ, Sodeifi A, Scrivani SJ, Kaban LB, Sonis ST (1998). The impact of mucositis on alpha-hemolytic streptococcal infection in patients undergoing autologous bone marrow transplantation for hematologic malignancies. *Cancer*, 82(11), 2275–81.

18 Awada A, van der Auwera P, Meunier F, et al. (1992). Streptococcal and enterococcal bacteremia in patients with cancer. *Clin Infect Dis*, 15, 33–48.

19 Quinn B, Potting CM, Stone R, et al. (2008). Guidelines for the assessment of oral mucositis in adult chemotherapy, radiotherapy and haematopoietic stem cell transplant patients. *Eur J Cancer* 44(1), 61–72.

20 National Cancer Institute Common Terminology Criteria for Adverse Events (CTCAE). Available from National Cancer Institute (US National Institutes of Health) website: http://www.cancer.gov/

21 Bensinger W, Schubert M, Ang KK, et al. (2008). NCCN Task Force Report. prevention and management of mucositis in cancer care. *J Natl Compr Canc Netw*, 6(Suppl 1), S1–21.

22 Blijlevens N, Sonis S (2006). Palifermin (recombinant keratinocyte growth factor-1): a pleiotropic growth factor with multiple biological activities in preventing chemotherapy- and radiotherapy-induced mucositis. *Ann Oncol*, 18(5), 817–26.

23 Lilleby K, Garcia P, Gooley T, et al. (2006). A prospective, randomized study of cryotherapy during administration of high-dose melphalan to decrease the severity and duration of oral mucositis in patients with multiple myeloma undergoing autologous peripheral blood stem cell transplantation. *Bone Marrow Transplant*, 37(11), 1031–5.

Chapter 16

Bisphosphonate-related osteonecrosis of the jaws

James Sciubba and Joel Epstein

Introduction

Bisphosphonates are an important class of drugs in the management of bony metastases from solid tumours including breast and prostate cancer, the management of multiple myeloma, and the management of tumour-related hypercalcaemia. Studies in certain subsets of cancer patients have emphasized reductions in skeletal pathology (i.e. bone pain, fracture of long bones, fracture of vertebrae, spinal cord compression), and improvements in quality of life, associated with use of these agents [1,2]. However, there is limited evidence to date demonstrating survival benefit. In addition, millions of patients worldwide are using oral bisphosphonates for the management of conditions such as osteopaenia, osteoporosis, and Paget's disease.

Bisphosphonates inhibit bone resorption via a number of different mechanisms, although the primary mechanism involves the inhibition of osteoclast function [3,4]. Bisphosphonates can inhibit the differentiation of stem cells to osteoclasts, affect the structure and function of osteoclasts, and cause apoptosis of osteoclasts. The latter actions rely on the bisphosphonate being taken up into the osteoclast by a process of endocytosis. Bisphosphonates also affect the interaction between ostoclasts and osteoblasts.

In addition, bisphosphonates can inhibit the growth of tumour cells, stimulate the immune system (against the tumour), and cause of apoptosis of tumour cells [3]. The inhibition of growth is achieved by a reduction in the adhesion of tumour cells to bone, a reduction in the secretion of tumour growth factors into the bone (secondary to a reduction in bone resorption), and an inhibition of tumour angiogenesis. It should be noted that different bisphosphonates have a different range of activities.

In 2003, case reports began to appear of the phenomenon now referred to as bisphosphonate-related osteonecrosis of the jaws (BRON) [5]. Subsequently, larger case series appeared confirming the emergence of this growing clinical problem [5,6]. These reports emphasized the association between the presence of BRON and the use of new-generation/more potent intravenous bisphosphonates (i.e. pamidronate, zoledronate).

Epidemiology

The incidence of BRON is difficult to determine given the likelihood of under-reporting during post-marketing surveillance, and the lack of specific prospective clinical trials. Nevertheless, the increase in the reporting of this condition supports the notion that BRON is not an uncommon phenomenon. Ninety-five percent of cases occur in patients with malignant skeletal disease. (Patients with cancer receive overall doses that are significantly higher than patients with benign conditions; patients with cancer also receive more potent bisphosphonates than patients with benign conditions.)

A large epidemiological study compared proxy measures of BRON in 16 073 cancer patients treated with intravenous bisphosphonates and 28 698 'matched controls' (i.e. cancer patients not treated with bisphosphonates) [7]. The proxy measures were inflammatory conditions, osteomyelitis, and surgery of the jaws/facial bones, and the absolute risk at 6 years for any of these problems was 5.48 events per 100 patients in the treatment group and 0.30 events per 100 patients in the control group.

Data from a Web-based survey of myeloma patients treated with pamidronate and zoledronate found that 6.8% had been diagnosed with BRON, while an additional 5.9% were demonstrating suspicious clinical features [8]. Wang and colleagues noted a 3.8% incidence of jawbone necrosis in a retrospective study of 447 patients treated with pamidronate or zoledronate. They found a 3.8% incidence in myeloma patients and a 3% incidence in those with solid tumours [9]. Investigators reported a 9.9% incidence in myeloma patients, and a 2.9% incidence in breast cancer patients over an 8-year period [10].

Aetiology

A summary of the risk factors for BRON are shown in Table 16.1 [11]. A risk of developing BRON exists with nearly all forms of bisphosphonate, although the degree of risk is especially dependent on the potency of the bisphosphonate, the route of administration, and the duration of treatment.

Potency of Bisphosphonate

BRON is particularly associated with the use of the potent bisphosphonates pamidronate and zoledronate. Pamidronate is 10 times more potent than clodronate, and zoledronate 10 000 times

Table 16.1a Risk factors for bisphosphonate-related osteonecrosis of the jaws (BRON) [11]

Category	Specific factors	Comments
Drug-related factors	Potency of bisphosphonate	Potent bisphosphonates are associated with an increased risk
	Route of administration	The risk is greater with the intravenous route of administration
	Duration of treatment	The risk is greater with a longer duration of treatment
Oral cavity-related factors	Dentoalveolar surgery (e.g. extractions, dental implant placement, periapical surgery, periodontal surgery involving osseous injury)	Patients that have dentoalveolar surgery have at least a seven times greater risk of developing BRON than patients that do not have such surgery
	Anatomical variations of mandible (e.g. lingual tori, mylohyoid ridge), or maxilla (e.g. palatal tori)	BRON is more likely to develop in patients with bony prominences with thin overlying mucosa
	Inflammatory dental disease (e.g. periodontal disease, dental abscess)	Patients that have inflammatory dental disease have a seven times greater risk of developing BRON than patients that do not have such disease
	Poor oral hygiene	Poor oral hygiene is thought to be a risk factor, although this needs to be confirmed by further studies

Table 16.1b Risk factors for bisphosphonate-related osteonecrosis of the jaws (BRON) [11]

Category	Specific factors	Comments
Demographic factors	Age	The risk is greater in older patients (in patients with myeloma treated with intravenous bisphosphonates)
	Ethnic origin	The risk is greater in patients of Caucasian origin
Systemic factors	Cancer diagnosis	Patients with myeloma are more likely to develop BRON than patients with breast cancer, who in turn are more likely to develop BRON than patients with other types of cancer
	Chemotherapy	Chemotherapy is thought to be a risk factor, although this needs to be confirmed by further studies
	Osteopenia/ osteoporosis	
	Corticosteroids	Corticosteroids are thought to be a risk factor, although this needs to be confirmed by further studies
	Diabetes	As above
	Smoking tobacco	As above
	Drinking alcohol	As above

more potent than clodronate (in terms of osteoclast inhibition) [12]. The frequency of BRON is higher with intravenous zoledronate than with any other form/type of bisphosphonate.

The mean time to developing BRON varies with the potency of the bisphosphonate, with a mean time of onset of 18 months with zoledronate versus 6 years with pamidronate (at the usual frequency of administration).[8] In another study, where 303 myeloma patients were receiving zoledronate, a 2-year time span was stated as a threshold for the development of clinical problems [13].

Route of Administration

The risk of BRON is much lower with oral bisphosphonates. Grbic and others conducted a 3-year prospective follow-up of 7714 women receiving bisphosphonates for post-menopausal osteoporosis, and only identified two cases of necrosis during this period [14].

Interestingly, an assessment of 714 217 medical claims for surrogates of necrosis of the jaws (pain and bone exposure) found no increase in risk with use of oral bisphosphonates, but a significant increase in risk with use of intravenous preparations (i.e. 4.0- to 6.8-fold increased risk) [15].

It should be noted that the level of risk for development of BRON for patients taking typical oral bisphosphonates for the management of osteopaenia, osteoporosis, and Paget's disease is very low. Indeed, the risk of developing BRON is so minimal that it has been suggested that systematic screening/prevention programmes, and the withholding of routine dental procedures, is not justified (see below) [16]. For example, the estimated of risk of developing BRON in association with oral alendronate administration is only 0.007% [17].

Duration of treatment

The duration of bisphosphonate administration is also of great importance with regard to risk potential. Thus, the level of risk may increase to 4% at 3–4 years, 6% at 4–5 years, 9% at 5–6 years, and 11% beyond 6 years of exposure[18].

Other factors

As discussed above, the main effect of bisphosphonates is the inhibition of osteoclast function. However, the anti-angiogenic properties of these agents contribute to their effect on bone metabolism, and so contribute to the evolution of the osteonecrosis. The predilection of this problem to affect the maxilla and mandible may involve several factors, but undoubtedly relates to the particularly high rate of alveolar bone turnover or metabolism in relation to bone at other anatomic sites. Indeed, it has been estimated that there is a 10-fold increase in the level of activity in this segment of the jaws. Other local predisposing factors include the performance of dentoalveolar surgery, and the presence of inflammatory dental disease (e.g. periodontal disease, dental abscess)[11].

Clinical features

The diagnosis of BRON relies upon having all of the following three clinical factors [11]:

1. Current or previous treatment with a bisphosphonate.

2. Exposed, necrotic bone in the maxillofacial region that has persisted for more than 8 weeks.

3. No history of radiotherapy/radiation therapy to the jaws.

The clinical features of BRON vary from case to case, and are somewhat dependent on the clinical stage of the disease (Table 16.2) [19]. BRON typically presents as a painless area of ulceration with exposed bone. Most cases are noted in the mandible (65%), while 26% cases affect the maxilla, and 9% of cases affect both sites. The onset of problems is preceded by the performance of a dental surgical procedure in 60% of cases, with the remainder of cases believed to result from other types of trauma and/or infection [20]. Sometimes, patients present with deep-seated, difficult-to-localize pain in the absence of exposed bone (or radiographic alterations). However, the presence of pain usually signifies the development of a complication of BRON (i.e. soft-tissue trauma, infection, fracture, or fistula). Other reported clinical features include tooth mobility, inflammation of the area, and altered sensation in the area[19].

The rate of progression of BRON is highly variable, and the condition can be stabilized with appropriate management. The evolution from initial discovery to sequestrum (separated piece of dead bone) formation can be rapid, although a time span of several months is more characteristic when antibiotic intervention is employed. The rate of progression of BRON is probably related to the same drug-related factors responsible for the development of BRON (see above).

Investigations

Imaging is an important component of diagnosing BRON. However, symptoms may presage demonstrable radiographic changes by weeks or months. Healthcare professionals, therefore,

Table 16.2 Clinical staging of bisphosphonate-related osteonecrosis of the jaws [11]

Stage	Clinical features
Stage 1	Exposed/necrotic bone in patients who are asymptomatic and have no evidence of infection
Stage 2	Exposed/necrotic bone associated with infection as evidenced by pain and erythema in the region of the exposed bone with or without purulent drainage
Stage 3	Exposed/necrotic bone in patients with pain, infection, and one or more of the following: pathological fracture, extra-oral fistula, or osteolysis extending to the inferior border

must maintain an index of suspicion in relevant groups of patients. Imaging can also aid in clinical decision-making.

Radiographic imaging, including routine intraoral, panoramic, and computed tomography (CT) images, will show initially subtle, and later more obvious, levels of osseous sclerosis or 'ground glass' appearance (Figure 16.1). The appearances are similar to those seen in benign fibro-osseous lesions of the jaws. The alveolar process is most commonly involved with variable lamina dura thickening or sclerosis. Occasionally, there is sclerosis of the full thickness of the dental alveolus. Less common alterations include poorly healing extraction sockets without evidence of remodelling or fill-in (Figure 16.2), periapical radiolucencies, periodontal membrane space widening, osteolysis, and sequestrum formation [21].

Recently, the usefulness of more sophisticated imaging techniques, including volumetric cone-beam tomography, has been described.[22] Nevertheless, routinely available imaging is usually adequate for defining the typical findings associated with BRON.

Management

Prevention

Prevention should be the primary goal in patients at risk of BRON. The initiation of BRON is often related to routine dentoalveolar surgery such as dental extractions, dental implant placement, and periapical surgery. Thus, the key to the preventive strategy is to establish optimal dental and oral health in anticipation of bisphosphonate treatment, and so to avoid future dentoalveolar surgery during bisphosphonate treatment. It is equally important to maintain optimal dental and oral health during exposure to these agents.

The initiation of bisphosphonate should, whenever possible, be delayed until optimal dental status is achieved. Furthermore, any invasive procedures should be completed in anticipation of treatment. There are no clear guidelines on the healing time required following dentoalveolar surgery (and prior to initiating bisphosphonates). Studies have suggested no increase in risk of

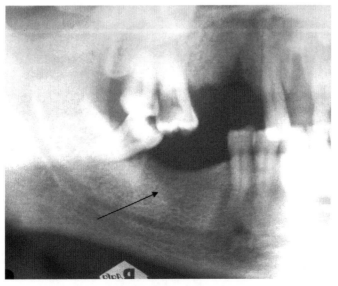

Fig. 16.1 Radiograph showing 'ground glass' appearance.

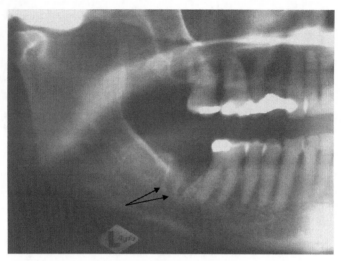

Fig. 16.2 Radiograph showing non-healing extraction socket.

delayed healing for some months following initiation of bisphosphonates, although a waiting time of 4–8 weeks has been suggested in one paper [23].

Patients require appropriate access to their dental providers, and rapid assessment/timely management, should they develop dental and oral problems while on bisphosphonate treatment. It has been suggested that termination of bisphosphonate drugs, assuming other health conditions allow, should occur 3 months prior to and 3 months following necessary dental surgery (although this is not evidence based). However, others experts have not recommended discontinuing bisphosphonates, due to the extended presence of these drugs in the bone (i.e. >10 years).

Management

Management of BRON remains problematic, with no routinely effective strategy currently available. Table 16.3 depicts the stage-specific management strategies recommended by the American Association of Oral and Maxillofacial Surgeons[11].

Chlorhexidine rinses 2–3 times daily is suggested in all stages of BRON. Orally administered antibiotics are advised during periods of active infection (Table 16.3). However, some experts recommend chronic oral antibiotic usage (once active infection is controlled). In cases of advanced BRON where control of bone destruction or infection is not possible, or in cases of pathological fracture, an alveolectomy or resection of affected bone may be necessary. The placement of a titanium reconstruction plate following resolution of the infection permits re-establishment of a normal contour and acceptable levels of function.

The decision concerning continuing/discontinuing bisphosphonates should be made in consultation with the treating medical oncologist. Thus, the significant risks of worsening of skeletal pathology should be balanced against the potential benefits of stabilization/improvement of BRON (Table 16.3). The strategy of 'drug holidays' is extremely questionable given the persistence of these agents once incorporated into bone.

Recently, a new management strategy has been described involving placement of platelet-derived growth factors into the defects created following resection of necrotic alveolar bone[24]. The technique, which was used in a small number of patients, resulted in complete healing of the bone defect in conjunction with mucosal coverage of the defect site.

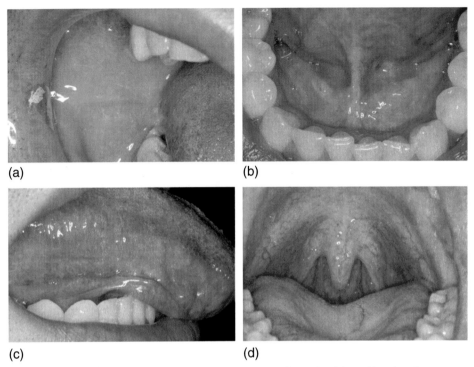

(a) (b)

(c) (d)

Fig. 3.1 Normal appearance of a) buccal mucosa; b) floor of mouth; c) lateral border of tongue; d) dorsal surface tongue, soft palate, and pharynx.

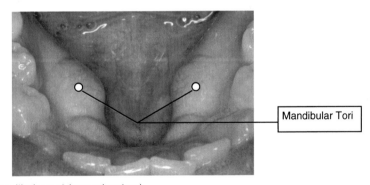

Mandibular Tori

Fig. 3.2 Mandibular tori (normal variant).

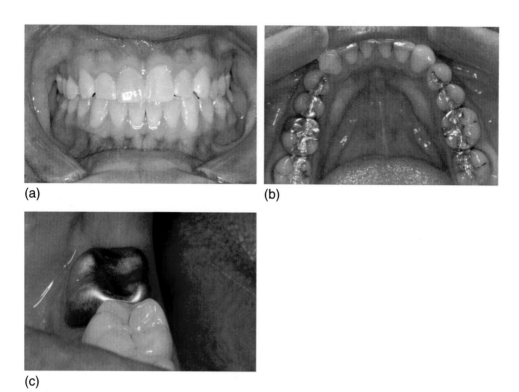

(a)

(b)

(c)

Fig. 3.3 a) Normal appearance of teeth and periodontal tissues; b) example of amalgam restorations; c) example of gold crown.

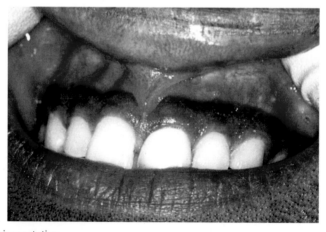

Fig. 4.1 Racial pigmentation.
Source: Reproduced with permission from Davies A and Finlay I (2005), Oral Care in Advanced Disease. Oxford University Press, Oxford

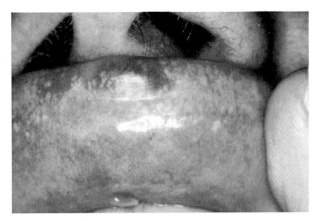

Fig. 4.2 Oral varicosity.
Source: Reproduced with permission from MP Sweeney and J Bagg (1997), Making Sense of the Mouth. Partnership in Oral Care, Glasgow

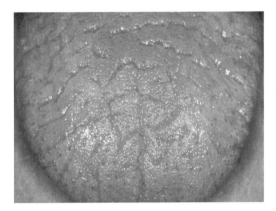

Fig. 4.3 Fissured tongue.
Source: Reproduced with permission from Davies A and Finlay I (2005), Oral Care in Advanced Disease. Oxford University Press, Oxford

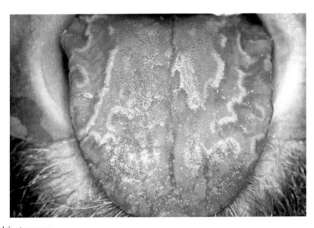

Fig. 4.4 Geographic tongue.
Source: Reproduced with permission from MP Sweeney and J Bagg (1997), Making Sense of the Mouth. Partnership in Oral Care, Glasgow

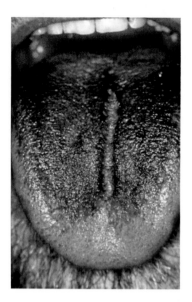

Fig. 4.5 Black hairy tongue.
Source: Reproduced with permission from MP Sweeney and J Bagg (1997), Making Sense of the Mouth. Partnership in Oral Care, Glasgow

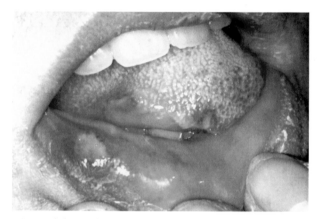

Fig. 4.6 Recurrent minor aphthous ulceration.
Source: Reproduced with permission from Davies A and Finlay I (2005), Oral Care in Advanced Disease. Oxford University Press, Oxford

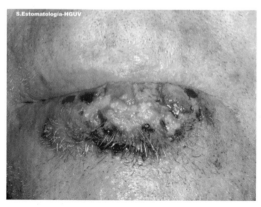

Figure 7.1 Squamous cell carcinoma of lip.

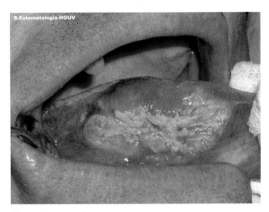

Figure 7.2 Squamous cell carcinoma of tongue.

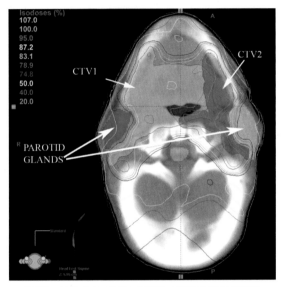

CTV1 - high dose region; CTV2 - elective dose region

Fig. 10.1 Axial image of IMRT plan for a right base of tongue tumour with sparing of both parotid glands.

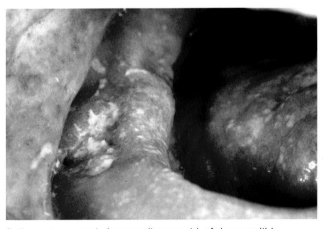

Fig. 12.1 Post-radiation osteonecrosis (osteoradionecrosis) of the mandible.

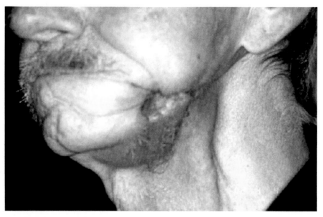

Fig. 12.3 Cutaneous fistula secondary to post-radiation osteonecrosis.
Source: Reproduced with permission from Davies A and Finlay I (2005), Oral Care in Advanced Disease. Oxford University Press, Oxford

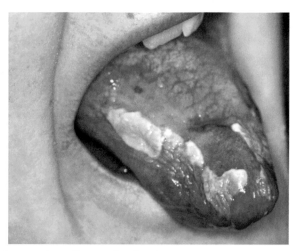

Fig. 14.1 Acute graft-versus-host disease of oral cavity.

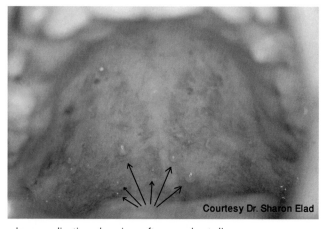

Fig. 14.2 Mucocoeles complicating chronic graft-versus-host disease.

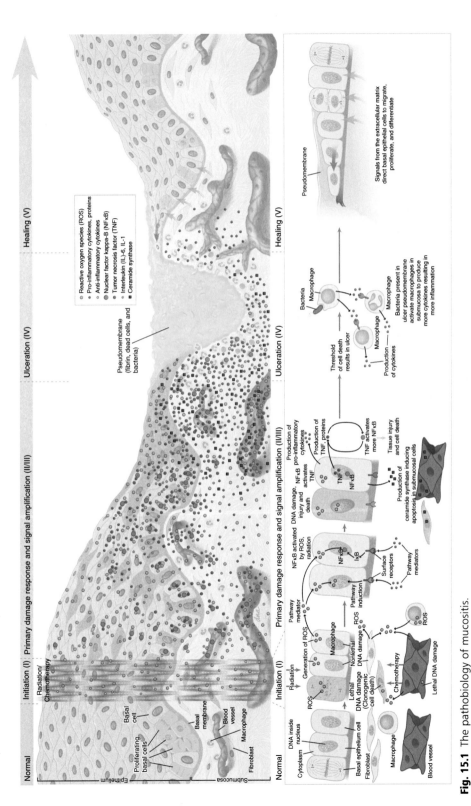

Fig. 15.1 The pathobiology of mucositis.

Source: Reproduced with permission from Sonis ST (2007). Pathobiology of oral mucositis: novel insights and opportunities. J Support Oncol, 5(9 Suppl 4), 3–11

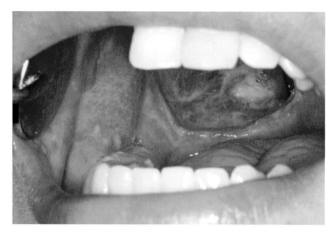

Fig. 15.2 Early mucositis with generalized erythema and spotty ulceration in a patient undergoing radiation therapy for carcinoma of palate.

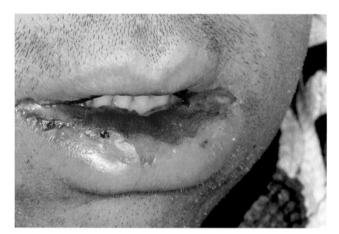

Fig. 15.3 Advanced mucositis with confluent ulceration of the lower lip in a patient undergoing induction chemotherapy for acute lymphoblastic leukaemia (ALL).

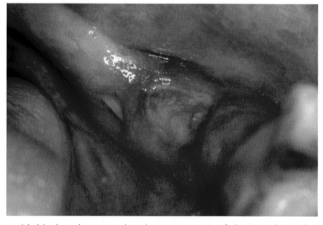

Fig. 16.3a Patient with bisphosphonate-related osteonecrosis of the jaws (BRON) at presentation: clinical photograph shows two sites of exposed alveolar bone (Stage 1 BRON).

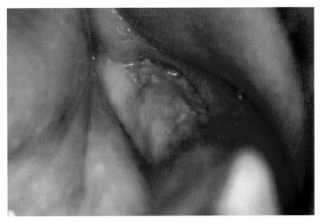

Fig. 16.4a Same patient four months after presentation: clinical photograph shows increased area of exposed alveolar bone.

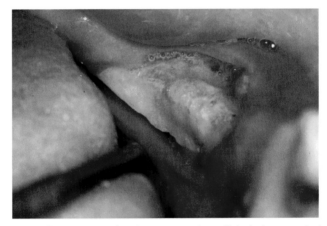

Fig. 16.5a Same patient fourteen months after presentation: clinical photograph shows the sequestrum.

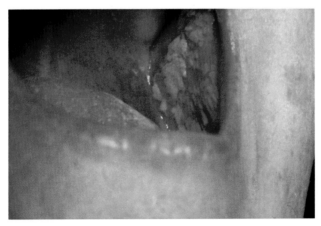

Fig. 18.1 Pseudomembranous candidosis.
Source: Reproduced with permission from Davies A and Finlay I (2005), Oral Care in Advanced Disease. Oxford University Press, Oxford

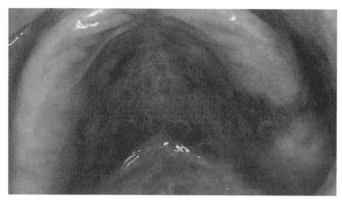

Fig. 18.2 Denture stomatitis.
Source: Reproduced with permission from Davies A and Finlay I (2005), Oral Care in Advanced Disease. Oxford University Press, Oxford

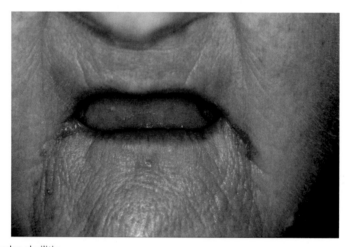

Fig. 18.3 Angular cheilitis.
Source: Reproduced with permission from Davies A and Finlay I (2005), Oral Care in Advanced Disease. Oxford University Press, Oxford

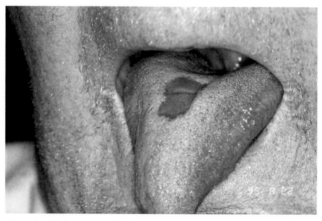

Fig. 18.4 Median rhomboid glossitis.
Source: Reproduced with permission from Davies A and Finlay I (2005), Oral Care in Advanced Disease. Oxford University Press, Oxford

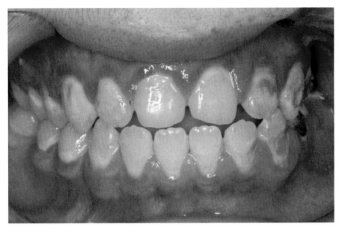

Fig. 19.1 Early dental caries.
Source: Reproduced with permission from Davies A and Finlay I (2005), Oral Care in Advanced Disease. Oxford University Press, Oxford

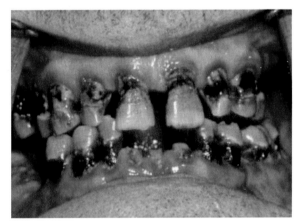

Fig. 19.2 Advanced dental caries.
Source: Reproduced with permission from Davies A and Finlay I (2005), Oral Care in Advanced Disease. Oxford University Press, Oxford

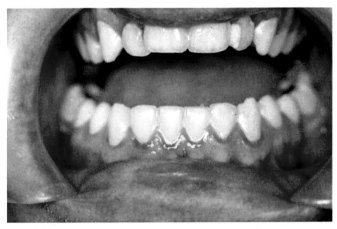

Fig. 19.3 Simple gingivitis.
Source: Reproduced with permission from Davies A and Finlay I (2005), Oral Care in Advanced Disease. Oxford University Press, Oxford

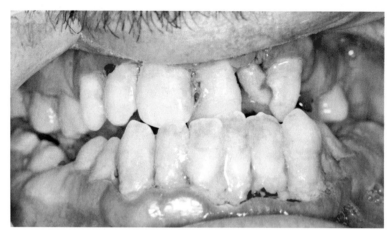

Fig. 19.4 Necrotizing gingivitis.
Source: Reproduced with permission from Davies A and Finlay I (2005), Oral Care in Advanced Disease. Oxford University Press, Oxford

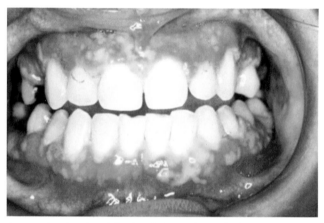

Fig. 20.1 Primary herpes simplex virus infection (primary herpetic gingivostomatitis).
Source: Reproduced with permission from MP Sweeney and J Bagg (1997), Making Sense of the Mouth. Partnership in Oral Care, Glasgow

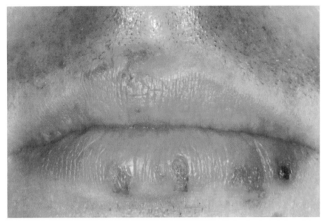

Fig. 20.2 Secondary herpes simplex virus infection (herpes labialis).
Source: Reproduced with permission from Davies A and Finlay I (2005), Oral Care in Advanced
Disease. Oxford University Press, Oxford

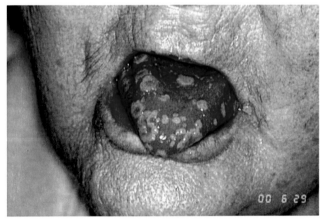

Fig. 20.3a Secondary herpes simplex infection in immunocompromised patient.
Source: Reproduced with permission from Davies A and Finlay I (2005), Oral Care in Advanced
Disease. Oxford University Press, Oxford

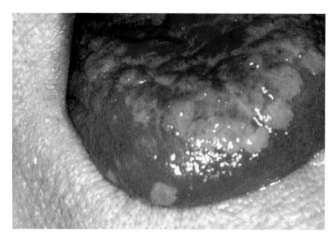

Fig. 20.3b Secondary herpes simplex infection in immunocompromised patient.
Source: Reproduced with permission from MP Sweeney and J Bagg (1997), Making Sense of the Mouth. Partnership in Oral Care, Glasgow

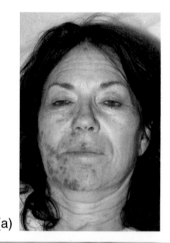

(a)

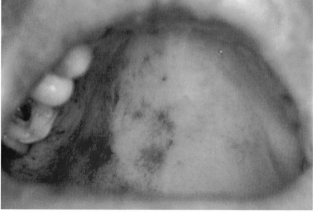

(b)

Fig. 20.4 Secondary varicella zoster infection ((a) facial and (b) oral components).

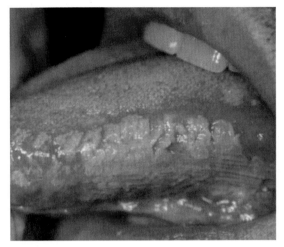

Fig. 20.5 Oral hairy leukoplakia.
Source: Reproduced with permission from Davies A and Finlay I (2005), Oral Care in Advanced Disease. Oxford University Press, Oxford

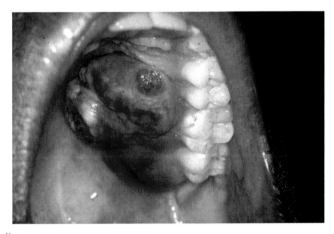

Fig. 20.6 Kaposi's sarcoma.
Source: Reproduced with permission from Davies A and Finlay I (2005), Oral Care in Advanced Disease. Oxford University Press, Oxford

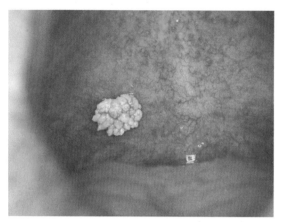
Fig. 20.7 Oral wart (HPV infection).
Source: Reproduced with permission from Davies A and Finlay I (2005), *Oral Care in Advanced Disease*. Oxford University Press, Oxford

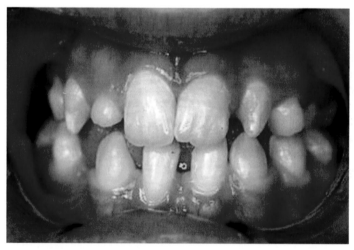
Fig. 26.6 Enamel hypoplasia following chemotherapy.

Table 16.3 Management of bisphosphonate-related osteonecrosis of the jaws [11]

Stage	Management
Stage 1	Patient education Antibacterial mouth rinse (e.g. chlorhexidine 0.12% twice daily) Quarterly follow up
Stage 2	Antibacterial mouth rinse Broad spectrum oral antibiotics (e.g. penicillin, cephalexin, clindamycin, 1st generation fluoroquinolone) Analgesia Superficial debridement of affected areas of bone (to relieve soft tissue irritation)
Stage 3	Antibacterial mouth rinse Broad spectrum oral antibiotics Analgesia Surgical debridement/resection of affected areas of bone
All stages	Review bisphosphonate treatment – discontinuation of oral bisphosphonates may lead to improvement of condition over time; discontinuation of IV bisphosphonates may lead to stabilization of condition over time Removal of bone sequestra – this should be considered as long as it does not expose unaffected areas of bone Removal of symptomatic teeth from affected areas of bone – this should be considered (and is unlikely to exacerbate the condition)

The role of hyperbaric oxygen administration, in a fashion similar to that used for management of radiation-related osteonecrosis, is also under investigation. The results of a recent clinical trial were encouraging, although continued improvement was associated with concomitant cessation of bisphosphonate therapy [25].

Finally, several studies are underway concerning the use of alternatives to the use of bisphosphonate agents (e.g. denosumab, strontium ranelate)[26,27].

Case report

The following case illustrates the presentation, progression, and management of an advanced case of BRON.

The concerned patient, a 61-year-old woman, presented with a several-month history of two painless, non-healing areas of exposed bone over an edentulous segment of the left mandibular body. She had had the teeth in the area extracted many years earlier, and stated that the partial denture she had been wearing had been ill-fitting (and recently had been adjusted).

Her past medical history included a 15-year diagnosis of breast cancer, with a 4-year diagnosis of metastatic lesions to multiple bony sites. She had been treated with intravenous pamidronate (Aredia®) for 1 year, prior to being switched to zoledronic acid (Zometa®) 3 years ago at the usual dosage (i.e. 4 mg per month administered intravenously). In addition, she was receiving docetaxel chemotherapy. Her metastatic disease was deemed to be stable on this treatment regimen.

At the initial examination, an ovoid area of exposed bone measuring 2.0×1.8 cm was present over the alveolar crest of the mandible (Figure 16.3a, see colour plate section). The exposed bone was well defined by an undermined mucosal margin. A smaller area of exposed bone was also noted in close proximity to this lesion. There was no tenderness, and no signs of drainage or suppuration. A panoramic radiograph suggested increased bone density in the area corresponding to the exposed bone (Figure 16.3b).

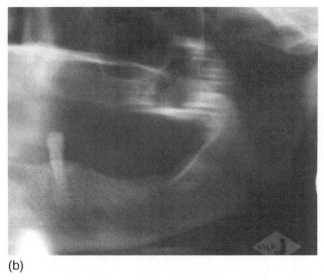

(b)

Fig. 16.3b Patient at presentation: radiograph shows subtle sclerosis ('ground glass' appearance) of the alveolar bone (Stage 1 BRON).

A working diagnosis of Stage 1 BRON was made, and she was treated with twice-daily chlorhexidine rinses. Discussions were held with the patient and her oncologist, and it was decided to empirically reduce the frequency of her zoledronic acid to quarterly infusions (at the usual dosage). The docetaxel chemotherapy was continued as per normal. She was reviewed every 3 months with regard to the BRON.

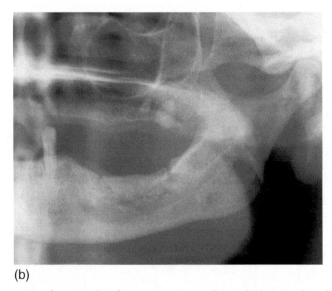

(b)

Fig. 16.4b Same patient four months after presentation: radiograph shows a clear delineation between the forming sequestrum and the underlying mandibular bone.

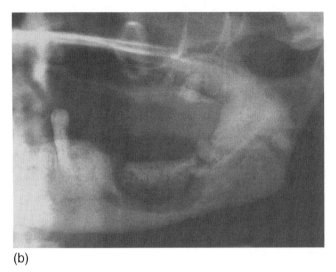

(b)

Fig. 16.5b Same patient fourteen months after presentation: radiograph shows separation of the established sequestrum from the underlying mandibular bone.

Over a period of months, the area of exposed bone slowly increased, as did the degree of bony sclerosis, with early indication of separation between the emerging sequestrum and the lower portion of the mandible (Figure 16.4a, see colour plate section and b). During this time, she developed pain that was managed with regular oral ibuprofen at a dose of 400 mg 3 times daily, and a suppurating infection that was managed with oral penicillin V at a dose of 500 mg 4 times daily.

The amount of exposed bone increased and the sequestrum continued to develop (Figure 16.5a, see colour plate section and b), until it was possible to simply remove the dead bone without the need for a formal surgical procedure. The bony destruction continued onwards, eventually leading to a spontaneous fracture 18 months after the initial presentation (Figure 16.6). A conservative resection was then performed with placement of a titanium fixation plate over the bone defect (Figure 16.7).

At present, the patient is free of pain and infection, although the areas of exposed bone remain.

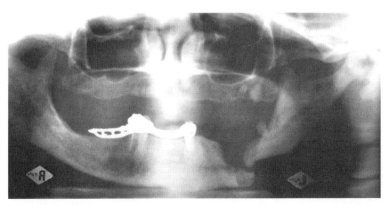

Fig. 16.6 Same patient eighteen months after presentation: radiograph shows a pathological fracture of the mandible.

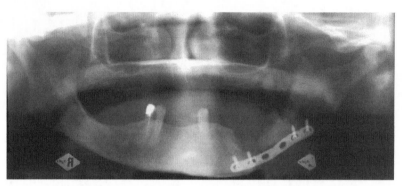

Fig. 16.7 Same patient post surgery: radiograph shows the titanium fixation plate *in situ*.

References

1 Berenson JR, Lichtenstein A, Porter L, et al. (1996). Efficacy of pamidronate in reducing skeletal events in patients with advanced multiple myeloma. *N Engl J Med*, 334(8), 488–93.

2 Hortobagyi GN, Theriault RL, Porter L, et al. (1996). Efficacy of pamidronate in reducing skeletal complications in patients with breast cancer and lytic bone metastases. *N Engl J Med*, 335(24), 1785–91.

3 Santini D, Vespasiani Gentilucci U, Vincenzi B, et al. (2003). The antineoplastic role of bisphosphonates: from basic research to clinical evidence. *Ann Oncol*, 14(10), 1468–76.

4 Green JR (2004). Bisphosphonates: preclinical review. *Oncologist*, 9 (Suppl 4), 3–13.

5 Ruggiero SL, Mehrotra B, Rosenberg TJ, Engroff SL (2004). Osteonecrosis of the jaws associated with the use of bisphosphonates: a review of 63 cases. *J Oral Maxillofac Surg*, 62(5), 527–34.

6 Marx RE (2003). Pamidronate (Aredia) and zoledronate (Zometa) induced avascular necrosis of the jaws: a growing epidemic. *J Oral Maxillofac Surg*, 61(9), 1115–17.

7 Wilkinson GS, Kuo YF, Freeman JL, Goodwin JS (2007). Intravenous bisphosphonate therapy and inflammatory conditions or surgery of the jaw: a population-based analysis. *J Natl Cancer Inst*, 99(13), 1016–24.

8 Durie BG, Katz M, Crowley J (2005). Osteonecrosis of the jaw and bisphosphonates. *N Engl J Med*, 353(1), 99–102.

9 Wang EP, Kaban LB, Strewler GJ, Raje N, Troulis MJ (2007). Incidence of osteonecrosis of the jaw in patients with multiple myeloma and breast or prostate cancer on intravenous bisphosphonate therapy. *J Oral Maxillofac Surg*, 65(7), 1328–31.

10 Bamias A, Kastritis E, Bamia C, et al. (2005). Osteonecrosis of the jaw in cancer after treatment with bisphosphonates: incidence and risk factors. *J Clin Oncol*, 23(34), 8580–7.

11 American Association of Oral and Maxillofacial Surgeons (2006). American Association of Oral and Maxillofacial Surgeons Position Paper on Bisphosphonate-Related Osteonecrosis of the Jaws. Available at: http://www.aaoms.org/docs/position_papers/osteonecrosis.pdf

12 Zahrowski JJ (2007). Comment on the American Association of Oral and Maxillofacial Surgeons statement on bisphosphonates. *J Oral Maxillofac Surg*, 65(7), 1440–1.

13 Zervas K, Vernou E, Teleioudis Z, et al. (2006). Incidence, risk factors and management of osteonecrosis of the jaw in patients with multiple myeloma: a single-centre experience in 303 patients. *Br J Haematol*, 134(6), 620–3.

14 Grbic JT, Landesberg R, Lin SQ, et al. (2008). Incidence of osteonecrosis of the jaw in women with postmenopausal osteoporosis in the health outcomes and reduced incidence with zolendronic acid once yearly pivotal fracture trial. *J Am Dent Assoc*, 139(1), 32–40.

15 Cartsos VM, Zhu S, Zavras AI (2008). Bisphosphonate use and the risk of adverse jaw outcomes: a medical claims study of 714,217 people. *J Am Dent Assoc*, 139(1), 23–30.

16 Bolland M, Hay D, Grey A, Reid I, Cundy T (2006). Osteonecrosis of the jaw and bisphosphonates-putting the risk in perspective. *N Z Med J*, 119 (1246), U2339.

17 American Dental Association. Expert Panel Recommendations: Dental Management of Patients on Oral Bisphosphonate Therapy. June 2006. Available at: http://ada.org/prof/resources/topics/osteonecrosis.asp

18 Marx RE (2006). *Oral & intravenous bisphosphonate-induced osteonecrosis of the jaws: history, etiology, prevention, and treatment.* Quintessence Publishing, Hanover Park

19 Ruggiero SL, Fantasia J, Carlson E (2006). Bisphosphonate-related osteonecrosis of the jaw: background and guidelines for diagnosis, staging and management. *Oral Surg Oral Med Oral Pathol Oral Radiol Endod*, 102(4), 433–41.

20 Woo SB, Hellstein JW, Kalmar JR (2006). Systematic review: bisphosphonates and osteonecrosis of the jaws. *Ann Intern Med*, 144(10), 753–61.

21 Phal PM, Myall RW, Assael LA, Weissman JL (2007). Imaging findings of bisphosphonate-associated osteonecrosis of the jaws. *Am J Neuroradiol*, 28(6), 1139–45.

22 Kumar V, Pass B, Guttenberg SA, et al. (2007). Bisphosphonate-related osteonecrosis of the jaws: a report of three cases demonstrating variability in outcomes and morbidity. *J Am Dent Assoc*, 138(5), 602–9.

23 Wade ML, Suzuki JB (2007). Issues related to diagnosis and treatment of bisphosphonate-induced osteonecrosis of the jaws. *Grand Rounds in Oral-Systemic Medicine*, 2(2), 46–53b.

24 Adornato MC, Morcos I, Rozanski J (2007). The treatment of bisphosphonate-associated osteonecrosis of the jaws with bone resection and autologous platelet-derived growth factors. *J Am Dent Assoc*, 138(7), 971–7.

25 Freiberger JJ, Padilla-Burgos R, Chhoeu AH, et al. (2007). Hyperbaric oxygen treatment and bisphosphonate-induced osteonecrosis of the jaw: a case series. *J Oral Maxillofac Surg*, 65(7), 1321–7.

26 McClung MR, Lewiecki EM, Cohen SB, et al. (2006). Denosumab in postmenopausal women with low bone mineral density. *N Engl J Med*, 354(8), 821–31.

27 Bruyere O, Roux C, Detilleux J, et al. (2007). Relationship between bone mineral density changes and fracture risk reduction in patients treated with strontium ranelate. *J Clin Endocrinol Metab*, 92(8), 3076–81.

Chapter 17

Oral infections – introduction

Susan Brailsford and David Beighton

Introduction

Oral microbial diseases are almost always due to endogenous organisms, which are part of the normal oral microbiota (i.e. commensal organisms). Thus, changes in environmental conditions (such as reduced salivary flow, prescription of antimicrobial agents, excess consumption of dietary sugars) may result in a shift in the normal oral microbiota with proliferation of organisms capable of causing oral disease (the so-called 'ecological plaque hypothesis') [1,2]. To date, no true pathogenic organisms have been identified in the mouth, although some organisms are strongly associated with oral disease (e.g. *Prevotella* species and periodontal disease).

The oral cavity supports a wide range of microbiota on the various intraoral surfaces (Table 17.1) [3]. Traditionally, organisms have been isolated by culture methods using appropriate media (non-selective or selective) and growth conditions (aerobic, microaerophilic, or anaerobic). More recently, the use of molecular techniques such as 16S rRNA sequencing has resulted in many new species being identified. At present, >700 different taxa have been isolated from the mouth using culture methods and molecular techniques [4]. Collaboration between the Forsyth Institute and King's College London has resulted in a website that contains the sequence data for all identified oral organisms [5].

Colonization of the oral cavity

The oral cavity is sterile at birth, but within a few hours it becomes colonized by bacteria, predominantly oral streptococci (i.e. *Streptococcus mitis, S. oralis, S. salivarius*) [6]. The eruption of the teeth provides a hard surface within the oral cavity, which leads to changes in the oral microbiota. For example, *S. mutans*, the organism classically associated with dental caries, is not usually detected prior to eruption of the teeth [7]. Following the eruption of the teeth, the oral microbiota remains relatively stable, although the frequency of isolation of *Staphylococcus* species and *Candida* species increases with age [8]. This phenomenon of a stable microbiota has been termed 'microbial homeostasis'[9].

The diversity of oral microbiota is due to the variety of colonization sites. Oral micro-organisms adhere to different sites as a result of the adhesins on the relevant cell surfaces[10]. For example, in a healthy mouth, the microbiota of the dorsum of the tongue consists predominantly of *S. salivarius*, with smaller numbers of other organisms such as *Rothia mucilaginosa* and *Eubacterium* species [4]. In general, the oral cavity is aerobic, and has a neutral pH (6.75–7.25). However, the gingival crevice is more anaerobic, and has an alkaline pH (7.5–8.5), which favours the growth of certain periodontal pathogens (e.g. *Prevotella* species).

The teeth, the gingival crevice, and the dorsum of the tongue are invariably covered with a biofilm. A biofilm is defined as a population or community of bacteria living in organized structures at an interface between liquid and solid[2]. However, other parts of the oral mucosa

Table 17.1 Commonly isolated oral microorganisms [3]

Group	Genus
Gram-positive cocci Aerobic or facultative†	Streptococcus Staphylococcus Enterococcus Micrococcus
Gram-positive cocci Obligate anaerobes††	Peptostreptococcus Peptococcus
Gram-positive rods Aerobic or facultative	Actinomyces Lactobacillus Corynebacterium Arachnia Rothia
Gram-positive rods Obligate anaerobes	Eubacterium Propionibacterium Bifidobacterium Bacillus Clostridium
Gram-negative cocci Aerobic or facultative	Neisseria / Branhamella
Gram-negative cocci Obligate anaerobes	Veillonella
Gram-negative rods Aerobic or facultative	Campylobacter Eikonella Actinobacillus Capnocytophaga Haemophilus Simonsiella
Gram-negative rods Obligate anaerobes	Bacteroides Fusobacterium Porphyromonas Prevotella Leptotrichia Wolinella / Selenomas
Other organisms	Mycoplasma Candida Spirochaetes Protozoa

† = prefers anaerobic conditions, but can tolerate aerobic conditions

†† = needs anaerobic conditions (cannot tolerate aerobic conditions)

(buccal mucosa, floor of mouth, palate, etc.) are rarely covered with a bioflim, because of the rapid rate of epithelial turnover/desquamation within the oral mucosa. Accumulation of micro-organisms within a biofilm allows them to survive by reducing their chance of removal by mechanical forces, and also by providing some protection from host defence mechanisms and exogenous antimicrobial agents[11]. It should be noted that, within a biofilm, there are areas with differing microenvironments, which encourage the proliferation of differing micro-organisms[12].

Moreover, micro-organisms within a biofilm may adopt a specific phenotype, and may express an array of different proteins (compared to 'planktonic'/non-biofilm organisms).

Dental plaque

The biofilm on the teeth is often referred to as 'dental plaque'. Dental plaque has been defined as 'the community of micro-organisms found on the surface as a biofilm, embedded in a matrix of polymers of salivary and bacterial origin'[13]. Colonization of the teeth occurs within minutes of them erupting/being cleaned. The salivary pellicle, which covers the teeth, forms the basis for the supragingival/subgingival biofilms. The salivary pellicle consists of salivary glycoproteins, which have binding sites for bacteria ('adhesins')[14].

The development of plaque is initiated by absorption of micro-organisms onto a surface. The main initial colonizers of the salivary pellicle are *Streptococci*, particularly *S. mitis, S. oralis,* and *S. salivarius.* These early colonizers are important in that they provide attachment sites for subsequent colonizers, and they may modify the environment of the biofilm. These organisms are able to avoid host defences; there is evidence that they possess IgA proteases which allow them to avoid the actions of salivary immunoglobulin A (IgA)[3]. Other initial colonizers of the salivary pellicle are predominantly *Actinomyces*, particularly *A. naeslundii.* The ability of these oral organisms to utilize salivary glycoproteins for growth ensures their survival when carbohydrates are not available[15].

The initial colonizers bind to the salivary glycoproteins, and to other bacteria, using their surface structures (pili, fimbriae)[16]. The initial period of bacterial adhesion/co-adhesion is followed by a period of bacterial growth. Saliva provides a source of nutrients for supragingival plaque, whilst gingival crevicular fluid provides a source of nutrients for subgingival plaque. The mouth of an individual tends to have a stable plaque community, although the microbiota within the biofilms is influenced by changing conditions of the mouth (e.g. pH, availability of substrates).

Maintenance of the oral microbiota

A variety of different homeostatic mechanisms maintains the normal commensal microbiota, and prevents the development of oral infection (Table 17.2). Some of these mechanisms are non-specific (affect all micro-organisms), whilst other mechanisms are specific (affect only certain micro-organisms).

Oral mucosa

The oral mucosa forms a physical barrier to invading organisms[17]. Furthermore, the rapid turnover of the surface cells of the oral mucosa prevents the establishment of a biofilm in many parts of the oral cavity. In addition, the surface layer of the oral mucosa is covered with a layer of saliva, and the deeper layers of the oral mucosa harbour immunoglobulins and lymphocytes.

Oral infections occur in patients with oral mucosal damage. For example, patients receiving head and neck radiotherapy invariably develop oral mucositis, and frequently develop secondary infections[18]. It should be noted that damage to the oral mucosa may lead not only to oral infections, but also to systemic infections (i.e. generalized septicaemia, localized distant infection)[19,20].

Commensal microbiota

Commensal organisms may use non-specific methods and/or specific methods to prevent colonization by pathogenic organisms. The non-specific methods involve competing with the

Table 17.2 Homeostatic mechanisms within the oral cavity

Non-specific factors*	Oral mucosa
	Commensal flora
	Saliva
	Gingival crevicular fluid
	Complement
	Phagocytes
Specific factors*	Secretory IgA
	Serum IgM, IgG, IgA
	Lymphocytes

* Many of these factors are inter-related

pathogenic organisms for occupancy of the oral mucosa, and utilization of the oral nutrients ('competitive inhibition')[2]. The specific methods involve actively suppressing the pathogenic organisms. For example, viridans streptococci can produce hydrogen peroxide, which inhibits periodontal pathogenic organisms[21]. Similarly, Gram-positive bacteria can produce bacteriocins (antibacterial factors), which inhibit certain pathogenic organisms[22]. Recent research suggests that contact dependent signalling might also be involved in the prevention of organisms binding to biofilms[23].

A number of factors can affect the commensal microbiota, including salivary dysfunction, ingestion of antibiotics, and ingestion of a high carbohydrate diet. For example, a high carbohydrate diet may cause a decrease in pH within the mouth, which favours the proliferation of acidophilic micro-organisms, many of which play a role in the development of dental caries[24].

Saliva

Saliva is very important for maintaining the normal commensal microbiota, and preventing the development of oral infections. Saliva has a number of different actions:

1. Flushing action' – the constant flow of saliva helps to prevent the adherence of micro-organisms, and to facilitate the removal of food/other oral debris (which act as substrate for micro-organisms).

2. Antimicrobial action – salivary gland secretions contain numerous antimicrobial factors, including secretory IgA, mucin, lysozyme, lactoferrin, the salivary peroxidase system, and histidine-rich polypeptides (see Table 17.3)[25]. The salivary factors act in a variety of different ways (Table 17.3)[26], and it is thought they may act synergistically (as well as individually)[27]. It should be noted that saliva is composed of salivary gland secretions, gingival crevicular fluid (see below), and various other components[28].

3. Maintenance of pH – saliva maintains a neutral pH within the mouth. The neutral pH within the mouth encourages the growth of commensal organisms, and discourages the growth of certain pathogenic organisms.

Salivary gland dysfunction is associated with significant changes in the oral microbiota[29]. Furthermore, salivary gland dysfunction is associated with increased prevalence of certain oral infections (e.g. dental caries, oral candidosis)[30]. Salivary gland dysfunction is discussed, in detail, in Chapter 21.

Table 17.3 Salivary proteins involved in homeostasis [26]

Salivary glycoprotein	Origin	Function	Comments
mUC5B (mucin MG1)	All mucous salivary glands	Physical barrier. Aggregation (bacteria, viruses)	5–20% total salivary protein
MUC7 (mucin MG2)	All mucous salivary glands	Physical barrier. Aggregation (bacteria, viruses)	5–20% total salivary protein
Immunoglobulins	B lymphocytes in all salivary glands	Inactivation and aggregation (bacteria, yeasts, viruses)	5–15% total salivary protein
Proline-rich glycoprotein	Parotid glands	Unknown (? aggregation)	1–10% total salivary protein
Cystatins	Submandibular > sublingual glands	Protease inhibitor (bacteria, viruses)	10% total salivary protein
Histatins	Parotid and submandibular glands	Broad spectrum killing (bacteria, yeasts)	5% total salivary protein
EP-GP (GCDFP15, SABP, PIP)	Submandibular and sublingual glands	Unknown	1–2% total salivary protein
Agglutinin (DMBT1, gp340)	Parotid > submandibular > sublingual glands	Aggregation (bacteria)	1–2% total salivary protein
Lysozyme	Sublingual > submandibular and parotid glands	Killing (bacteria, yeasts)	1–2% total salivary protein
Lactoferrin	All salivary glands (mucous > serous)	Growth inhibition (bacteria, yeasts, viruses)	1–2% total salivary protein
Lactoperoxidase	Parotid > submandibular glands	Growth inhibition (bacteria, yeasts, viruses)	<1% total salivary protein
Cathelicidin (hCAP18, LL37)	Salivary glands and neutrophils	Broad spectrum killing (bacteria)	1–2% total salivary protein
Defensins	Salivary glands, epithelial cells and neutrophils	Broad spectrum killing (bacteria, yeasts)	1–2% total salivary protein

Gingival crevicular fluid

Gingival crevicular fluid is a serum transudate: the fluid passes from the systemic circulation, through the junctional epithelium of the gingiva, and into the gingival crevice/oral cavity. Gingival crevicular fluid contains a variety of antimicrobial agents, including complement, immunoglobulins (IgG, IgM, IgA), phagocytes (polymorphonuclear leucocytes, macrophages), and lymphocytes (B cells and T cells).[17] Moreover, the constant flow of gingival crevicular fluid may help to prevent the adhesion of micro-organisms.

Immune system

The innate/non-specific immune system within the mouth includes phagocytes (polymorphonuclear leucocytes, macrophages), and complement[31]. Phagocytes engulf and destroy a variety of different pathogens. They are derived from the blood, and enter the oral cavity in the gingival crevicular fluid. Complement has a number of functions including lysing/destroying Gram-negative bacteria, enhancing the action of phagocytes ('opsonization'), and promoting the migration of lymphocytes. Complement is derived from the blood, and also enters the oral cavity in the gingival crevicular fluid.

The acquired/specific immune system within the mouth consists of immunoglobulins (antibodies), and cell-mediated immunity (T cells)[17]. The immunoglobulins include secretory IgA, and serum IgG, IgM, and IgA. Secretory IgA is derived from lymphoid tissue within the salivary glands, and reaches the oral cavity in the saliva. Secretory IgA acts by preventing microbial adherence to host surfaces[3]. Serum IgG, IgM, and IgA are derived from systemic lymphoid tissue, and reach the oral cavity in the gingival crevicular fluid. The serum immunoglobulins act in a number of ways – preventing microbial adherence to host surfaces, inhibiting microbial metabolism, or promoting microbial phagocytosis. T cells occur in a variety of different forms, which have a variety of different roles – stimulating B cells (TH2/T helper cells), and killing infected cells (TC/cytotoxic T cells).

Immunodeficiency is associated with changes in the oral microbiota, and an increased prevalence of certain oral infections[32]. The pattern of oral infection is influenced somewhat by the nature of the immunodeficiency. For example, human immunodeficiency virus (HIV) infection/acquired immune deficiency syndrome (AIDS), which is characterized by a reduction in CD4+ cells (T cells), is associated with oral candidosis, periodontal disease, and oral hairy leucoplakia[33]. The development of these oral infections is strongly correlated with the CD4+ cell count (and the viral load)[34].

References

1   Marsh PD (1991).The significance of maintaining the stability of the natural microflora of the mouth. *Br Dent J*, 171(6), 174–7.

2   Marsh PD (1994). Microbial ecology of dental plaque and its significance in health and disease. *Adv Dent Res*, 8(2), 263–71.

3   Marcotte H, Lavoie MC (1998). Oral microbial ecology and the role of salivary immunoglobulin A. *Microbiol Mol Biol Rev*, 62(1), 71–109.

4   Aas JA, Paster BJ, Stokes LN, Olsen I, Dewhirst FE (2005). Defining the normal bacterial flora of the oral cavity. *J Clin Microbiol*, 43(11), 5721–32.

5   Human Oral Microbiome Database website: http://www.homd.org/

6   Pearce C, Bowden GH, Evans M, et al. (1995). Identification of pioneer viridans streptococci in the oral cavity of human neonates. *J Med Microbiol*, 42(1), 67–72.

7   Kononen E, Jousimies-Somer H, Bryk A, Kilp T, Kilian M (2002). Establishment of streptococci in the upper respiratory tract: longitudinal changes in the mouth and nasopharynx up to 2 years of age. *J Med Microbiol*, 51(9), 723–30.

8   Percival RS, Challacombe SJ, Marsh PD (1991). Age-related microbiological changes in the salivary and plaque microflora of healthy adults. *J Med Microbiol*, 35(1), 5–11.

9   Alexander M (1971). Biochemical ecology of microorganisms. *Annu Rev Microbiol*, 25, 361–92.

10 Gibbons RJ, Spinell DM, Skobe Z (1976). Selective adherence as a determinant of the host tropisms of certain indigenous and pathogenic bacteria. *Infect Immun*, 13(1), 238–46.

11 Bowden GH (1999). Oral biofilm an archive of past events? in Newman HH, Wilson M, (eds) *Dental Plaque Revisited – Oral Biofilms in Health and Disease*, pp. 211–35. BioLine Publications, Cardiff.

12 Vroom JM, De Grauw KJ, Gerritsen HC, et al. (1999). Depth penetration and detection of pH gradients in biofilms by two-photon excitation microscopy. *Appl Environ Microbiol*, 65(8), 3502–11.

13 Marsh P, Martin MV (1999). *Oral microbiology*, 4th edn. Wright, Oxford.

14 Liljemark WF, Bloomquist C (1996). Human oral microbial ecology and dental caries and periodontal diseases. *Crit Rev Oral Biol Med*, 7(2), 180–98.

15 Frandsen EV (1994). Carbohydrate depletion of immunoglobulin A1 by oral species of gram-positive rods. *Oral Microbiol Immunol*, 9(6), 352–8.

16 Kolenbrander PE (2000). Oral microbial communities: biofilms, interactions, and genetic systems. *Annu Rev Microbiol*, 54, 413–37.

17 Bagg J, MacFarlane TW, Poxton IR, Miller CH, Smith AJ (1999). *Essentials of microbiology for dental students*. Oxford University Press, Oxford.

18 Redding SW, Zellars RC, Kirkpatrick WR, et al. (1999). Epidemiology of oropharyngeal Candida colonization and infection in patients receiving radiation for head and neck cancer. *J Clin Microbiol*, 37(12), 3896–900.

19 Meurman JH, Pyrhonen S, Teerenhovi L, Linqvist C (1997). Oral sources of septicaemia in patients with malignancies. *Oral Oncol*, 33(6), 389–97.

20 Fiehn NE, Gutschik E, Larsen T, Bangsborg JM (1995). Identity of streptococcal blood isolates and oral isolates from two patients with infective endocarditis. *J Clin Microbiol*, 33 (5), 1399–401.

21 Hillman JD, Socransky SS, Shivers M (1985). The relationships between streptococcal species and periodontopathic bacteria in human dental plaque. *Arch Oral Biol*, 30(11–12), 791–5.

22 Balakrishnan M, Simmonds RS, Tagg JR (2001). Diverse activity spectra of bacteriocin-like inhibitory substances having activity against mutans streptococci. *Caries Res*, 35(1), 75–80.

23 Jenkinson HF, Lamont RJ (2005). Oral microbial communities in sickness and in health. *Trends Microbiol*, 13(12), 589–95.

24 Marsh PD (2003). Are dental diseases examples of ecological catastrophes? *Microbiology*, 149(Pt 2), 279–94.

25 Amerongen AV, Veerman EC (2002). Saliva – the defender of the oral cavity. *Oral Dis*, 8(1), 12–22.

26 Van Nieuw Amerongen A, Bolscher JG, Veerman EC (2004). Salivary proteins: protective and diagnostic value in cariology? *Caries Res*, 38(3), 247–53.

27 Rudney JD, Hickey KL, Ji Z (1999). Cumulative correlations of lysozyme, lactoferrin, peroxidase, S-IgA, amylase, and total protein concentrations with adherence of oral viridans streptococci to microplates coated with human saliva. *J Dent Res*, 78(3), 759–68.

28 Anonymous (1992). Saliva: Its role in health and disease. FDI Working Group 10 of the Commission on Oral Health, Research and Epidemiology (CORE). *Int Dent J*, 42 (4 Suppl 2), 291–304.

29 Almstahl A, Wikstrom M (1999). Oral microflora in subjects with reduced salivary secretion. *J Dent Res*, 78(8), 1410–16.

30 Sreebny LM (1996). Xerostomia: diagnosis, management and clinical complications, in Edgar WM, O'Mullane DM (eds) *Saliva and Oral Health*, 2nd edn, pp. 43–66. British Dental Association, London.

31 Smith DJ, Taubman MA (1992). Ontogeny of immunity to oral microbiota in humans. *Crit Rev Oral Biol Med*, 3(1–2), 109–33.

32 Atkinson JC, O'Connell A, Aframian D (2000). Oral manifestations of primary immunological diseases. *J Am Dent Assoc*, 131(3), 345–56.

33 Chapple IL, Hamburger J (2000). The significance of oral health in HIV disease. *Sex Transm Infect*, 76(4), 236–43.

34 Campo J, Del Romero, J, Castilla J, Garcia S, Rodriguez C, Bascones A (2002). Oral candidiasis as a clinical marker related to viral load, CD4 lymphocyte count and CD4 lymphocyte percentage in HIV-infected patients. *J Oral Pathol Med*, 31(1), 5–10.

Chapter 18

Oral fungal infections

Lakshman Samaranayake and Mohaideen Sitheeque

Introduction

Fungi are eukaryotes as opposed to bacteria that are prokaryotic (i.e. fungi consist of cells that are organized into complex structures, and that are enclosed within membranes). Fungi may exhibit two distinct structural forms (i.e. yeast form and mould form). Yeasts are unicellular organisms, while moulds consist of multicellular filaments or hyphae. A mass of hyphae is referred to as a mycelium. Some fungi exist only in the yeast form, while others may occur in both forms at different times (and are referred to as dimorphic).

Several fungal species cause human oral infections, also known as oral mycoses (Table 18.1). However, the predominant fungal infection to affect the oral mucosa is caused by yeasts belonging to the genus *Candida* (termed either 'oral candidosis' or 'oral candidiasis'). Other fungi mainly cause superficial or invasive mycoses in immunocompromised hosts. All fungal infections of the oral mucosa, including those caused by the genus *Candida*, are deemed to be opportunistic infections.

Fungal infections, in general, and oral fungal infections, in particular, are a source of significant morbidity in cancer patients [1]. Indeed, these infections can even lead to fatalities in cancer patients.[2] With the ever-increasing numbers of cancer patients, and the more aggressive forms of cancer therapy, increasing incidences of fungal infections are being encountered[3]. In the discussion that follows, oral candidosis and other fungal infections are described, prior to delving into issues pertaining to these infections in the cancer patient.

Oral candidal infections

Candida albicans is the predominant species to cause the different clinical variants of oral candidosis (~90% *Candida* infections). Other species such as *C. glabrata*, *C. tropicalis*, *C. krusei*, *C. parapsilosis*, and *C. guilliermondii* have been reported to cause disease in a small number of cases. Candidal oral infections are endogenous in origin, as *Candida* species are indigenous to the oral cavity, with *C. albicans* being the commonest species encountered as a commensal in the mouth. The clinical features do not differ with the species of *Candida* causing the infection.

Classification

Oral candidosis is generally classified as follows[1]:

- Primary oral candidosis – localized candidosis affecting only the oral and perioral tissues.
- Secondary oral candidosis – generalized candidal infections of the oral and other mucous membranes, as well as of the cutaneous surfaces of the body (mucocutaneous candidosis). This group is seen mostly in patients with primary immune deficiencies such as congenital thymic aplasia and candidosis endocrinopathy syndrome.

Table 18.1 Fungal species of medical importance

Fungal species	Fungal disease
Yeasts	
Candida species	Candidosis
Cryptococcus species	Cryptococcosis
Moulds	
Aspergillus species	Aspergillosis
Blastomyces species	Blastomycosis
Coccidioides species	Coccidioidomycosis
Geotrichum species	Geotrichosis
Histoplasma species	Histoplasmosis
Mucor species	Mucormycosis, zygomycosis
Paracoccidioides species	Paracoccidioidomycosis
Penicillium species	Penicilliosis
Sporothrix species	Sporotrichosis

Clinically, oral candidosis may present as three main variants (i.e. pseudomembranous, erythematous, and hyperplastic lesions). Primary oral candidosis exists in all three variants, while secondary oral candidosis presents mostly as the hyperplastic variant.

Clinical features

The clinical variants of oral candidosis are listed in Table 18.2, and described in detail in the following sections. Table 18.2 also lists the recognized predisposing factors for these clinical variants of oral candidosis.

Pseudomembranous candidosis

Pseudomembranous candidosis, which is also known as 'oral thrush', presents as curd-like white patches (pseudomembranes) on the oral mucosa of the hard and soft palate, tongue, and buccal mucosa (Figure 18.1, see colour plate section). These patches can easily be rubbed off leaving an erythematous or bleeding base. Patients do not usually complain of any symptoms, although sometimes there may be a mild burning sensation. Extension of the pseudomembranes into the upper respiratory and oesophageal mucosa is often seen.

Erythematous (atrophic) candidosis

Erythematous candidosis may involve most areas of the oral mucosa. The condition is usually asymptomatic, although it may be accompanied by a burning sensation. Some cases of erythematous candidosis follow the shedding of pseudomembranes in the pseudomembranous variant. Another subtype is found among denture wearers, and is categorized as a candida-associated lesion ('denture stomatitis' – see below).

Chronic hyperplastic candidosis

Chronic hyperplastic candidosis is, sometimes, referred to as candidal leucoplakia[4]. Chronic hyperplastic candidosis appears as unilateral or bilateral, clearly demarcated, raised, white, or

Table 18.2 Main predisposing factors for oral candidosis

Clinical variant	Predisposing factors
Pseudomembranous candidosis	◆ Salivary gland dysfunction
	◆ Systemic/inhaled corticosteroid therapy
	◆ Extremes of age (young, old)
	◆ Acquired Immune Deficiency Syndrome (AIDS)
	◆ Chronic systemic diseases
	◆ Diabetes mellitus
	◆ Malignant diseases
	◆ Radiotherapy for head and neck malignancy
	◆ Neutropenia
	◆ Severe blood dyscrasias
Erythematous candidosis	◆ Pseudomembranous candidosis (after shedding of pseudomembranes)
	◆ Systemic corticosteroid therapy
	◆ Systemic/topical broad spectrum antibiotic therapy
	◆ Acquired Immune Deficiency Syndrome
	◆ Denture wearing (see below)
Chronic hyperplastic candidosis	◆ Heavy smoking
	◆ Oral epithelial dysplasia
Chronic mucocutaneous candidosis	◆ Primary immunodeficiency disorders
	◆ Endocrine disorders
Candida-associated lesions:	
◆ Chronic erythematous candidosis ('denture stomatitis')	◆ Inadequate hygiene of denture/appliance
	◆ Ill-fitting denture/appliance
	◆ Chronic local irritants
	◆ Salivary gland dysfunction
	◆ Diabetes mellitus
	◆ Carbohydrate rich diet
◆ Angular stomatitis	◆ Denture-induced stomatitis
	◆ Acquired Immune Deficiency Syndrome
	◆ Anaemia
	◆ Haematinic deficiency
◆ Median rhomboid glossitis	◆ (Controversial)
	◆ Developmental anomaly (depapillated area)
	◆ Smoking

speckled (mixed white and red) plaques on the buccal mucosa usually involving the areas immediately adjacent to the commissures. These plaques feel hard to the touch, and cannot be rubbed off. At times, the white areas of the speckled plaque may adopt a nodular appearance. Chronic hyperplastic candidosis lesions have a high degree of malignant transformation to squamous cell carcinoma (i.e. 9–40%).

Chronic mucocutaneous candidosis

Chronic mucocutaneous candidosis appears early in life in children who have inherited immune defects or endocrine disorders. Hyperplastic plaque-like lesions occur on the oral mucosa and on the skin. Nail defects may also be seen (candidal paronychia).

Candida-associated lesions

Candida-associated lesions have multiple aetiologies, one of which may be candidal infection.

Chronic erythematous candidosis (denture stomatitis, 'denture sore mouth') This is a common problem amongst denture wearers, or children wearing orthodontic appliances with poor hygiene. The upper denture-bearing palatal mucosa exhibits oedema and a variable degree of erythema ranging from pinpoint areas (Newton's type 1) to the whole area covered by the denture or appliance (Newton's type 2) (Figure 18.2, see colour plate section). Sometimes, the central palatal area may display papillary hyperplasia (Newton's type 3). Affected individuals are usually symptom free, and are unaware of the presence of the lesion. Angular cheilitis often accompanies the condition (see below). The condition is extremely rare under the lower denture.

Angular cheilitis (angular stomatitis) This is often seen in denture wearers affected by denture stomatitis. It presents as unilateral or bilateral soreness at the corners of the mouth accompanied by redness and fissuring (Figure 18.3, see colour plate section). The lesion may involve a symbiotic infection of *Candida* and *Staph. aureus*. (The presence of yellow crusting indicates the involvement of *Staph. aureus*).

Median rhomboid glossitis (glossal central papillary atrophy) This condition presents as an oval or rhombus shaped area of papillary atrophy, 2–3 cm in length, in the midline of the dorsum of the tongue just anterior to the circumvallate papillae (Figure 18.4, see colour plate section). Although the lesion is usually flat, it may present as a raised, lobulated, or even exophytic lesion. The patient is usually asymptomatic.

Diagnosis

The diagnosis of oral candidosis is largely based on the clinical features. However, occasionally, confirmatory laboratory investigations are required. Table 18.3 summarizes the specimens suitable for the laboratory diagnosis of oral candidosis.

Management

Measures that can be taken to try to prevent fungal infections include generic oral hygiene measures and elimination of well-known sources of infection (e.g. decontamination of dentures).

Table 18.3 Specimens for laboratory diagnosis of oral candidosis

Variant	Smear (& Microscopy)	Swab (& Culture)	Biopsy
Pseudomembranous candidosis	Yes	Yes	Not appropriate
Erythematous candidosis	May be	May be	Not appropriate
Hyperplastic candidosis	Yes	May be	Yes
Denture stomatitis	Yes	Yes	Not appropriate
Angular stomatitis	Yes	Yes	Not appropriate
Median rhomboid glossitis	Yes	Yes	Not appropriate

The drug treatment of oral candidosis in patients with cancer is described in Table 18.4. Oropharyngeal candidosis usually responds to topical antifungal therapy with amphotericin, nystatin, or miconazole. However, if the infection is unresponsive, fluconazole is generally effective when taken by mouth.

Non-candidal oral fungal infections

The important human non-candidal oral fungal infections are: aspergillosis, blastomycosis (North American blastomycosis), coccidioidomycosis, cryptococcosis, geotrichosis, histoplasmosis, mucormycosis (zygomycosis), paracoccidioidomycosis (South American blastomycosis), penicilliosis, and sporotrichosis.

These infections are very uncommon in comparison to oral candidosis. Rarely, healthy individuals may become infected, particularly in endemic areas (see below); these infections largely remain asymptomatic and resolve spontaneously. However, these mycoses can cause fulminant disease in immunocompromised persons, with systemic dissemination frequently proving fatal.

Aspergillosis

Aspergillosis is the most common non-candidal human mycoses. Aspergillosis has a worldwide distribution. *Aspergillus* species are common saprophytes present in the environment in soil and decaying vegetation. *Aspergillus fumigatus* is the most common species, while *A. flavus* is the most virulent species. Inhalation of airborne spores is difficult to avoid. However, unless the inhalation dose is very heavy, or the subject is immunocompromised, clinical disease is exceedingly uncommon. In the latter circumstances, inhalation of the spores results in their germination/colonization within the respiratory and oral mucosae. Macrophages and neutrophils, which constitute the main defence against the fungus, can be weakened by toxins produced by the fungus.

In the otherwise healthy individual, an aspergilloma (hyphal ball) occurs within the maxillary sinus. In the immunocompromised host, invasive aspergillosis of the maxillary antrum associated

Table 18.4 Management of oral candidosis

Clinical variant	Treatment	Comments
Pseudomembranous candidosis	Amphotericin lozenge 10mg 4 times/day for 10-14 days *Or:* Nystatin pastille/suspension 100,000 U 4 times/day *Or:* Miconazole gel (24mg/ml) 5–10ml 4 times/day *Or:* Fluconazole 50–100 mg daily for 7 days	Continue treatment for 48hr after lesions have resolved. Apply after food. Continue treatment for 48hr after lesions have resolved. Clotrimazole is an alternative option (USA)
Erythematous candidosis	As above	
Chronic hyperplastic candidosis	Fluconazole 50 mg daily for 14 days	
Denture stomatitis	Miconazole gel	Apply to fitting surface of denture. Decontamination of denture is also required.
Angular cheilitis	Miconazole cream	Decontamination of denture is also required.

with chronic sinusitis and oral lesions may develop. The patient affected by invasive aspergillosis may develop antral pain, swelling, proptosis, and impaired vision from orbital invasion, or headache and signs of meningism due to intracranial extension. Invasive aspergillosis has a high degree of mortality (30–95%). Oral lesions of aspergillosis are seen mainly in immunocompromised individuals with invasive disease. Necrotic ulcers that are yellow or black in colour may develop on the palate, or, rarely, on the posterior parts of the tongue.

Blastomycosis

The term blastomycosis is now restricted to North American blastomycosis, which is caused by *Blastomyces dermatitidis*. Blastomycosis is endemic in many parts of the United States, and some parts of Canada. However, the disease has a global distribution, and is also encountered in Africa, the Middle East, India, and Australia. Serotype 1 of *Blastomyces dermatitidis* is seen in North America, and serotype 2 is seen in Africa and other regions. The organism is a dimorphic fungus, and enters the body by inhalation of fungal conidia. In an immunocompetent individual, natural resistance is offered by the alveolar macrophages, which inhibit the germination of the conidia into the yeast form. Although subclinical disease may occur in some immunocompetent persons, overt disease tends to occur in immunocompromised individuals.

Oral blastomycosis is usually secondary to pulmonary involvement, and presents as ulcerating lesions of the oral mucosa. Occasionally, an oral mucosal lesion represents an extension from mandibular involvement (disseminated disease). Cutaneous blastomycosis may spread to involve the lips.

Coccidioidomycosis

Coccidioidomycosis is an endemic fungal disease in the arid areas of southwestern USA and northwestern Mexico. It is caused by *Coccidioides immitis*, or occasionally *C. posadasii*. The former is a saprophytic fungus resident in the soil in the relevant geographic regions. The fungus remains dormant during dry spells, and develops into a mould with the advent of first rains. Spores from these moulds may become airborne (and inhaled) during farming or construction activity.

The disease is usually mild with fever and other flu-like symptoms accompanied by a skin rash. However, in vulnerable people, a severe pulmonary disease develops, which may become disseminated producing multi-system involvement. Fatalities are not uncommon. Oral lesions of coccidioidomycosis are rare, and are often secondary to pulmonary involvement although may arise from infection of the jaw bone. Oral mucosal lesions tend to be verrucous in nature.

Cryptococcosis

Cryptococcosis is a worldwide infection caused by the capsulated yeast *Cryptococcus neoformans*. Two subtypes of the fungus have been identified namely *C. neoformans* var *neoformans* (capsular serotypes A, D, and AD), and the less common *C. neoformans* var *gattii* (capsular serotypes B and C). The former is found in the excreta of pigeons, parrots, budgerigars, and canaries, rotting vegetables, and fruits and vegetables (and hence is ubiquitous as a soil contaminant). Infection occurs through inhalation of spores. Cryptococcosis is an AIDS-defining condition and is also increasingly seen in other immunocompromised patients.

Cryptococcosis may vary between a cutaneous form and a pulmonary type. Dissemination of pulmonary disease may lead to cryptococcal menigitits. Oral cryptococcal lesions may present as non-healing extraction wounds, or chronic ulceration on the palate or tongue.

Histoplasmosis

Histoplasmosis is encountered worldwide, and is endemic in some states of USA. The disease is caused by *Histoplasma capsulatum*, a saprophytic fungus found in soil contaminated by bird and bat droppings. The fungus is dimorphic, remaining in the mould form at ambient temperature, and in the yeast form at body temperature. Infection occurs when airborne conidia or mycelial fragments are inhaled. Most residents in endemic areas are sub-clinically infected, and symptoms usually occur if the host is immunocompromised.

Histoplasmosis is classified into three forms: (1) Primary acute pulmonary form; (2) Chronic pulmonary form; and (3) Disseminated form – may progress to fatal involvement of multiple organ systems. Oral lesions are usually the local manifestation of pulmonary or disseminated forms. (Oral lesions are the earliest sign in 30–66% patients with disseminated histoplasmosis.) Occasionally, oral lesions may be the main or the only presentation of the disease, and they may be encountered in apparently healthy individuals. The oral lesions may be ulcerative, nodular, indurated, or granular, and are found on the tongue, palate, buccal mucosa, or gingivae. Occasionally, the mucosal lesions may invade the mandible or maxilla.

Geotrichosis

This is a rarely reported fungal infection caused by the fungi of the genus *Geotrichum*. The fungus is found in the environment, and rarely in human sputum and faeces. *G. candidum* and *G. capitatum* are the species usually implicated. The organism can cause invasive and disseminated disease in immunocompromised individuals.

Oral lesions consist of sharply defined, purplish-red swellings with ulceration on the soft palate or tongue.

Mucormycosis (zygomycosis)

Although mucormycosis is mainly caused by *Mucor* and *Rhizopus* species of the order *Mucorales*, several other fungal species belonging to the class Zygomycetes are also involved in the causation of this condition. Hence, it is also referred to as zygomycosis. These fungi are found worldwide as saprophytes in soil, manure, and decaying organic matter. Some *Mucor* and *Rhizopus* species are found in the nose, mouth, throat, and faeces of healthy persons, but infection is extremely rare in immunocompetent individuals.

Mucormycosis is a deep fungal infection affecting mainly the face and oropharynx. Mucormycosis commonly starts in the nasal cavity or the maxillary antrum leading to pain, nasal discharge, and fever. The lesion may spread to the palate destroying the intervening bone and presenting as black, necrotic ulcers that may discharge black pus. Some forms of zygomycosis may first appear in the palate.

Paracoccidioidomycosis

Paracoccidioidomycosis is endemic in Brazil and adjoining countries in South America. The disease is caused by the fungus *Paracoccidioides brasiliensis*. The causative fungus is found in the soil in these regions. *P. brasiliensis* has a dimorphic character, remaining in the mould form at ambient temperature and in the yeast form at body temperature. Infection is acquired by inhalation of spores. Subclinical infection is frequently seen in the endemic areas.

Paracoccidioidomycosis affects the mucous membranes, lungs, and bone (and also causes lymphadenopathy). Oral lesions are seen predominantly in males. The majority of patients have multiple lesions in the mouth, involving the lips, palate, buccal mucosa, and (particularly) gingivae.

Oral lesions are painful, and have a violaceous, hyperplastic/ulcerative ('mulberry-like') appearance. Involvement of the lips causes a pronounced increase in thickness and consistency. Oral paracoccidioidomycosis can result in perforation of the hard palate. The juvenile form can cause alveolar bone destruction and tooth loss.

Penicilliosis

This disease is found almost exclusively in Southeast Asian countries, and is caused by the fungus *Penicillium marneffei*.

Penicilliosis is a systemic fungal infection, with involvement of the skin, reticuloendothelial system, respiratory tract, and gastrointestinal tract. Oral lesions are very common, with erosions or superficial ulcers that are usually covered with white slough affecting the palate, gingivae, tongue, labial mucosa, and oropharynx. Facial lesions are also very common.

Sporotrichosis

This disease is caused by the fungus *Sporothrix schenkii*, which is found in rose plants, hay, soil, and infected cats. It is usually acquired by entry of the fungus through cuts or abrasions on the hands or arms. Veterinarians may contract the disease from infected cats.

The common form of infection seen in immunocompetent individuals is the cutaneous form of the disease. A pulmonary form of the disease may develop if spores of the organism are inhaled. Disseminated disease can involve bones, joints, and the central nervous system. Oral lesions have been reported, and consist of painful ulcerated lesions with superficial granulation on the soft palate.

Diagnosis

The differential diagnoses that should be considered for these infections are shown in Table 18.5. The diagnosis of these mycoses is based on the following: (1) clinical features; (2) medical history; (3) social history (e.g. residence/travel in endemic areas); (4) laboratory investigations; and (5) other investigations (e.g. radiological imaging). The laboratory tests that may be useful for these infections are shown in Table 18.6.

Management

The drug treatment of non-candidal oral fungal infections in patients with cancer is shown in Table 18.7.

In invasive fungal diseases of the paranasal sinuses, drug treatment should be supplemented by surgical debridement (e.g. aspergillosis, zygomycosis)[5]. In mucormycosis, adjunct measures are important in the management. For instance, neutropaenia should be reversed with the use of colony-stimulating factors, and the withdrawal of cytotoxic chemotherapy. Furthermore, corticosteroids and other immunosuppressive drugs may have to be curtailed (depending on circumstances). If the patient is on desferrioxamine therapy, then this must be discontinued: the fungus has an affinity for iron, and iron-chelating drugs such as desferrioxamine can enhance the growth of the fungus. There is some evidence that hyperbaric oxygen therapy is useful in conjunction with surgical debridement in management of some fungal infections[6].

Oral fungal infections in the cancer patient

The cancer patient may be affected by oral fungal infections prior to, during, and following anti-cancer therapy.

Table 18.5 Differential diagnoses of important non-Candidal fungal infections

Aspergillosis	Mucormycosis (zygomycosis)	Blastomycosis	Histoplasmosis	Coccidioidomycosis	Paracoccidioidomycosis	Cryptococcosis
Mucormycosis	Dental abscess	Actinomycosis	Aspergillosis	Actinomycosis	Carcinoma	Basal cell carcinoma
Mycetoma	Chronic sinusitis	Aspergillosis	Blastomycosis	Aspergillosis	Lymphoma	Histoplasmosis
Sarcoidosis	Migraines	Brain Abscess	Coccidioidomycosis	Blastomycosis	Tuberculosis	Lipomas
Tuberculosis	Thyrotoxicosis	Cryptococcosis	Sarcoidosis	Histiocytosis	Sarcoidosis	Molluscum contagiosum
Wegener's granulomatosis	Bacterial orbital cellulitis Cavernous sinus thrombosis	Histoplasmosis	Paracoccidioido-mycosis	Histoplasmosis	Syphilis	Syphilis
Zygomycosis	Aspergillosis	Metastatic cancer (unknown primary site)	Cryptococcosis	Lymphadenopathy	Wegener's granulomatosis	Toxoplasmosis
Histoplasmosis	Orbital tumor	Sporotrichosis		Lymphoproliferative disorders	Actinomycosis	Tuberculosis
	Other causes of eye pain	Tuberculosis		Osteomyelitis	Histoplasmosis	
	Blepharitis	Paracoccidioido-mycosis		Sarcoidosis	Cryptococcosis	
	Preseptal cellulitis			Toxoplasmosis	Blastomycosis	
	Orbital cellulitis			Tuberculosis	Coccidioidomycosis	
	Other causes of proptosis			Wegener's Granulomatosis	Mucocutaneous leishmaniasis	
	Posttraumatic subperiosteal hematoma			Paracoccidioidio-mycosis		
	Inflammatory pseudotumor					
	Antral malignancy					

Table 18.6 Laboratory investigations for important non-Candidal fungal infections

Aspergillosis	Mucormycosis (zygomycosis)	Blastomycosis	Histoplasmosis	Coccidioido-mycosis	Paracoccidioido-mycosis	Cryptococcosis
Microscopy of smear	Microscopy of smear	Microscopy of smear	Microscopy of smear	Biopsy demonstrates granulomas with spherules containing endospores	Microscopy of wet mount of sputum in 10% potassium hydroxide - demonstrates 'pilot wheel' arrangement of budding yeasts around mother cell	Microscopy of smear (with India ink or nigrosin)
Biopsy with PAS staining or Gomori methenamine silver staining may show the fungus in tissue (beware of confusion with similar fungi)	Biopsy with PAS staining or Gomori methenamine silver staining demonstrates tissue invasion by characteristic hyphae	Biopsy with PAS staining, Gomori methenamine silver staining or Fontana-Masson staining may show fungus in tissue with granulomas (beware of confusion with similar fungi)	Biopsy may show granulomas and microabscesses with necrosis. PAS staining may show spores with a narrow halo in macrophages	DNA probes	Biopsy with Gomori methenamine silver staining demonstrates suppurative granulomas with giant cells and blastospores that range from 2–30 μm in diameter, and show "pilot wheel" or "mickey mouse" arrangement	Biopsy with PAS, Gomori methenamine silver or Mucicarmine demonstrates fungus in granulomas.
Immunostaining.	(Culture difficult)	Culture on Sabouraud's dextrose agar (beware of confusion with similar fungi)	Culture on Sabouraud's dextrose agar	Serology for Coccidioidal IgM (latex agglutination test, enzyme immunoassay, immunodiffusion, tube precipitins, immunoelectro-phoresis)	Culture very slow	Fluorescent microscopy (yeasts fluoresce under UV light)
Culture on Sabouraud's or Mycosel agar		Immunostaining (most useful)	Complement fixation tests (possible cross reactivity with blastomycosis and coccidioidomycosis)	Spherulin or Coccidioidin skin tests.	(Serology (immuno-diffusion))	Culture on Sabouraud's dextrose agar
Assay of serum precipitin and IgG		Culture may be slow	DNA probes	Culture (may be hazardous to laboratory staff)	(Complement fixation tests)	Serology for capsular antigen and antibody (latex agglutination test)
Assay of IgE antibody levels		Urine blastomyces antigen testing (commercially available)			(Paracoccidioidin skin tests)	
Assay of serum galactomannan		DNA probes				

Table 18.7 Management of important non-Candidal fungal infections

Fungal disease	Treatment	Comments
Aspergillosis	Amphotericin IV infusion of 1mg over 20–30min test dose, then 250mcg/kg daily and if tolerated increase to 1mg/kg daily. Maximum 1.5mg/kg daily on prolonged basis ***When nephrotoxicity is feared, or high dose required:*** Amphotericin lipid formulation 1mg over 10min test dose, then 5mg/kg daily for at least 14days ***Or:*** Itraconazole ***Or:*** Voriconazole ***Or:*** Posaconazole ***Or:*** Caspofungin	
Mucormycosis	Amphotericin IV infusion of 1mg over 20–30min test dose, then 250mcg/kg daily and if tolerated increase to 1mg/kg daily. Maximum 1.5mg/kg daily on prolonged basis ***When nephrotoxicity is feared, or high dose required:*** Amphotericin lipid formulation 1mg over 10min test dose, then 5mg/kg daily for at least 14days ***Or:*** Posaconazole	
Blastomycosis	Itraconazole orally 200mg daily or bd until successful outcome ***For severe infections:*** Amphotericin IV infusion of 1mg over 20–30min test dose, then 250mcg/kg daily and if tolerated increase to 1mg/kg daily. Maximum 1.5mg/kg daily until successful outcome	
Histoplasmosis	Itraconazole orally 200mg daily or bd until successful outcome ***Or:*** Ketoconazole ***For severe infections:*** Amphotericin IV infusion of 1mg over 20–30min test dose, then 250mcg/kg daily and if tolerated increase to 1mg/kg daily. Maximum 1.5mg/kg daily until successful outcome	After successful outcome, itraconazole can be continued as a prophylactic measure
Coccidioidomycosis	Fluconazole 50–400mg oral/iv daily depending on degree of risk ***Or:*** Itraconazole ***Or:*** Ketoconazole	

(continued)

Table 18.7 (continued)

Fungal disease	Treatment	Comments
Paracoccidioidomycosis	Itraconazole orally 200mg daily for 6 months *Or:* Fluconazole *Or:* Ketoconazole *For refractory infections:* Amphotericin	Complete destruction of the fungus may not be achieved even after prolonged therapy, and maintenance therapy for as long as 3 years with sulphonamides may be required
Cryptococcosis	Amphotericin IV infusion of 1mg over 20-30min test dose, then 250mcg/kg daily and if tolerated increase to 1mg/kg daily. Maximum 1.5mg/kg daily on prolonged basis *With or without:* Flucytosine IV infusion 200mg/kg daily in 4 divided doses for 7 days (longer period for cryptococcal meningitis) *Or:* Fluconazole	After successful outcome, fluconazole can be continued as a prophylactic measure (until recovery of immunity)

Patients affected by cancer may present with one or more of the three major variants of oral candidosis even before therapeutic interventions. Haematogenous malignancies may directly compromise the immunity of the patient. Such patients may develop oral pseudomembranous or erythematous candidosis, and, not infrequently, candidal septicaemia[7]. Invasive fungal infections such as aspergillosis [5] and mucormycosis [8,9] have also been reported in patients with acute leukaemia even prior to therapeutic interventions (causing invasive disease of the palate and other orofacial tissues).

Radiotherapy for head and neck cancers may cause oral mucositis and salivary gland dysfunction. These complications result in an ideal environment for oral yeast proliferation, leading particularly to the pseudomembranous and erythematous variants of oral candidosis. It has been estimated that >90% of patients undergoing radiotherapy for head and neck malignancies have oral mucosal colonization with *Candida*, and has been shown that 17–29% of patients have evidence of clinical infection[10].

Cytostatic chemotherapy often causes oral mucosal ulceration and neutropaenia. If the neutropenia is persistent, it may lead to the development of invasive fungal infections[11]. Invasive fungal infections are a leading cause of morbidity and mortality in patients with haematological malignancies[11]. High doses of corticosteroids further compromise immunity by depressing the production of T lymphocytes[12].

Patients receiving haematopoietic stem cell transplantation often develop salivary gland dysfunction leading to candidal colonization (particularly in conjunction with aggressive chemotherapy). Bone marrow transplantation can result in graft-versus-host disease (GVHD), which may also induce salivary gland dysfunction. GVHD may also lead to lichenoid reactions, which may render the oral mucosa susceptible to candidal colonization[13].

Several reports have shown that antifungal drugs administered prophylactically to patients receiving chemotherapy can prevent oral candidosis and other invasive fungal diseases (and so contribute to a reduction in mortality)[14,15]. There is evidence from randomized controlled trails that drugs that are absorbed or partially absorbed should be selected in preference to those that are not absorbed from the gastrointestinal tract, as the former are significantly better at preventing oral candidosis[14]. In general, an oral imidazole or triazole antifungal will be the drug of choice for prophylaxis for immunocompromised patients. Fluconazole has been the traditional choice, because of its good absorption, low toxicity, and good patient adherence (due to once daily administration).

References

1 Samaranayake LP, MacFarlane TW (1990). *Oral candidosis*. Wright, London.

2 Saral R (1991). Candida and aspergillus infections in immunocompromised patients: an overview. *Rev Infect Dis*, 13(3), 487–92.

3 Ribaud P (1997). Fungal infections and the cancer patient. *Eur J Cancer*, 33 (Suppl 4), S50–4.

4 Sitheeque MA, Samaranayake LP (2003). Chronic hyperplastic candidosis/candidiasis (candidal leukoplakia). *Crit Rev Oral Biol Med*, 14(4), 253–67.

5 Karabulut AB, Kabakas F, Berkoz O, Karakas Z, Kesim SN (2005). Hard palate perforation due to invasive aspergillosis in a patient with acute lymphoblastic leukemia. *Int J Pediatr Otorhinolaryngol*, 69(10), 1395–8.

6 Segal E, Menhusen MJ, Shawn S (2007). Hyperbaric oxygen in the treatment of invasive fungal infections: a single-center experience. *Isr Med Assoc J*, 9(5), 355–7.

7 Gonzalez Gravina H, Gonzalez de Moran E, Zambrano O, et al. (2007) Oral candidiasis in children and adolescents with cancer. Identification of Candida spp. *Med Oral Patol Oral Cir Bucal*, 12(6), E419–23.

8 Mohammed S, Sahoo TP, Jayshree RS, Bapsy PP, Hema S (2004). Sino-oral zygomycosis due to Absidia corymbifera in a patient with acute leukemia. *Med Mycol*, 42(5), 475–8.

9 Ryan M, Yeo S, Maguire A, Webb D, et al. (2001). Rhinocerebral zygomycosis in childhood acute lymphoblastic leukaemia. *Eur J Pediatr*, 160(4), 235–8.

10 Ramirez-Amador V, Silverman S Jr, Mayer P, Tyler M, Quivey J (1997). Candidal colonization and oral candidiasis in patients undergoing oral and pharyngeal radiation therapy. *Oral Surg Oral Med Oral Pathol Oral Radiol Endod*, 84(2), 149–53.

11 Glasmacher A, Cornely O, Ullmann AJ, et al. (2006). An open-label randomized trial comparing itraconazole oral solution with fluconazole oral solution for primary prophylaxis of fungal infections in patients with haematological malignancy and profound neutropenia. *J Antimicrob Chemother*, 57(2), 317–25.

12 Stanbury RM, Graham EM (1998) Systemic corticosteroid therapy – side effects and their management. *Br J Ophthalmol*, 82(6), 704–8.

13 Sato M, Tokuda N, Fukumoto T, Mano T, Sato T, Ueyama Y(2006). Immunohistopathological study of the oral lichenoid lesions of chronic GVHD. *J Oral Pathol Med*, 35(1), 33–6.

14 Clarkson JE, Worthington HV, Eden TO (2007). Interventions for preventing oral candidiasis for patients with cancer receiving treatment. *Cochrane Database Syst Rev*, (1), CD003807.

15 Robenshtok E, Gafter-Gvili A, Goldberg E, et al. (2007). Antifungal prophylaxis in cancer patients after chemotherapy or hematopoietic stem-cell transplantation: systematic review and meta-analysis. *J Clin Oncol*, 25(34), 5471–89.

Chapter 19

Oral bacterial infections

Anthony Chow

Introduction

Bacterial infections of the oral cavity most commonly arise from the indigenous microflora that colonize unique niches in the mouth such as the teeth, gingival sulcus, tongue, buccal mucosa, or the saliva. Under normal conditions, they exist as commensal flora in a symbiotic relationship with the host, serving the important function of preventing colonization and invasion by exogenous pathogens. However, under certain pathological conditions such as poor oral hygiene, systemic disease, immunodeficiency, or mucosal injury from irradiation or chemotherapy, these micro-organisms can undergo adaptations that predispose to pathogenicity [1].

It is important to recognize that these endogenous infections do not fit the pattern of classical infectious diseases caused by exogenous pathogens. Hence, these endogenous infections are often caused by a microflora that is often polymicrobial (rather than monomicrobial), and involve both aerobic and anaerobic bacteria. Furthermore, there is an orderly bacterial succession from initiation events to established disease, such that the flora of the advanced lesion may bear little resemblance to the flora of the incipient lesion[2]. Additionally, in a polymicrobial infection, it is often difficult to determine which constituents are the initiators of infection, which are the perpetuators of infection, and which are simply innocent bystanders.

The oral bacterial microflora is discussed in detail in Chapter 17.

Aetiology

Several risk factors for oral infections have been identified in the cancer patient, including poor oral/dental health, oral mucositis, myelosuppression, and salivary gland dysfunction. These risk factors represent impairment of the oral host-defence mechanisms. The oral host-defence mechanisms are discussed in detail in Chapter 17.

Clinical features

Bacterial infections are a major cause of morbidity and mortality in cancer patients receiving local irradiation, systemic chemotherapy, or haematopoietic stem cell transplantation[3,4]. A variety of endogenous bacterial infections are encountered, including exacerbations of dental caries or periodontal disease, necrotizing gingivitis or stomatitis, odontogenic deep space infections, and bacterial overgrowth and secondary infections complicating oral mucositis. Furthermore, the oral cavity is an important source of bacteraemia and sepsis, particularly in patients with neutropaenia[5]. It should be noted that, in the immunocompromised patient, the classical manifestations of an inflammatory response to an infection are frequently muted (and so the presence of infection may be missed).

Odontogenic infections

Dental caries

There is growing awareness of the infectious nature of dental caries, and that only certain micro-organisms residing within dental plaques are cariogenic (the 'specific' plaque hypothesis)[2]. Dental caries are primarily caused by micro-organisms within the supragingival plaque, which is composed mainly of facultative anaerobic and microaerophilic Gram-positive cocci and rods. The mutans streptococci group, notably *Streptococcus mutans* and *S. sobrinus*, are the primary organisms associated with dental caries[6]. Root caries are also associated with *Actinomyces* species, including *A. naeslundii* and *A. viscosus*. Plaque-bacteria ferment sugar, leading to acid production which penetrates the tooth surface and causes demineralization.

The earliest clinical finding is the presence of pits and fissures on the affected tooth surface, which gradually become stained because of demineralization of the enamel and dentine (Figure 19.1, see colour plate section). The lesions have a soft-to-rubbery texture. Progressive demineralization leads to collapse and cavitation, until the enamel surface is destroyed and the dental pulp becomes exposed (Figure 19.2, see colour plate section). Clinically, root caries are more difficult to diagnose than coronal caries, since they tend to occur on the interproximal tooth surfaces where gingival recession has occurred. They are also more common, because of retained food debris and relative inaccessibility to brushing. Coronal caries are more likely to present as recurrent lesions around existing restorations.

Pulpal infection

Pulp tissue that is exposed to oral bacteria invariably becomes infected. Pulpal infections are usually caused by a polymicrobial flora of obligate anaerobes, primarily *Bacteroides* species, *Porphyromonas endodontalis*, *Eubacterium* species, *Fusobacterium nucleatum*, and *Peptostreptococcus micros*[1]. The pressure builds rapidly within the pulp chamber once inflammation is established. This usually elicits excruciating pain along branches of cranial nerve V; the pain may worsen in response to heat or cold in the oral environment. Eventually, ischaemia and necrosis of the pulp tissue develops due to occlusion of blood vessels entering at the apical foramen. When this occurs, the sensory nerve endings are no longer viable, and so dental pain ceases to be a problem. Infection may extend through the necrotic apical root canal causing a localized periodontitis or dentoalveolar abscess. Chronic infection leads to osteitis and occasionally osteomyelitis of the jaws.

Pericoronitis

Pericoronitis is an acute localized infection caused by the entrapment of food particles and micro-organisms under the gum flaps of a partially erupted or an impacted molar tooth. The mandibular molars are most commonly involved. Prominent symptoms include pain, limitation of mouth opening (trismus), discomfort on mastication and swallowing, and facial swelling. Clinically, the pericoronal tissues are swollen and erythematous, and digital pressure can often express an exudate from under the infected flap. The breath is usually malodorous, and painful lymphadenopathy may be noted in the submandibular region.

Persistent periapical dental infection may lead to chronic osteomyelitis of the jaws [7]. Similarly, periapical infections arising from anterior maxillary teeth may perforate the Schneidarian membrane to cause chronic or recurrent maxillary sinusitis.

Periodontal disease

Periodontal disease affects the connective tissues supporting the tooth, including the gingiva, periodontal ligament, and alveolar bone. The process can be confined to the soft tissues supporting the tooth causing gingivitis, or involve deeper structures with loss of alveolar support for the tooth, eventually leading to tooth loss. Periodontal disease is mainly caused by micro-organisms within the subgingival dental plaque, which penetrate the gingival epithelium and elicit an inflammatory response[8]. The microflora is predominated by *Actinomyces* species such as *A. viscosus* and *A. naeslundii*, and *Porphyromonas gingivalis*. Other organisms such as *S. sanguis* and *S. anginosus* are also found. As periodontal disease advances, *Porphyromonas gingivalis*, *Prevotella intermedia*, *Tannerella forsythia*, and *Treponema denticola* become predominant[2]. In addition to plaque-induced inflammation, other conditions that can trigger gingival inflammation include hormonal changes (e.g. pregnancy), and medications (e.g. ciclosporin, phenytoin). Periodontal infection is a major source for fever and sepsis in cancer patients, and causes considerable morbidity especially in patients with neutropaenia.[3] However, gingival infection can be missed, because signs of gingival inflammation such as redness and swelling may be muted as a result of neutropaenia. Radiological investigation (e.g. bite-wing X-ray, orthopantogram) is an essential aspect of making the diagnosis (Figure 19.3, see colour plate section).

Necrotizing gingivitis/stomatitis

Necrotizing gingivitis

Necrotizing gingivitis (also known as acute necrotizing ulcerative gingivitis, 'trench mouth', and Vincent's angina) is an aggressive form of periodontitis associated with rapid progression and tissue destruction. The gingival connective tissues are invaded by a polymicrobial microflora dominated by *Treponema denticola*, *Prevotella intermedia*, and *Fusobacterium nucleatum*[9]. Herpesviruses (i.e. herpes simplex virus-1 (HSV-1), Epstein–Barr virus (EBV), and cytomegalovirus (CMV)) are frequently found to coexist with periodontopathic bacteria, and so have been suggested to play a role in the pathogenesis of necrotizing gingivitis[10]. However, a causal relationship remains to be determined. Necrotizing gingivitis is associated with severe impairment of immune responses due to underlying disease, and may be one of the first signs of acute leukaemia or the acquired immune deficiency syndrome (AIDS)[11]. It may also occur in patients undergoing haematopoietic stem cell transplantation. Necrotizing gingivitis is characterized by ulceration, bleeding, and necrosis of the interdental soft tissues (Figure 19.4, see colour plate section). The onset is abrupt, and the patient usually complains of pain and systemic manifestations of infection.

Necrotizing stomatitis

Necrotizing stomatitis (also known as gangrenous stomatitis, noma, and cancrum oris) bears some resemblance to necrotizing gingivitis, but is more focal and destructive, involving deeper tissues to the gingiva. Cultures and molecular analysis from advancing lesions reveal a diverse microflora dominated by fusospirochaetal organisms such as *Treponema vincentii*, *Fusobacterium nucleatum*, and *Prevotella melaninogenica*[12]. It has been described following irradiation of the head and neck (in the absence of significant periodontal disease)[13]. The earliest lesion is a small, painful red spot or vesicle on the attached gingiva in the premolar or molar region of the mandible. A necrotic ulcer rapidly develops and undermines the deeper tissue. Painful cellulitis of the cheeks and lips is observed as the lesion extends outwards in a cone-like fashion. Within a short period, sloughing of necrotic soft tissues occurs, exposing the underlying deep tissues (e.g. bone).

Bacterial sialoadenitis

Sialoadenitis, or infection of salivary tissue, most commonly involves the parotid gland. However, the submandibular and sublingual glands can also be affected. Common pathogens include

Staphylococcus aureus, Enterobacteriaceae, and anaerobic Gram-negative rods such as *Prevotella* and *Fusobacterium* species[14]. Risk factors for infection include myelosuppression and ductal obstruction caused by calculi, irradiation, and salivary gland hypofunction. Clinically, the patient presents with a sudden onset of pain and swelling over the affected gland. Thus, parotitis is characterized by swelling of the pre- and post-auricular areas, which may extend towards the angle of the mandible. In addition, suppuration may be noted at the orifice of the Stenson's duct. Systemic features of infection are generally present (e.g. fever, chills). Progression of the infection may lead to massive swelling of the neck (resulting in respiratory obstruction), osteomyelitis of adjacent facial bones, and septicaemia.

Odontogenic deep-space infections

Odontogenic deep-space infections tend to involve the more superficial masticator, buccal, canine, submental, and infratemporal spaces. Extension may occur to involve the deeper fascial spaces of the head and neck, such as the submandibular, sublingual, lateral pharyngeal, and retropharyngeal spaces[15]. The third mandibular molars are the most common sources for odontogenic deep-space infections[16]. Infections involving the mandibular molars may extend into the submandibular and sublingual spaces resulting in massive swelling of the base of the tongue and acute airway obstruction (Ludwig's angina), while those involving maxillary premolars may extend infratemporally into the orbit. Similarly, infections arising from the masticator spaces may extend into the lateral pharyngeal space and eventually invade the carotid sheath and the internal jugular vein (Lemierre syndrome). Finally, infection involving the retropharyngeal space may dissect directly into the posterior mediastinum resulting in an acute necrotizing mediastinitis. The clinical features of these deep-space infections are summarized in Table 19.1[17].

Oral mucositis

Although oral mucositis is not generally considered an infectious disease, there is considerable support for secondary bacterial overgrowth, and invasion of the submucosa during the so-called ulcerative phase[18]. Patients with ulceration associated with mucositis have a significantly increased risk of bacteraemia and septicaemia compared to patients without ulceration[19,20]. Oral mucositis is discussed in detail in Chapter 15.

Bacteraemia and sepsis

Bacteraemia and sepsis is a serious complication in patients with neutropaenia, particularly among those with a haematological malignancy. Bacteraemia in these patients are predominantly (~70% cases) caused by Gram-positive cocci, particularly viridans streptococci and staphylococci[7,21]. Molecular analysis has revealed that bacteraemia with viridans stretpotocci is most likely derived from the oral cavity[22], whereas bacteraemia with coagulase-negative staphylococci most likely arises from the nasopharynx or the skin (i.e. intravenous catheters)[23]. Indeed, oropharyngeal colonization with viridans streptococci of a given ribotype has been shown to precede bacteraemia with the same ribotype[24]. Patients with viridans streptococcal bacteraemia are more likely to have poor dental health or oral mucositis than patients without streptococcal bacteraemia[20]. Bacteraemia associated with viridans streptococci is especially common in children, and causes considerable morbidity and mortality[22]. Thus, almost one-third of infected patients develop a shock syndrome[25].

Table 19.1 Clinical features of odontogenic deep space infections [17]

Deep space infection	Usual site of origin	Clinical features				
		Pain	Trismus	Swelling	Dysphagia	Dyspnoea
Masticator	Molars (especially 3rd)	Present	Prominent	May not be evident (deep)	Absent	Absent
◆ Masseteric & Pterygoid	Posterior maxillary molars	Present	None	Face, orbit (late)	Absent	Absent
◆ Temporal						
Buccal	Biscuspids, molars	Minimal	Minimal	Cheek (marked)	Absent	Absent
Canine	Maxillary canines, incisors	Moderate	None	Upper lip, canine fossa	Absent	Absent
Infratemporal	Posterior maxillary molars	Present	None	Face, orbit (late)	Occasional	Occasional
Submental	Mandibular incisors	Moderate	None	Chin (firm)	Absent	Absent
Parotid	Masseteric spaces	Intense	None	Angle of jaw (marked)	Absent	Absent
Submandibular	Mandibular molars (2nd, 3rd)	Present	Minimal	Submandibular	Absent	Absent
Sublingual	Mandibular incisors	Present	Minimal	Floor of mouth (tender)	Present if bilateral	Present if bilateral
Lateral pharyngeal	Masticator spaces	Intense	Prominent	Angle of jaw	Present	Occasional
◆ Anterior	Masticator spaces	Minimal	Minimal	Posterior pharynx	Present	Severe
◆ Posterior						
Retropharyngeal	Lateral pharyngeal space	Present	Minimal	Posterior pharynx (midline)	Present	Present

Investigation

Microbiological investigation

A major challenge in the microbiological investigation of oral infections is how to distinguish true pathogens from commensal flora. The mere presence of an organism is insufficient to ascribe a causal role in a polymicrobial endogenous infection. This underscores the importance of proper specimen collection, and the need to correlate clinical information with laboratory data. Imaging techniques may also be useful in certain circumstances.

Aerobic and anaerobic blood cultures should always be obtained. Surface cultures obtained from mucosal sites are regularly contaminated by resident commensal flora and are generally not recommended. Direct microscopic examination of stained smears often provides more useful information. For closed-space infections, needle aspiration of pus is desirable, but is often not feasible due to neutropaenia and/or thrombocytopaenia. Specimens should be collected in appropriate transport medium and delivered as soon as possible to the laboratory under anaerobic conditions.

Occasionally, biopsy of specific lesions may be required in order to arrive at a histopathological diagnosis. Immunofluorescence staining and DNA probes or polymerase chain reaction (PCR) are increasingly available for pathogens that are fastidious or non-cultivable[26,27]. The benzoyl-DL-arginine-naphthylamide (BANA) test detects a trypsin-like enzyme produced by periodonto-pathic bacteria including *Porphomonas gingivalis, Treponema denticola*, and *Tannerella forsythia*. A positive BANA test correlates both qualitatively and quantitatively with the presence of these micro-organisms and is useful for the diagnosis of anaerobic periodontal infections[28].

Management

The management of odontogenic and other oromucosal infections in the cancer patient requires a multidisciplinary approach. A proactive approach is necessary for all patients, involving routine oral hygiene measures, and regular dental check ups/care. Chapter 5 discusses pretreatment screening/treatment in detail, whilst Chapter 6 discusses routine oral hygiene in detail.

Endogenous oral pathogens are no longer universally susceptible to penicillin. Thus, β-lactamase-producing anaerobic Gram-negative bacteria have been increasingly recognized[29]. They include *Prevotella* species, *Porphyromonas* species, *Fusobacterium* species, and others[30,31]. Indeed, failure of penicillin therapy in odontogenic infections due to these micro-organisms is well documented[32]. Thus, a β-lactam/β-lactamase-inhibitor combination should be considered if the clinical response to penicillin is suboptimal (and there is no evidence for loculated infection requiring surgical drainage). There are also increasing reports of *in vitro* resistance to metronidazole and azithromycin amongst *Fusobacterium* species and other anaerobic Gram-negative bacteria isolated from odontogenic infections[33]. However, the clinical significance of these findings is unclear at this time. Nevertheless, the emergence of resistance among oral bacteria is disconcerting, and is probably due to selection pressure from widespread and inappropriate use of broad-spectrum antibiotics.

The recommended antimicrobial regimens for various odontogenic and oromucosal infections in normal and immunocompromised hosts are summarized in Table 19.2. The selection of antimicrobial agents should be guided by their predicted antibacterial spectrum, and the bioavailability of oral or parenteral formulations. Since immunocompromised patients are particularly at risk for rapidly spreading orofacial infections, empirical broad-spectrum antimicrobial therapy is usually warranted. The antibiotic regimen must be broad-spectrum, bactericidal, and appropriate in dose and schedule. In hospitalized patients, and those with severe neutropaenia, it is prudent

Table 19.2 Antimicrobial regimens for odontogenic and oromucosal infections

Clinical entity	Unique microbial species	Antimicrobial regimen
Supragingival dental plaque and dental caries	*Streptococcus mutans* Other streptococci *Actinomyces* spp.	Fluoride-containing dentifrices or oral rinses (e.g. sodium fluoride 1.1% or stannous fluoride 0.4%) used 2 or 3 times daily. Fluoride-containing varnishes (e.g. sodium fluoride 5%) applied 3 or 4 times yearly Chlorhexidine 0.12% oral rinses
Subgingival dental plaque and simple gingivitis	Streptococci, *Actinomyces* spp Spirochaetes	Penicillin G 1-4 MU IV q4-6h (or penicillin V 500 mg PO q8h) **plus** metronidazole 500 mg PO or IV q8h Ampicillin-sulbactam 1.5-3 g IV q6h (or amoxicilin-clavulanate 500 mg PO q8h) Clindamycin 450 mg PO or 600 mg IV q6-8 h
Periodontitis, early-onset, 'aggressive' or 'localized juvenile'	*Actinobacillus actinomycetemcomitans Porphyromonas gingivalis Treponema denticoli Prevotella intermedia*	Tetracycline 500 mg PO q6h or 1 g IV q12h Doxycycline 200 mg PO or IV q12h Metronidazole 500 mg PO or IV q8h
Periodontitis, adult or 'established'	*Treponema denticoli* Other oral spirochaetes *Porphyromonas gingivalis Prevotella intermedia Tannerella forsythia*	Topical minocycline microspheres Topical doxycycline hyclate periodontal extended-release liquid
Necrotizing gingivitis/ stomatitis	*Prevotella intermedia Fusobacterium* spp *Tannerella forsythia Treponema denticoli* Other oral spirochaetes	Ampicillin-sulbactam 1.5-3 g IV q6h (or amoxicillin-clavulanate 500 mg PO q8h) Metronidazole 500 mg PO or IV q8h Clindamycin 450 mg PO or 600 mg IV q6-8h
Bacterial sialoadenitis	*Staphylococcus aureus* Mixed anaerobes	Cloxacillin 2 g IV q4 h (or nafcillin 2 g IV q4h) **plus either** metronidazole 500 mg IV or PO q6h, **or** clinamycin 600 mg IV or PO q6-8h (For methicillin-resistance *S. aureus*, substitute cloxacillin or nafcillin with vancomycin 15-20 mg/kg IV to maintain trough serum concentrations ~ 10-15 μg/mL **or** linezolid 600 mg IV or PO q12h **or** daptomycin 4-6 mg/kg IV q24 h)
Odontogenic deep space infections	*Streptococcus viridans* Other streptococci *Peptostreptococcus* spp *Bacteroides* spp Other oral anaerobes	**Normal hosts** Penicillin G 2-4 MU IV q4-6h, **plus** metronidazole 0.5 g IV q6h Ampicillin-sulbactam 2 g IV q4h Clindamycin 600 mg IV q6h Doxycycline 200 mg IV q12h Cefoxitin 1-2 g IV q6h Moxifloxacin 400 mg IV q24h **Immunocompromised hosts** Cefotaxime 2 g IV q6h Ceftizoxime 4 g IV q8h Ticarcillin-clavulanate 3 g IV q4h Piperacillin-tazobactam 3 g IV q4h Imipenem 500 mg IV q6h Meropenem 1 g IV q8h

to cover for facultative Gram-negative bacilli as well as strepotococci and oral anaerobes. In addition, coverage for methicillin-resistant *S. aureus* (MRSA) may be required.

References

1 Ruby J, Barbeau J (2002). The buccale puzzle: the symbiotic nature of endogenous infections of the oral cavity. *Can J Infect Dis*, 13(1), 34–41.

2 Loesche W (2007). Dental caries and periodontitis: contrasting two infections that have medical implications. *Infect Dis Clin North Am*, 21(2), 471–502, vii.

3 Raber-Durlacher JE, Epstein JB, Raber J, et al. (2002). Periodontal infection in cancer patients treated with high-dose chemotherapy. *Support Care Cancer*, 10(6), 466–73.

4 Heimdahl A (1999). Prevention and management of oral infections in cancer patients. *Support Care Cancer*, 7(4), 224–8.

5 Lockhart PB, Loven B, Brennan MT, Fox PC (2007). The evidence base for the efficacy of antibiotic prophylaxis in dental practice. *J Am Dent Assoc*, 138(4), 458–74.

6 Marsh PD (1999). Microbiologic aspects of dental plaque and dental caries. *Dent Clin North Am*, 43(4), 599–614, v–vi.

7 Lerman MA, Laudenbach J, Marty FM, Baden LR, Treister NS (2008). Management of oral infections in cancer patients. *Dent Clin North Am*, 52(1), 129–53, ix.

8 Van Dyke TE, Serhan CN (2003). Resolution of inflammation: a new paradigm for the pathogenesis of periodontal diseases. *J Dent Res*, 82(2), 82–90.

9 Bermejo-Fenoll A, Sanchez-Perez A (2004). Necrotising periodontal diseases. *Med Oral Patol Oral Cir Bucal*, 9(Suppl), 114–19.

10 Slots J (2007). Herpesviral-bacterial synergy in the pathogenesis of human periodontitis. *Curr Opin Infect Dis*, 20(3), 278–83.

11 Robinson PG (2002). The significance and management of periodontal lesions in HIV infection. *Oral Dis*, 8(Suppl 2), 91–7.

12 Paster BJ, Falkler JW Jr, Enwonwu CO, et al. (2002). Prevalent bacterial species and novel phylotypes in advanced noma lesions. *J Clin Microbiol*, 40(6), 2187–91.

13 Mayorca A, Hazime N, Dekeister C, Paoli JR (2002). Necrotizing stomatitis after radiotherapy in a patient with AIDS: case report. *J Oral Maxillofac Surg*, 60(1), 100–1.

14 Brook I (2003). Acute bacterial suppurative parotitis: microbiology and management. *J Craniofac Surg*, 14(1), 37–40.

15 Reynolds SC, Chow AW (2007). Life-threatening infections of the peripharyngeal and deep fascial spaces of the head and neck. *Infect Dis Clin North Am*, 21(2), 557–76, viii.

16 Chow AW (1992). Life-threatening infections of the head and neck. *Clin Infect Dis*, 14(5), 991–1002.

17 Hull MW, Chow AW (2005). An approach to oral infections and their management. *Curr Infect Dis Rep*, 7(1), 17–27.

18 Treister N, Sonis S (2007). Mucositis: biology and management. *Curr Opin Otolaryngol Head Neck Surg*, 15(2), 123–9.

19 Rondinelli PI, Ribeiro KC, de Camargo B (2006). A proposed score for predicting severe infection complications in children with chemotherapy-induced febrile neutropenia. *J Pediatr Hematol Oncol*, 28(10), 665–70.

20 Bochud PY, Eggiman P, Calandra T, Van Melle G, Saghafi L, Francioli P (1994). Bacteremia due to viridans streptococcus in neutropenic patients with cancer: clinical spectrum and risk factors. *Clin Infect Dis*, 18(1), 25–31.

21 Kurt B, Flynn P, Shenep JL, et al. (2008). Prophylactic antibiotics reduce morbidity due to septicemia during intensive treatment for pediatric acute myeloid leukemia. *Cancer*, 113(2), 376–82.

22 Reilly AF, Lange BJ (2007). Infections with viridans group streptococci in children with cancer. *Pediatr Blood Cancer*, 49(6), 774–80.

23   Costa SF, Barone AA, Miceli MH, et al. (2006). Colonization and molecular epidemiology of coagulase-negative Staphylococcal bacteremia in cancer patients: a pilot study. *Am J Infect Control*, 34(1), 36–40.

24   Wisplinghoff H, Reinert RR, Cornely O, Seifert H (1999). Molecular relationships and antimicrobial susceptibilities of viridans group streptococci isolated from blood of neutropenic cancer patients. *J Clin Microbiol*, 37(6), 1876–80.

25   Gamis AS, Howells WB, DeSwarte-Wallace J, Feusner JH, Buckley JD, Woods WG (2000). Alpha hemolytic streptococcal infection during intensive treatment for acute myeloid leukemia: a report from the Children's cancer group study CCG-2891. *J Clin Oncol*, 18(9), 1845–55.

26   Roscoe DL, Hoang L (2007). Microbiologic investigations for head and neck infections. *Infect Dis Clin North Am*, 21(2), 283–304, v.

27   Slots J, Ashimoto A, Flynn MJ, Li G, Chen C (1995). Detection of putative periodontal pathogens in subgingival specimens by 16S ribosomal DNA amplification with the polymerase chain reaction. *Clin Infect Dis*, 20(Suppl 2), S304-7: S304–7.

28   Loesche WJ, Bretz WA, Kerschensteiner D, et al. (1990). Development of a diagnostic test for anaerobic periodontal infections based on plaque hydrolysis of benzoyl-DL-arginine-naphthylamide. *J Clin Microbiol*, 28(7), 1551–9.

29   Brook I (1988). Beta-lactamase producing bacteria in head and neck infection. *Laryngoscope*, 98(4), 428–31.

30   Brook I (1993). Infections caused by beta-lactamase-producing Fusobacterium spp. in children. *Pediatr Infect Dis*, 12(6), 532–3.

31   Brook I (2002). Antibiotic resistance of oral anaerobic bacteria and their effect on the management of upper respiratory tract and head and neck infections. *Semin Respir Infect*, 17(3), 195–203.

32   Heimdahl A, von Konow L, Nord CE (1980). Isolation of beta-lactamase producing Bacteroides strains associated with clinical failures with penicillin treatment of human orofacial infections. *Arch Oral Biol*, 25(10), 689–92.

33   Bresco-Salinas M, Costa-Riu N, Berini-Aytes L, Gay-Escoda C (2006). Antibiotic susceptibility of the bacteria causing odontogenic infections. *Med Oral Patol Oral Cir Bucal*, 11(1), E70–5.

Chapter 20

Oral viral infections

Deborah Lockhart and Jeremy Bagg

Introduction

Viruses are strict intracellular parasites that require a host cell for replication. They consist of nucleic acid (DNA or RNA) surrounded by a protein coat (capsid), and may be encased in a lipid envelope. Although a variety of viruses may infect the oro-facial region[1], the herpes group of viruses predominates (Table 20.1). Cell-mediated immunity is an important defence mechanism, and consequently cancer patients deficient in T cells are more susceptible to viral infections.

Oral viral infections are a significant cause of morbidity amongst cancer patients, resulting in both oropharyngeal symptoms (e.g. pain), and systemic symptoms (e.g. malaise). Atypical presentations may be seen in immunocompromised patients[2]. Usually, these infections represent a reactivation of latent viruses, although *de novo* infections may also occur in this group of patients. The oral cavity provides a potential portal for systemic dissemination (with resultant morbidity/mortality).

Laboratory results must be interpreted in conjunction with clinical findings. Traditional diagnostic methods include electron microscopy, immunofluorescence, tissue culture, and serology. Polymerase chain reaction (PCR)-based assays for the detection of viral nucleic acid in clinical specimens are likely to emerge as the 'gold standard' investigation. In urgent situations requiring rapid diagnosis, the turnaround time may be 2–3 h for immunofluorescence, and 6 h for PCR.

Herpes virus infections

The human herpes viruses are double-stranded, enveloped DNA viruses. Most herpes viruses have oro-facial manifestations (with the salivary secretions being a common mode of transmission).

Herpes viruses may cause:

+ Primary infection – the first encounter with the virus (seroconversion).

+ Latent infection – refers to the persistent presence of viral genome but not infectious virus. Herpes viruses characteristically establish lifelong latent infections.

+ Reactivation – refers to asymptomatic viral shedding (often in saliva).

+ Secondary infection – refers to evidence of clinical disease ('recurrence'/'recrudescence').

Herpes Simplex Virus (HSV)

Epidemiology

Primary herpetic gingivostomatitis is the most common viral infection of the mouth, and the majority of the adult population are seropositive for HSV (i.e. 70–80%). The virus remains latent in the trigeminal ganglion, and approximately one-third of people develop secondary infections due to reactivation of the virus.

Table 20.1 Viral infections involving the oral cavity [2,4]

Family	Virus	Oro-facial manifestation
Human herpes viruses	Herpes simplex type I/II virus	Primary herpetic gingivostomatits Herpes labialis ('cold sore') Atypical intra-oral recurrences in immunocompromised
	Varicella zoster virus	Chickenpox Shingles
	Epstein Barr virus	Infectious mononucleosis Oral hairy leukoplakia Nasopharyngeal carcinoma Burkitt's lymphoma Hodgkin's lymphoma Post-transplantation lymphoproliferative disorder
	Cytomegalovirus	Non-specific ulcers
	Human herpes virus 6 & 7	Roseola infantum (childhood disease)
	Human herpes virus 8	Kaposi's sarcoma
Papilloma viruses	Human papilloma virus	Oral wart Associated with oral squamous cell carcinoma
Paramyxoviruses	Measles virus Mumps virus	Koplik's spots on buccal mucosa Salivary gland inflammation
Picornaviruses	Coxsackie group A viruses	Hand, foot and mouth disease Herpangina
Retroviruses	Human immunodeficiency virus	Numerous oral manifestations (relating to associated immunosuppression)

Recurrence is a particular concern in cancer patients. Following high-dose chemotherapy or haematopoietic stem cell transplantation (HSCT), around 75% of patients develop clinical disease in the absence of prophylaxis[3]. Lower rates of HSV recurrence occur in less intensively treated patients (e.g. 38–68% in Non-Hodgkin's lymphoma, 15–20% in head and neck cancer [3]).

Traditionally, HSV type I was associated with oro-facial lesions, whereas HSV type II was associated with infection of the genital tract. However, HSV type II may also cause oral infections. Numerous factors have been reported to reactivate HSV including stress, hormonal changes, and ultraviolet light. Deficiencies in cell-mediated immunity account for the manifestations seen in immunocompromised patients.

Clinical features

Primary herpetic gingivostomatitis

In young children the infection is often subclinical or attributed to 'teething', while clinical disease is more pronounced in adolescents and young adults. Typical features include fever, cervical lymphadenopathy, and intra-oral discomfort making eating and swallowing difficult. Classic intra-epithelial vesicles develop on the oral mucosa, including the gingivae, tongue, and buccal mucosa. These subsequently rupture resulting in superficial ulcers with erythematous margins and a greyish-yellow base (Figure 20.1, see colour plate section). The lips may become swollen and covered in a blood-stained crust. The disease is self-limiting, and the lesions resolve without scarring within 10 days.

Secondary infection (immunocompetent patients)

Herpes labialis or 'cold sore' is the most common type of recurrence, and usually affects the vermillion border or the skin adjacent to the nostril (Figure 20.2, see colour plate section). The presence of vesicles is often heralded by a prodrome of tingling or burning in the preceding 24 h. Within 10–14 days the vesicles have ruptured, crusted, and healed without scarring. Intra-oral reactivations are rare in the immunocompetent, and may present as small crops of lesions on the palatal mucosa[4].

Secondary infection (immunocompromised patients)

The presentation is often atypical, and may be mistaken for oral mucositis or aphthous ulceration. However, the degree of pain may be considerably greater in recurrent HSV infection. Extensive intra-oral lesions may affect any part of the oral mucosa either as small crops of ulcers (Figure 20.3a, see colour plate section), or as a more florid reaction (Figure 20.3b, see colour plate section). The lesions may become co-infected with other viral, bacterial, and/or fungal pathogens. The lesions may persist for months without adequate therapy.

Diagnosis

Most infections are diagnosed clinically in the immunocompetent patient. Atypical presentations necessitate prompt laboratory investigation of suspicious lesions in immunocompromised patients. (Any acute, painful oral ulceration must be considered a potential HSV recurrence in this group of patients.) Clinicians should liaise with their local microbiology laboratory regarding the optimal diagnostic specimens.

Management

In all cases, adequate oral hygiene should be maintained to minimize bacterial co-infection.

Primary herpetic gingivostomatitis

Symptomatic remedies such as rest, antipyretics, and adequate fluid intake are the mainstay of treatment. Aciclovir may shorten the duration and severity of symptoms if prescribed early enough (Table 20.2)[5].

Secondary infection (immunocompetent patients)

Antiviral treatment may reduce the severity of the lesions, and should be initiated during the premonitory phase. 1% penciclovir cream has been shown to be more beneficial than 5% aciclovir cream[6], although both regimens require multiple applications and good patient adherence. A short-course of high-dose oral antiviral therapy combined with topical corticosteroids offers an alternative strategy. Immunomodulatory drugs may have a role in future management[7].

Secondary infection (immunocompromised patients)

Owing to the potential serious complications of disseminated disease, systemic antiviral therapy should be immediately commenced on suspicion of infection. There have been several evidence-based reviews regarding the optimal treatment (Table 20.2) [8–10]. Lesions should be monitored to ensure resolution, and, if not improving within 7–10 days, evaluated for co-infection[2].

Antiviral prophylaxis should be considered to prevent secondary infections in this patient group, although there is no consensus on the duration of therapy[8,9]. Aciclovir resistance is rare,

Table 20.2 Management of herpes simplex virus and varicella zoster virus infections [8,9,13]

Infection	Drug	Comment
Primary herpetic gingivostomatitis	Aciclovir – oral; 200 mg; 5 times daily for 5–7 days	Increase dose in immunocompromised.
Recurrent herpes labialis	Aciclovir – topical; 5% cream; every 3–4 hr for 5 days	
	Aciclovir – oral; 200 mg; 5 times daily for 5–7 days	
	Penciclovir – topical; 1% cream; every 2 hr for 5 days	May be more effective than topical aciclovir.
	Valaciclovir – oral; 1–2 g; twice daily for 1 day	
	Famciclovir – oral; 1.5g; once daily for 1 day	May be given as two doses of 750 mg.
Recurrent herpes infection in the immunocompromised	Aciclovir – oral; 400mg; 3–5 times daily for 10 days or longer	Often up to several weeks.
	Aciclovir – IV; 5mg/kg; every 8 hr for 5 days	Severe infection.
	Valaciclovir – oral; 0.5–1g; 2–3 times daily for 10 days or longer	Often up to several weeks.
	Famciclovir – oral; 500mg; twice daily	Prolonged duration.
Prophylaxis for recurrent herpes infection in the immunocompromised	Aciclovir – oral; 200–800mg; 3–4 times daily	May be given IV
	Valaciclovir – oral; 0.5–1g; twice daily	
	Famciclovir – oral; 0.5–1g; twice daily	
Herpes zoster	Aciclovir – oral; 800mg; 5 times daily for 7 days	IV in immunocompromised
	Valaciclovir – oral; 1g; 3 times daily for 7 days	
	Famciclovir – oral; 250mg; 3 times daily for 7 days	Increase dose in immunocompromised
	Famciclovir – oral; 750 mg; once daily for 7 days	

but has been reported amongst leukaemic patients[11]. Intravenous foscarnet can be used as an alternative agent in proven aciclovir resistance.

Varicella Zoster Virus (VZV)

Epidemiology

Approximately 6% of the adult population remain susceptible to VZV[12]. In the United States, a live-attenuated vaccine is now part of the childhood immunisation schedule, but it is not routinely given in the United Kingdom and elsewhere.

Primary infection with VZV causes varicella ('chickenpox'), with the virus establishing latency in the sensory nerve-root ganglia. Reactivation of VZV causes herpes zoster ('shingles'), and is more common in those over the age of 60 years. In addition, it may be triggered by immuno-deficiency-associated conditions, such as non-Hodgkin's lymphoma or HSCT.

Clinical features

Varicella

Oral lesions may precede the skin rash, and consist of ulcers of approximately 2–4 mm in diameter surrounded by an erythematous halo. Ulcers may be detectable on the hard palate, the pillars of the fauces, and the uvula.

Herpes zoster

The trigeminal nerve is involved in about 15% of cases. Both the facial skin and oral mucosa may demonstrate lesions if the mandibular and/or maxillary branches are affected (Figure 20.4a and b, see colour plate section). Skin eruptions are often preceded by several days of localised paraesthesia and (severe) pain. The skin lesions typically present as unilateral clusters of vesicles/ulcers solely involving the area of skin supplied by a particular dermatome. The lesions form scabs within a few days, and heal without scarring.

Diagnosis

Clinical examination normally suffices, but laboratory confirmation may be advocated for the immunocompromised (when the infection may be disseminated).

Management

VZV is intrinsically less sensitive to aciclovir, and so higher doses are required for therapeutic effects (Table 20.2).

Varicella

Aciclovir administered within 24 h of the onset of rash may reduce the duration and severity of symptoms[13].

Herpes zoster

Systemic antivirals should be prescribed as soon as possible (and certainly within 72 h). This may reduce the likelihood of complications such as post-herpetic neuralgia. In addition, it reduces viral shedding and the severity and duration of pain. Corticosteroids and analgesics may also be given as adjunct therapies[13].

Epstein Barr Virus (EBV)

Epidemiology

Approximately 90% of the population are seropositive for EBV. The virus establishes latency in B lymphocytes and oropharyngeal epithelial cells.

Clinical features

Most people experience a subclinical infection rather than overt infectious mononucleosis. Infectious mononucleosis is characterized by fever, cervical lymphoadenopathy, pharyngitis, and malaise.

EBV is also associated with oral hairy leucoplakia and lymphoproliferative malignancies (Table 20.1). Oral hairy leucoplakia is usually asymptomatic and typically presents as bilateral, vertical, striated white plaques on the lateral surface of the tongue (Figure 20.5, see colour plate section). Occasionally, the ventral and dorsal surfaces may be affected, and the lesions can become co-infected with *Candida* species[14]. Oral hairy leucoplakia is indicative of immunosuppression.

Diagnosis

EBV-specific serology for infectious mononucleosis may be unreliable in the immuno-compromised, necessitating the use of EBV-specific PCR assays. Accurate diagnosis of oral hairy leucoplakia requires a biopsy of the lesion demonstrating the presence of EBV using *in situ* hybridization or other methods.

Management

Infectious mononucleosis is self-limiting, and requires no specific treatment. Oral hairy leucoplakia is also usually self-limiting. Topical application of 25% podophyllum resin has been suggested for oral hairy leucoplakia, but there are insufficient data to support this form of treatment[15].

Cytomegalovirus (CMV)

Epidemiology

Approximately 50–80% of the population have latent virus in their salivary glands, endothelial cells, and leucocytes[16].

Clinical features

CMV may present with a mononucleosis-like illness, but symptoms are generally only seen in infants and the immunocompromised. Oral manifestations of recurrence may rarely be seen during HSCT, with non-specific painful ulcers on mucosal surfaces or major salivary gland infections. Co-infection with other bacterial, fungal, or viral pathogens may complicate the diagnosis.

Management

Ganciclovir can be used for life-threatening infections.

Human herpes virus 8 (Kaposi's sarcoma associated herpes virus)

Kaposi's sarcoma is the commonest human immunodeficiency virus (HIV)-associated tumour, although its incidence has declined following introduction of highly active antiretroviral treatment (HAART). The tumour arises from endothelial cells of vascular and lymphatic origin. Kaposi's sarcoma has been linked with infection with human herpes virus 8 (HHV-8).

Clinical features

The tumour may affect any tissue system, but particularly involves the skin. Around 50% patients have oral manifestations commonly involving the palatal mucosa and the anterior maxillary gingivae (Figure 20.6, see colour plate section). Initially, the lesion presents as an asymptomatic purplish macule, which may cause pain as it becomes raised and ulcerated.

Diagnosis

Histological examination is required for a definitive diagnosis of Kaposi's sarcoma.

Management

Management options include surgical excision, cryotherapy, and radiotherapy.

Kaposi's sarcoma is discussed in detail in Chapter 8.

Human papillomavirus (HPV) infections

HPV is a non-enveloped double-stranded DNA virus that specifically infects epithelia and mucous membranes. Over 100 types have been identified with HPV-16/18 having oncogenic potential, and forming the basis of the recently approved HPV cervical cancer vaccines[17]. HPV-6/11 are associated with benign genital warts.

Investigators have found an association between HPV and oral squamous cell carcinoma (OSCC)[18]. HPV papillomas may be seen in post-HSCT patients as painless, pink, papillary masses on the gingivae, tongue, or labial mucosa (Figure 20.7, see colour plate section). These are usually excised, but they often recur[2].

References

1 Bagg J, MacFarlane TW, Poxton IR, Smith AJ (2006). *Essentials of microbiology for dental students*, 2nd edn. Oxford University Press, Oxford.

2 Lerman MA, Laudenbach J, Marty FM, Baden LR, Treister NS (2008). Management of oral infections in cancer patients. *Dent Clin North Am*, 52(1), 129–53.

3 Khan SA, Wingard JR (2001). Infection and mucosal injury in cancer treatment. *J Natl Cancer Inst Monogr*, 29, 31–6.

4 Bagg J (2005). Viral infections, in Davis A, Findlay I (eds) *Oral Care in Advanced Disease*, pp. 87–96. Oxford University Press, Oxford.

5 Amir J (2001). Clinical aspects and antiviral therapy in primary herpetic gingivostomatitis. *Paediatr Drugs*, 3(8), 593–7.

6 Femiano F, Gombos F, Scully C (2001). Recurrent herpes labialis: efficacy of topical therapy with penciclovir compared with acyclovir (aciclovir). *Oral Dis*, 7(1), 31–3.

7 Gilbert S, Corey L, Cunningham A, et al. (2007). An update on short-course intermittent and prevention therapies for herpes labialis. *Herpes*, 14(Suppl1), 13A–18A.

8 Arduino PG, Porter SR (2006). Oral and perioral herpes simplex virus type 1 (HSV-1) infection: review of its management. *Oral Dis*, 12(3), 254–70.

9 Woo SB, Challacombe SJ (2007). Management of recurrent herpes simplex infections. *Oral Surg Oral Med Oral Pathol Oral Radiol Endod*, 103(Suppl), S12–18.

10 Glenny AM, Fernandez Mauleffinch LM, Pavitt S, Walsh T (2009). Interventions for the prevention and treatment of herpes simplex virus in patients being treated for cancer. *Cochrane Database Syst Rev*, (1), CD006706.

11 Chilukuri S, Rosen T (2003). Management of acyclovir-resistant herpes simplex virus. *Dermatol Clin*, 21(2), 311–20.

12 Kudesia G, Partridge S, Farrington CP, Soltanpoor N (2002). Changes in age related seroprevalence of antibody to varicella zoster virus: impact on vaccine strategy. *J Clin Pathol*, 55(2), 154–5.

13 Anonymous (2008). British National Formulary 55. BMJ Group and RPS Publishing, London.

14 Wray D, Lowe GD, Dagg JH, Felix DH, Scully C (1999). *Textbook of general and oral medicine*. Churchill Livingstone, Edinburgh.

15 Sroussi HY, Epstein JB (2007). Changes in the pattern of oral lesions associated with HIV infection: implications for dentists. *J Can Dent Assoc*, 73(10), 949–52.

16 Doumas S, Vladikas A, Papagianni M, Kolokotronis A (2007). Human cytomegalovirus-associated oral and maxillo-facial disease. *Clin Microbiol Infect*, 13(6), 557–9.

17 Villa LL (2006). Prophylactic HPV vaccines: reducing the burden of HPV-related diseases. *Vaccine*, 24(Suppl1), S23–8.

18 Scully C (2005). Oral cancer; the evidence for sexual transmission. *Br Dent J*, 199(4), 203–7.

Chapter 21

Salivary gland dysfunction

Andrew Davies

Introduction

The salivary glands are divided into two main groups[1]:

Major salivary glands

There are six major salivary glands: two parotid glands, two submandibular glands, and two sublingual glands (Figure 2.5).

Minor salivary glands

There are hundreds of minor salivary glands, situated in the tongue, the palate, the buccal mucosa, and the labial mucosa.

The secretion of saliva is predominantly controlled by the parasympathetic nervous system [1]. Thus, stimulation of the parasympathetic nervous system leads to an increase in the secretion of saliva, whilst inhibition of the parasympathetic nervous system leads to a decrease in the secretion of saliva. The sympathetic nervous system can also affect saliva secretion. The sympathetic nervous system is mainly concerned with the composition of saliva secreted, rather than with the volume of saliva secreted.

The 'unstimulated' (resting) salivary flow rate is affected by a number of factors, including[1]:

- Degree of hydration – subjects who are dehydrated have a decreased salivary flow rate. Indeed, if the total body water content falls by 8%, then the salivary flow rate falls to zero.

- Body posture – salivary flow rate is highest when standing, intermediate when sitting, and lowest when lying down.

- Exposure to light – salivary flow rate decreases by 30–40% when subjects are placed in the dark.

- Circadian rhythms – salivary flow rate is highest in the late afternoon, and is lowest in the night.

Eating is the predominant cause of salivary gland stimulation, i.e. increased secretion of saliva[1]. Food stimulates gustatory, touch, and pressure receptors in the mouth, which feedback to the parasympathetic nervous system. Furthermore, mastication of the food stimulates pressure and proprioception receptors in the surrounding tissues (periodontal ligament, muscles of mastication, temporomandibular joint, etc), which also feedback to the parasympathetic nervous system. Other relevant stimuli include the smell (via olfactory receptors in the nose) and the sight of food (via higher centres in the brain).

The 'stimulated' salivary flow rate is affected by a number of factors, including[1]:

- Consistency of food – food with a firm consistency causes a greater increase in salivary flow than food with a soft consistency.

- Taste of food – food with strong flavours causes a greater increase in salivary flow than food with bland flavours.
- Other characteristics of food, e.g. pH.

It has been calculated that the average person produces 500–600 ml of saliva per day[2]. At rest, the submandibular glands contribute ~65%, the parotid glands contribute ~20%, the sublingual glands ~7–8%, and the minor salivary glands ~7–8% of the salivary gland output. However, during periods of stimulation, the parotid gland contribution increases to ~50% of the total. The individual salivary glands produce secretions with a slightly different protein composition. For example, the minor salivary glands produce secretions rich in mucin. Indeed, the minor salivary glands contribute ~70% of the total mucin content of whole saliva.

Ninety-nine percent of saliva is water[2]. The remaining 1% consists of a variety of electrolytes, small organic molecules, and large organic molecules. The diverse constituents of saliva reflect the diverse functions of saliva (see below). The composition of saliva is affected by a number of factors, including the salivary flow rate, and the composition of plasma. It should be noted that there are a number of other components of saliva, including gingival crevicular fluid, epithelial cells, serum, blood cells, various organisms, and food debris.

Definitions

Xerostomia is defined as 'the subjective sensation of dryness of the mouth'[1].

Salivary gland hypofunction is defined as 'any objectively demonstrable reduction in either whole and/or individual gland flow rates'[3].

Salivary gland dysfunction (SGD) has been defined as 'any alteration in the qualitative or quantitative output of saliva caused by an increase (hyperfunction) or decrease (hypofunction) in salivary output'[4]. However, SGD is more often used as an umbrella term to describe patients with xerostomia and/or salivary gland hypofunction[2].

Epidemiology

The prevalence of xerostomia is 22–26% in the general population[5,6], whereas the prevalence of xerostomia is 54–55% in mixed oncology populations[7,8], and 78–82% in advanced oncology populations[9,10]. Thus, xerostomia is one of the most common symptoms experienced by all groups of oncology patients[7–10]. Xerostomia is extremely common in patients that have received conventional radiotherapy to the head and neck region[11].

Investigators have found a disparity between the recorded prevalence of xerostomia and the true prevalence of xerostomia[12]. It is unclear why there is such a disparity, but this probably reflects both healthcare professional-related factors (e.g. perception that the symptom is unimportant) and patient-related factors (e.g. perception that other symptoms are more important)[13]. It should be noted that the aforementioned figures are based on studies where patients were specifically asked about the presence of xerostomia, rather than studies where patients were expected to spontaneously report the presence of xerostomia.

The prevalence of salivary gland hypofunction has been reported to be 82–83% in advanced oncology populations[14,15]. In the study by Davies et al., 82% of the patients had a low unstimulated whole salivary flow rate (UWSFR), whilst 42% of the patients had a low stimulated whole salivary flow rate (SWSFR)[15]. There are no analogous studies involving less advanced oncology populations. Salivary gland hypofunction is extremely common in patients that have received conventional radiotherapy to the head and neck region[16].

Aetiology

There are numerous causes of SGD in the general population[17], with the most common cause being drug treatment[18]. SGD is a side effect of many drugs[19], including many of the drugs used in day-to-day clinical practice[20]. Drugs cause SGD via a number of different mechanisms[21]: the direct effects usually relate to interference with the autonomic nervous supply of the salivary glands; the indirect effects may relate to interference with the production of saliva (e.g. diuretics causing dehydration), or to the secretion of saliva (e.g. antibiotics causing taste disturbance). Similarly, there are numerous causes of SGD in the oncology population (Table 21.1)[9,16,21–32], with the most common cause again being drug treatment[9]. SGD is a side effect of many of the drugs used in supportive care/palliative care (e.g. analgesics, anti-emetics)[9].

Pathophysiology

Xerostomia is usually the result of a decrease in the volume of saliva secreted (i.e. salivary gland hypofunction). Indeed, normal subjects usually complain of a dry mouth when their UWSFR falls by 50%[33]. However, xerostomia may also result from a change in the composition of the saliva secreted [34]. Indeed, Davies et al., reported that 15% of advanced cancer patients with

Table 21.1 Aetiology of cancer-related salivary gland dysfunction

Cancer-related
- Tumour infiltration*
- Paraneoplastic syndrome* [22]

Cancer treatment-related
- Surgery* [21]
- Radiotherapy [16]
- Radionuclide therapy (e.g. I^{131} therapy) [23]
- Chemotherapy [16]
- Biological therapy (e.g. interleukin-2) [24]
- Graft versus host disease [25]

Other causes
- Drug treatment** [9]
- Dehydration [26]
- Malnutrition
- Decreased oral intake (e.g. PEG feeding)
- Decreased mastication (e.g. liquid diet) [27]
- Anxiety [28]
- Depression [29]
- Sjögren's syndrome [30]
- Other disorders of salivary glands [31]
- Neurological disorders [32]

* Uncommon causes

**Most common cause

xerostomia had a 'normal' UWSFR (i.e. UWSFR $\geq$ 0.1 ml/min), and that 53% of advanced cancer patients with xerostomia had a 'normal' SWSFR (i.e. SWSFR $\geq$ 0.5 ml/min) [9].

Clinical features

The clinical features of SGD are very variable (Table 21.2)[5,9,11,35–48], and reflect the differing functions of saliva[17]. SGD is associated with a number of oral problems, but is also associated with more generalized problems. Indeed, SGD is associated with a significant negative impact on quality of life (Box 21.1)[44]. This chapter will not discuss these clinical features in any detail since many of them are discussed in other chapters in the book.

The clinical features of SGD vary from individual to individual, and may vary within an individual over time. Patients with xerostomia may have some or none of the aforementioned

Table 21.2 Complications of salivary gland dysfunction

General problems	Oral discomfort [9,11]
	Lip discomfort [35]
	Cracking of lips [5]
Eating-related problems	Anorexia [9]
	Taste disturbance [9,35]
	Difficulty chewing [9,35]
	Difficulty swallowing [9,35]
	Decreased intake of nutrition [36,37]
Speech-related problems	Difficulty speaking [9,35]
Oral hygiene	Poor oral hygiene
	Halitosis [38]
Oral infections	Oral candidosis [39]
	Dental caries [40]
	Periodontal disease [41]
	Salivary gland infections [42]
Systemic infections	Secondary to oral infection (e.g. pneumonia, septicaemia)
Dental/denture problems	Dental erosion (leading to dental sensitivity/trauma to oral mucosa) [41]
	Poorly fitting dentures (leading to trauma to oral mucosa) [43]
Psychosocial problems	Embarrassment [44]
	Anxiety [11,44]
	Depression [11]
	Social isolation [44]
Miscellaneous problems	Sleep disturbance [44,45]
	Difficulty using oral transmucosal medication (i.e. sublingual/buccal medication) [46,47]
	Oesophagitis [48]
	Urinary frequency (secondary to increased intake of fluid)

Box 21.1 Quotations from cancer patients with xerostomia [44]

"It's so dry and sticky, my mouth glues, sometimes I have difficulties even opening my mouth".

"Eating takes a long time, I stayed there at the table for 30–45 minutes after everybody else. I had to sip before each swallowing, totally about 1 litre of water".

"My voice disappears totally as a consequence of dryness of the mouth, and it is very tiresome to talk".

"We were to celebrate my birthday and I had helped to prepare salmon and looked forward to have dinner with the family. The taste alteration was incredible, the food tasted of absolutely nothing or possibly of wheat flour; I was disappointed and depressed and felt sorry for myself, I couldn't feel or share happiness with my family during that occasion".

"...the problems are there constantly, my illness is there constantly, I am never free".

clinical features. In addition, the xerostomia may be of varying frequency, varying severity and lead to varying levels of distress (Table 21.3)[9]. Similarly, patients with salivary gland hypofunction may have some or none of the aforementioned clinical features (including xerostomia).

It is important to emphasize that there may be a discrepancy between the symptoms experienced by patients and the signs identified by healthcare professionals. The 'classic' signs of salivary gland hypofunction include dryness of the oral mucosa, dryness of the lips, absence of a 'pool' of saliva in the floor of the mouth, fissuring of the oral mucosa (especially of the tongue), and cracking of the lips[3]. However, patients with xerostomia, and some patients with salivary gland hypofunction, may have no obvious abnormalities on examination. Hence, a normal oral examination does not preclude a diagnosis of SGD (see Section on Assessment).

Table 21.3 Clinical features of xerostomia in patients with advanced cancer [9]

Characteristic	Descriptor	Percentage
Frequency	'Rarely'	4%
	'Occasionally'	20%
	'Frequently	40%
	'Almost constantly'	36%
Severity	'Slight'	14%
	'Moderate'	37%
	'Severe'	33%
	'Very severe'	16%
Distress	'Not at all'	16%
	'A little bit'	21%
	'Somewhat'	23%
	'Quite a bit'	26%
	'Very much'	14%

Assessment

A wide range of investigations may be employed in the management of SGD in the general population[31]. Some of these investigations are used to diagnose SGD (e.g. measurement of salivary flow rates), whilst other investigations are used to determine the cause of the SGD (e.g. detection of auto-antibodies). However, most of these investigations are not indicated in the assessment of SGD in the cancer population. Indeed, a diagnosis of SGD can invariably be made on the basis of routine clinical skills, i.e. taking a history and performing an examination[3].

Various techniques have been developed to measure unstimulated salivary flow rates (resting salivary flow rates), stimulated salivary flow rates, salivary flow from all of the glands ('whole' salivary flow rates), and salivary flow from the individual glands. The most clinically relevant salivary flow rates are the UWSFR, and the SWSFR. The UWSFR is more closely related to the presence of xerostomia than the SWSFR[9,49]. Nevertheless, sialometry (measurement of salivary flow rates) is generally not indicated in day-to-day clinical practice.

A number of assessment tools have been developed for use in clinical practice and/or clinical trials. In clinical practice, the assessment of SGD can be done using everyday assessment tools (e.g. verbal rating scales – 'none', 'mild', 'moderate', and 'severe'). However, in clinical trials, the assessment of SGD should be done using relevant validated assessment tools (e.g. Xerostomia Inventory, Xerostomia Questionnaire; Figure 21.1 and 21.2)[50,51].

Dry Mouth Questionnaire

Please circle the answer which <u>best</u> applies to you during the last 4 weeks:

I sip liquids to aid in swallowing food	NEVER	HARDLY EVER	OCCASIONALLY	FAIRLY OFTEN	VERY OFTEN
My mouth feels dry when eating a meal	NEVER	HARDLY EVER	OCCASIONALLY	FAIRLY OFTEN	VERY OFTEN
My lips feel dry	NEVER	HARDLY EVER	OCCASIONALLY	FAIRLY OFTEN	VERY OFTEN
I have difficulties swallowing certain foods	NEVER	HARDLY EVER	OCCASIONALLY	FAIRLY OFTEN	VERY OFTEN
My mouth feels dry	NEVER	HARDLY EVER	OCCASIONALLY	FAIRLY OFTEN	VERY OFTEN
I get up at night to drink	NEVER	HARDLY EVER	OCCASIONALLY	FAIRLY OFTEN	VERY OFTEN
My eyes feel dry	NEVER	HARDLY EVER	OCCASIONALLY	FAIRLY OFTEN	VERY OFTEN
I have difficulty in eating dry foods	NEVER	HARDLY EVER	OCCASIONALLY	FAIRLY OFTEN	VERY OFTEN
The inside of my nose feels dry	NEVER	HARDLY EVER	OCCASIONALLY	FAIRLY OFTEN	VERY OFTEN
I suck sweets or cough lollies to relieve dry mouth	NEVER	HARDLY EVER	OCCASIONALLY	FAIRLY OFTEN	VERY OFTEN
The skin of my face feels dry	NEVER	HARDLY EVER	OCCASIONALLY	FAIRLY OFTEN	VERY OFTEN

Figure 21.1 The Xerostomia Inventory (XI)[50].
Source: Reproduced with permission of Prof Murray Thompson

Below are several questions that will help describe the dryness in your mouth and how that dryness affects your daily life. Please encircle the number that corresponds to your condition during the last week in each of the following questions:

1. Rate the difficulty you experience in speaking due to dryness of your mouth and tongue:

0	1	2	3	4	5	6	7	8	9	10
Easy								Extremely Difficult		

2. Rate the difficulty you experience in chewing food due to dryness:

0	1	2	3	4	5	6	7	8	9	10
Easy								Extremely Difficult		

3. Rate the difficulty you experience in swallowing food due to dryness:

0	1	2	3	4	5	6	7	8	9	10
Easy								Extremely Difficult		

4. Rate the dryness your mouth feels when eating a meal:

0	1	2	3	4	5	6	7	8	9	10
Easy								Extremely Difficult		

5. Rate the dryness in your mouth while not eating or chewing:

0	1	2	3	4	5	6	7	8	9	10
Easy								Extremely Difficult		

6. Rate the frequency of sipping liquids to aid in swallowing food:

0	1	2	3	4	5	6	7	8	9	10
Easy								Extremely Difficult		

7. Rate the frequency of fluid intake required for oral comfort when not eating:

0	1	2	3	4	5	6	7	8	9	10
Easy								Extremely Difficult		

8. Rate the frequency of sleeping problems due to dryness:

0	1	2	3	4	5	6	7	8	9	10
Easy								Extremely Difficult		

Figure 21.2 The Xerostomia Questionnaire (XQ)[51].
Source: Reproduced with permission of Prof Avraham Eisbruch

Table 21.4 shows the relevant National Cancer Institute Common Terminology Criteria for Adverse Events (CTCAE) relating to cancer treatment[52]. These criteria are widely used in clinical practice/clinical trials, and are recommended by organizations such as the Food and Drug Administration (United States of America). However, research suggests that similar observer-completed assessment tools may have poor inter-observer reliability, may not correlate with objective measures of SGD, and (particularly) may not correlate with subjective measures of SGD[53].

Management

SGD is a heterogeneous condition, and so requires individualized management. The management of SGD depends on a variety of different factors, including the aetiology/pathophysiology of

Table 21.4 National Cancer Institute Common Toxicity Criteria for Adverse Events (CTCAE) version 3 [adapted from 50]

Adverse event (AE)	Grade 1 –'mild' AE	Grade 2 –'moderate' AE	Grade 3 – 'severe' AE	Grade 4 – life threatening/ disabling AE	Grade 5 – death due to AE
Dry mouth/salivary gland (xerostomia) Short name – dry mouth	Symptomatic (dry or thick saliva) without significant dietary alteration; unstimulated salivary flow >0.2 ml/min	Symptomatic and significant oral intake alteration (e.g. copious water, other lubricants, diet limited to purees and/or soft, moist foods); unstimulated saliva 0.1 to 0.2 ml/min	Symptoms leading to inability to adequately aliment orally, IV fluids, tube feedings, or TPN indicated; unstimulated saliva <0.1 ml/min	–	–
Salivary gland changes/saliva Short name – salivary gland changes	Slightly thickened saliva; slightly altered taste (e.g. metallic)	Thick ropy, sticky saliva; markedly altered taste; alteration in diet indicated; secretion-induced symptoms not interfering with ADL	Acute salivary gland necrosis; severe secretion-induced symptoms interfering with ADL	Disabling	–

the SGD, the clinical features of the SGD, the general condition of the patient, the dental status of the patient, the treatment preferences of the patient, the availability of specific interventions, and the affordability of specific interventions[2]. The management of SGD involves a number of different strategies, including: (1) the prevention of SGD; (2) the treatment of the cause of SGD; (3) the symptomatic treatment of SGD; (4) the prevention of the complications of SGD; and (5) the treatment of the complications of SGD[2].

Prevention of salivary gland dysfunction

As discussed above, SGD is extremely common in patients that have received conventional radiotherapy to the head and neck region. A number of strategies have been used to try to prevent radiotherapy-related SGD, including surgical transfer of salivary glands, use of novel radiotherapy techniques (e.g. intensity modulated radiotherapy), use of radioprotectors (e.g. amifostine), and use of other agents (e.g. pilocarpine)[54].

Surgical transfer of salivary glands

The surgical transfer of salivary glands has been pioneered by the group at the University of Alberta. The so-called 'Seikaly & Jha method' involves surgical transfer of a submandibular gland into the submental space prior to radiotherapy (with appropriate shielding of the submental space during radiotherapy) [55]. The technique is used in selected patients who are undergoing primary surgery for either squamous cell carcinoma of oropharynx, hypopharynx, larynx, or an unknown primary with neck nodes, and who are expected to receive postoperative radiotherapy encompassing the major salivary glands (i.e. a dose of >50 Gy to the parotid glands and the other submandibular gland)[56]. The technique appears to be effective in preventing SGD, and does not appear to be associated with significant short-term/long-term morbidity (including local recurrence of the cancer)[57,58].

Novel radiotherapy techniques

Over the last 20 years, radiotherapy techniques have become increasingly more sophisticated (e.g. three-dimensional conformal radiotherapy, intensity-modulated radiotherapy (IMRT)). These new techniques have allowed clinical oncologists to optimize the dose of radiation delivered to the tumour, whilst minimizing the dose of radiation delivered to the normal tissues (e.g. major salivary glands). Several uncontrolled studies suggest that IMRT is effective in preventing/limiting the development of SGD. However, a recent randomized controlled study reported a disparity between the objective and subjective endpoints used to assess SGD, i.e. IMRT was not effective in preventing/limiting the development of xerostomia[59]. The reason for this disparity is probably related to the fact that the IMRT 'spared' the parotid glands that produce much of the fluid content of saliva, but did not spare the minor salivary glands that provide most of the mucin (lubricant) content of saliva[2,60]. The use of novel radiotherapy techniques is discussed, in detail, in Chapter 10.

Radioprotectors

Amifostine, an inorganic thiophosphate, has been used in an attempt to prevent/ameliorate radiotherapy-related SGD. A recent systematic review concluded that 'amifostine significantly reduces the side effects of radiation therapy'[61]. Indeed, the use of amifostine was associated with a 76% reduction in Grades 2–3 acute xerostomia, and a 67% reduction in Grades 2–3 late xerostomia[61]. However, the widespread use of amifostine has been limited by the dosing schedule of the drug, the toxicity of the drug, and ongoing concerns about radioprotection of the tumour[62]. It should be noted that the systematic review also concluded that 'the efficacy of radiotherapy was not itself affected by the use of this drug', and that 'patients receiving amifostine were able to achieve higher rates of complete response'[61].

Other agents

Other pharmacological agents have also been used to prevent/ameliorate radiotherapy-related SGD, including pilocarpine (muscarinic agonist)[63,64], biperiden (muscarinic antagonist)[65], and a coumarin/toroxutine combination[66]. These interventions are the subject of an ongoing Cochrane Collaboration systematic review. The provisional findings of the review are that pilocarpine does not prevent the development of radiation-induced xerostomia (the primary end point of the review), and that there is insufficient data to assess the effects of other pharmacological agents (Anne-Marie Glenny, personal communication).

Treatment of the cause of salivary gland dysfunction

Table 21.1 shows the main causes of cancer-related SGD. Some of these causes may be amenable to a specific intervention, although most are not amenable to any intervention. Drug treatment is the most common cause of cancer-related SGD[9]. In theory, it is possible to discontinue or substitute the relevant drugs. However, it is often difficult to discontinue these drugs, since they are needed to manage the underlying cancer or another serious condition. Similarly, it is usually futile to substitute these drugs, since the SGD is a side effect of the class of drug, rather than a side effect of the individual drug[19].

It should be noted that researchers are starting to investigate novel techniques to repair damaged salivary glands, including the utilization of gene therapy and tissue engineering[67].

Symptomatic treatment of salivary gland dysfunction

The symptomatic treatment of SGD involves the use of saliva stimulants (agents that promote saliva secretion) and saliva substitutes (agents that replace missing saliva). There are good reasons for prescribing saliva stimulants rather than saliva substitutes[2]. Thus, saliva stimulants increase the secretion of 'normal' saliva, and so will ameliorate xerostomia and the other clinical features of SGD. In contrast, saliva substitutes, which are very different from normal saliva (i.e. physically, chemically), will usually only ameliorate xerostomia. Moreover, in studies that have compared saliva stimulants with saliva substitutes, patients have generally expressed a preference for the saliva stimulants[68,69]. Nevertheless, some patients do not respond to treatment with saliva stimulants, and so will require treatment with saliva substitutes (e.g. some patients with radiation-induced SGD).

Saliva stimulants

Chewing gum

Chewing gum increases salivary flow by two mechanisms; ~85% of the increase is related to stimulation of chemoreceptors within the oral cavity (i.e. taste effect), whilst ~15% of the increase is related to stimulation of mechanoreceptors in/around the oral cavity (i.e. chewing effect)[70]. Patients with SGD should use 'sugar-free' chewing gum, and patients with dental prostheses should use 'low-tack' (less sticky) chewing gum.

Chewing gum has been reported to be effective in the management of xerostomia in various groups of patients[71], including patients with radiation-induced SGD [69] and advanced cancer patients with drug-induced SGD[72]. Moreover, chewing gum has been reported to be more effective than organic acids and artificial saliva in studies involving mixed groups of patients with SGD[68,69]. It should be noted that studies involving patients with radiation-induced SGD have produced variable results, with some reporting good results [69] and others less good results[68].

Chewing gum is generally well tolerated. However, side effects can occur, and may be related to: (1) chewing, e.g. jaw discomfort, headache; (2) inappropriate ingestion, e.g. respiratory tract obstruction, gastrointestinal obstruction; (3) non-allergic reactions to additives, e.g. oral discomfort, flatulence; and (4) allergic reactions to additives, e.g. stomatitis, perioral dermatitis[72]. Chewing gum is an acceptable form of treatment for most patients, including most elderly patients[72,73].

Organic acids

Various organic acids have been used as saliva stimulants, including ascorbic acid (vitamin C), citric acid (the acid in citrus fruits), and malic acid (the acid in apples and pears)[71]. Organic acids increase salivary flow through stimulation of chemoreceptors within the oral cavity.

Ascorbic acid has been reported to be relatively ineffective in a study involving a mixed group of patients with SGD[68]. Thus, only 33% of the patients rated ascorbic acid as either 'good' or 'very good', and only 23% of patients wanted to continue with it after the study. Indeed, ascorbic acid received the lowest ranking of all the products tested in this study.

Studies suggest that citric acid can provide symptomatic improvement for some groups of patients with SGD, although not patients with radiation-induced SGD[69,74]. However, in the study by Stewart et al., only 24% patients expressed a preference for the citric acid product, compared with 46% for the chewing gum and 30% for the artificial saliva[69].

Malic acid has been reported to be relatively more effective in a study involving a mixed group of patients with SGD[68]. Thus, 51% of the patients rated malic acid as either 'good' or 'very good', and 44% of patients wanted to continue with it after the study. Indeed, malic acid received the second highest ranking of all the products tested in this study, and was the most highly ranked product by patients with radiation-induced SGD. Similarly, a lozenge containing malic acid (and citric acid) has been reported to be effective in a study involving patients with radiation-induced SGD[75].

The use of organic acids is associated with the development of oral discomfort[68,69]. Thus, organic acids should not be used in patients with dry mucosae, cracked mucosae, stomatitis, and/or mucositis. Moreover, the use of organic acids may be associated with the exacerbation of certain pH-related complications of SGD (i.e. demineralization of the teeth, dental caries, oral candidosis, etc.)[2,76]. Thus, organic acids should not be used in patients with teeth, and should be used with caution in patients with dental prostheses.

Parasympathomimetic drugs

Parasympathomimetic drugs stimulate the part of the autonomic nervous system responsible for the secretion of saliva from the salivary glands. The parasympathomimetic drugs include choline esters (e.g. pilocarpine, cevimeline) that have a direct effect, and cholinesterase inhibitors (e.g. distigmine, pyridostigmine) that have an indirect effect by inhibiting the metabolism of endogenous acetylcholine.

Pilocarpine has been used to treat xerostomia for generations by South American Indians, and for over 100 years by European physicians[77]. It has been reported to be effective in the management of SGD due to salivary gland disease (e.g. Sjögren's syndrome)[78], drug treatment[79], radiotherapy[80, 81], and graft-versus-host disease[82,83]. Indeed, it has been reported to be more effective than artificial saliva in the management of SGD secondary to drug treatment[79], and radiotherapy[84]. It should be noted that although pilocarpine acts primarily on muscarinic receptors, it also acts on beta-adrenergic receptors[77].

A recent Cochrane systematic review investigated the role of parasympathomimetic drugs in the management of radiation-induced SGD[85]. The reviewers concluded that 'there is limited evidence to support the use of pilocarpine hydrochloride in the treatment of radiation-induced salivary gland dysfunction', and that 'currently, there is little evidence to support the use of other parasympathomimetic drugs in the treatment of this condition'. It should be noted that the efficacy of pilocarpine appears to be somewhat greater/quicker in other groups of patients, although the tolerability of pilocarpine appears to be similar in these groups of patients[78,79].

The systematic review found that 49–52% patients respond to pilocarpine[80,81]. However, the response rate in the included studies may not reflect the response rates in the general population. Thus, one of the inclusion criteria for the two main included studies was 'some evidence of residual salivary function'[80,81], which is clearly not a universal finding in patients with radiation-induced SGD. It is reasonable to suppose that patients with evidence of salivary gland functioning would be more likely to respond to pilocarpine, since such findings confirm that the salivary glands are still functioning to an extent, and so still capable of responding to a stimulant.

Overall, the response rates were similar for patients taking the standard (5 mg tds) and the higher dose (10 mg tds) in the main fixed-dose study [80]. Nevertheless, some patients only appeared to respond to the higher doses (10 mg tds) in the main dose-titration study[81]. There are two possible explanations for the latter finding: (1) some patients improved because of the increase in dose; or (2) some patients improved because of the increase in time on the drug, i.e. some patients had a delayed response to the drug. It is difficult to determine the importance of these two factors, although it is clear from the data that some patients do have a delayed response to the drug, i.e. up to 12 weeks[80].

The systematic review also found that many patients develop side effects. The side effects are usually related to generalized parasympathetic stimulation, and include sweating, headache, urinary frequency, and vasodilatation. The incidence of side effects is dose related, i.e. the higher the dose of pilocarpine the higher the incidence of side effects. However, the systematic review found that few (6%) patients discontinue pilocarpine due to side effects at the standard dose of 5 mg tds[80].

The other choline esters that have been used in clinical practice include bethanechol, carbacholine[86], and cevimeline. Bethanechol has been reported to be effective in the management of drug-induced SGD[87], and of radiotherapy-induced SGD[88,89]. Similarly, cevimeline has been reported to be effective in the management of Sjögren's syndrome[90], radiotherapy-induced SGD[91,92], and graft-versus-host disease[93]. The cholinesterase inhibitors that have been used in practice include distigmine [94], and pyridostigmine [95].

Acupuncture

Acupuncture has been reported to be useful in the management of SGD secondary to benign salivary gland disease[96], drug treatment[97], and radiotherapy[98,99],]. Nevertheless, a recent systematic review concluded that (at present) 'there is no evidence for the efficacy of acupuncture in the management of xerostomia', and stated that 'there is a need for future high quality randomized controlled trials'[100].

Investigators have reported the use of diverse acupuncture points (number/type of points) and diverse treatment schedules (number/duration of treatments). The effect of acupuncture often increases during a course of treatment[97], and often continues for some time following the end of the course of treatment[98,99]. Moreover, the effect of acupuncture may be maintained by single treatments given on an as-required basis (e.g. 1–2 monthly)[101]. The mechanism of action of acupuncture has yet to be elucidated, although increases in relevant neuropeptide secretion and intra-oral blood flow have been reported[97].

Acupuncture is generally well tolerated, although it can cause local haemorrhage[96,98], and also local/systemic infection[102]. Hence, acupuncture should be used with caution in patients with bleeding diatheses, and in patients that are immunocompromised. Some patients report feeling tired following treatment[96,98], whilst other patients report coincidental health-related benefits from the treatment[96,98].

Other strategies

A number of other pharmacological means have been reported to be useful, including anetholetrithione[103], nicotinamide (B group vitamin)[68], and yohimbine (alpha 2 adrenoreceptor antagonist)[104]. Similarly, a number of other non-pharmacological means have been reported to be useful, including 'sugar-free' breath mints [70], anhydrous crystalline maltose lozenges [105], herbal medicines [106], Chinese medicines [107], and homeopathic treatments[108]. In addition, there are a number of reports in the literature of the successful use of intra-oral electrostimulating devices [109,110], and one report of the successful use of an 'acupuncture-like' transcutaneous electrical nerve-stimulation device [111].

Saliva substitutes

Water

Patients often use water to treat dryness of the mouth. However, in studies, patients have reported that water is less effective than 'artificial saliva'[112,113]. Moreover, in one study, patients reported that the mean duration of improvement of dryness of the mouth was only 12 min (range: 4–29 min)[114].

In spite of the above, many patients choose to use water rather than other saliva substitutes[115]. The reasons for this phenomenon include familiarity, efficacy (moderate), tolerability, availability, and affordability[115]. The use of water is not associated with side effects *per se*, although polydipsia is inevitably associated with polyuria (and nocturia)[2].

'Artificial saliva'

It is common practice for healthcare professionals to prescribe 'artificial saliva' for the treatment of SGD. A number of commercial products have been developed, which differ in formulation (e.g. spray, gel, lozenge), lubricant (e.g. carboxymethylcellulose, hydroxyethylcellulose, mucin), and additives (e.g. flavourings, fluoride, antimicrobial factors)[116]. It should be noted that most of these commercial products have not been formally tested in cancer patients with SGD, or indeed in any group of patients with SGD.

The 'ideal' artificial saliva should be easy to use, pleasant to use, effective, and well tolerated[115]. Moreover, it should have a neutral pH (to prevent demineralization of the teeth), and contain fluoride (to enhance remineralization of the teeth). Unfortunately, some commercial products have an acidic pH, and these should definitely not be prescribed in dentate patients, and should probably not be prescribed in any patient with SGD[34].

A commercial mucin-based spray (Saliva Orthana®) has been reported to be relatively effective/well tolerated in patients with radiation-induced SGD[117,118], and in cancer patients with drug-induced SGD[72,79]. Indeed, Saliva Orthana® was reported to be more effective/better tolerated than a carboxymethylcellulose-based artificial saliva in patients with radiation-induced SGD[117,118]. However, the duration of effect of the Saliva Orthana® was only ~30 min, which necessitated repeated use of the product during the day and night[117]. (The duration of effect of the carboxymethylcellulose-based artificial saliva was ~10 min.) [117].

Similarly, two commercial hydroxethylcellulose-based gels containing lactoperoxidase, lysozyme, and lactoferrin (Oral Balance®, BioXtra®) have been reported to be relatively effective/ well tolerated in patients with radiation-induced SGD[119, 120]. Indeed, the Oral Balance® gel and associated toothpaste was reported to be more effective/better tolerated than a carboxymethylcellulose-based artificial saliva and conventional toothpaste in patients with radiation-induced SGD[119]. It should be noted that there is little evidence that the presence of antimicrobial factors in these products actually prevents/ameliorates the infectious complications of SGD (Table 21.2)[121]. Other products that have shown promise in patients with radiation-induced SGD, include one based on linseed extract (Salinum®) [122], and another one based on hydroxyethylcellulose with citric acid (Optimoist®)[123].

Artificial saliva is generally well tolerated, although some patients report local problems (e.g. oral irritation, taste disturbance), whilst some patients even report systemic problems (e.g. nausea, diarrhoea)[79,115]. The duration of effect of artificial saliva is invariably short, which necessitates the repeated use of these products during the day and night. Indeed, the short duration of effect is one of the main reasons why patients do not continue to use artificial saliva. In an attempt to overcome this problem, a number of investigators have developed intra-oral artificial saliva reservoirs. Reservoirs can be incorporated into new (purpose built) dental prostheses [124], or into existing (standard) dental prostheses[125]. Moreover, reservoirs can be incorporated into bite guards, that may be worn throughout the day[126], or simply at night time [127].

Other agents

Other agents that have been suggested/utilized as saliva substitutes include milk[128], butter[129], margarine[129], vegetable oil[129,130], and glycerine (and lemon)[131]. However, margarine has been shown to be less effective than three commercial artificial saliva products in a mixed group of patients[132]. Similarly, glycerine has been shown to be less effective than a non-commercial artificial saliva product in patients with Sjögren's syndrome[133]. Moreover, glycerine actually appears to cause dryness of the mouth[134].

Prevention of the complications of salivary gland dysfunction

The main complications of SGD are shown in Table 21.2. Adequate management of SGD may prevent the development of these complications. Nevertheless, the following preventative strategies should be considered in all patients with SGD:

1. Maintenance of oral hygiene – dentate patients need to clean their teeth at least twice a day, and edentulous patients need to clean their dentures at least once a day and to remove their dentures at night-time[135].

2. Use of fluoridated toothpaste – all dentate patients should use a toothpaste with at least 1000 ppm fluoride, whilst dentate patients with radiation-induced SGD should use a specialist toothpaste with 5000 ppm fluoride.

3. Avoidance of acidic drinks/foods/medication – acidic products will contribute to complications such as dental erosion, dental caries, and oral candidosis.

4. Avoidance of sugar sweetened drinks/foods/medication – sugar-sweetened products will contribute to complications such as dental caries and oral candidosis.

5. Avoidance of xerostomic medication – it should be noted that some oral care products contain alcohol, which may further aggravate the situation.

6. Regular dental review – patients should have regular dental reviews (with a dentist/dental hygienist). It should be noted that the dental management of a patient with xerostomia is somewhat different from that of a patient without xerostomia [43].

Treatment of the complications of salivary gland dysfunction

Again adequate management of SGD may resolve some or all of the complications. The treatment of the complications of SGD is discussed in detail in a number of the other chapters in the book.

References

1 Edgar WM, O'Mullane DM (1996). *Saliva and oral health*, 2nd edn. British Dental Association, London.

2 Davies A (2005). Salivary gland dysfunction, in Davies A, Finlay I (eds) *Oral Care in Advanced Disease*, pp. 97–113. Oxford University Press, Oxford.

3 Navazesh M, Christensen C, Brightman V (1992). Clinical criteria for the diagnosis of salivary gland hypofunction. *J Dent Res*, 71(7), 1363–9.

4 Millard HD, Mason DK (1998). Third World Workshop on Oral Medicine. University of Michigan, *Ann Arbor*

5 Billings RJ, Proskin HM, Moss ME (1996). Xerostomia and associated factors in a community-dwelling adult population. *Community Dent Oral Epidemiol*, 24(5), 312–16.

6 Nederfors T, Isaksson R, Mornstad H, Dahlof C (1997). Prevalence of perceived symptoms of dry mouth in an adult Swedish population – relation to age, sex and pharmacotherapy. *Community Dent Oral Epidemiol*, 25(3), 211–16.

7 Portenoy RK, Thaler HT, Kornblith AB, et al. (1994). Symptom prevalence, characteristics and distress in a cancer population. *Qual Life Res*, 3(3), 183–9.

8 Chang VT, Hwang SS, Feuerman M, Kasimis BS, Thaler HT (2000). The Memorial Symptom Assessment Scale Short Form (MSAS-SF). *Cancer*, 89(5), 1162–71.

9 Davies AN, Broadley K, Beighton D (2001). Xerostomia in patients with advanced cancer. *J Pain Symptom Manage*, 22(4), 820–5.

10 Tranmer JE, Heyland D, Dudgeon D, Groll D, Squires-Graham M, Coulson K (2003). Measuring the symptom experience of seriously ill cancer and noncancer hospitalized patients near the end of life with the Memorial Symptom Assessment Scale. *J Pain Symptom Manage*, 25 (5), 420–9.

11 Dirix P, Nuyts S, Vander Poorten V, Delaere P, Van den Bogaert W (2008). The influence of xerostomia after radiotherapy on quality of life. *Support Care Cancer*, 16(2), 171–9.

12 Shah S, Davies AN (2001). Medical records vs. patient self-rating. *J Pain Symptom Manage*, 22(4), 805–6.

13 Shorthose K, Davies A (2003). Symptom prevalence in palliative care. *Palliat Med*, 17(8), 723–4.

14 Chaushu G, Bercovici M, Dori S, Waller A, Taicher S, Kronenberg J, et al. (2000). Salivary flow and its relation with oral symptoms in terminally ill patients. *Cancer*, 88(5), 984–7.

15 Davies AN, Broadley K, Beighton D (2002). Salivary gland hypofunction in patients with advanced cancer. *Oral Oncol*, 38(7), 680–5.

16 Jensen SB, Pedersen AM, Reibel J, Nauntofte B (2003). Xerostomia and hypofunction of the salivary glands in cancer therapy. *Support Care Cancer*, 11(4), 207–25.

17 Anonymous (1992). Saliva: Its role in health and disease. FDI Working Group 10 of the Commission on Oral Health, Research and Epidemiology (CORE). *Int Dent J*, 42 (4 Suppl 2), 291–304.

18 Sreebny LM, Valdini A, Yu A (1989). Xerostomia. Part II: Relationship to nonoral symptoms, drugs, and diseases. *Oral Surg Oral Med Oral Pathol*, 68(4), 419–27.

19 Sreebny LM, Schwartz SS (1997). A reference guide to drugs and dry mouth – 2nd edn. *Gerodontology*, 14(1), 33–47.

20 Smith RG, Burtner AP (1994). Oral side-effects of the most frequently prescribed drugs. *Spec Care Dentist*, 14(3), 96–102.

21 Schubert MM, Izutsu KT (1987). Iatrogenic causes of salivary gland dysfunction. *J Dent Res*, 66 (Spec Iss), 680–8.

22 Folli F, Ponzoni M, Vicari AM (1997). Paraneoplastic autoimmune xerostomia. *Ann Intern Med*, 127(2), 167–8.

23 Solans R, Bosch JA, Galofre P, et al. (2001). Salivary and lacrimal gland dysfunction (sicca syndrome) after radioiodine therapy. *J Nucl Med*, 42(5), 738–43.

24 Nagler RM, Gez E, Rubinov R, et al. (2001). The effect of low-dose interleukin-2-based immunotherapy on salivary function and composition in patients with metastatic renal cell carcinoma. *Arch Oral Biol*, 46(6), 487–93.

25 Nagler R, Marmary Y, Krausz Y, Chisin R, Markitziu A, Nagler A (1996). Major salivary gland dysfunction in human acute and chronic graft-versus-host disease (GVHD). *Bone Marrow Transplant*, 17(2), 219–24.

26 Gregersen MI, Bullock LT (1933). Observations on thirst in man in relation to changes in salivary flow and plasma volume. *Am J Physiol*, 105, 39–40.

27 Johansson I, Ericson T (1989). Effects of a 900-kcal liquid or solid diet on saliva flow rate and composition in female subjects. *Caries Res*, 23(3), 184–9.

28 Bergdahl M, Bergdahl J (2000). Low unstimulated salivary flow and subjective oral dryness: association with medication, anxiety, depression, and stress. *J Dent Res*, 79(9),1652–8.

29 Antilla SS, Knuuttila ML, Sakki T K (1998). Depressive symptoms as an underlying factor of the sensation of dry mouth. *Psychosom Med*, 60(2), 215–18.

30 Vitali C, Bombardieri S, Jonsson R, et al. (2002). Classification criteria for Sjögren's syndrome: a revised version of the European criteria proposed by the American – European Consensus Group. *Ann Rheum Dis*, 61(6), 554–8.

31 Porter SR, Scully C, Hegarty AM (2004). An update of the etiology and management of xerostomia. *Oral Surg Oral Med Oral Pathol Oral Radiol Endod*, 97(1), 28–46.

32 Ship JA (2002). Diagnosing, managing, and preventing salivary gland disorders. *Oral Diseases*, 8(2), 77–89.

33 Dawes C (1987). Physiological factors affecting salivary flow rate, oral sugar clearance, and the sensation of dry mouth in man. *J Dent Res*, 66(Spec Iss), 648–53.

34 Pankhurst CL, Smith EC, Rogers JO, Dunne SM, Jackson SHD, Proctor G (1996a). Diagnosis and management of the dry mouth: part 1. *Dent Update*, 23(2), 56–62.

35 Sreebny LM, Valdini A (1988). Xerostomia. Part I: Relationship to other oral symptoms and salivary gland hypofunction. *Oral Surg Oral Med Oral Pathol*, 66(4), 451–8.

36 Rhodus NL, Brown J (1990). The association of xerostomia and inadequate intake in older adults. *J Am Diet Assoc*, 90(12), 1688–92.

37 Backstrom I, Funegard U, Andersson I, Franzen L, Johansson I (1995). Dietary intake in head and neck irradiated patients with permanent dry mouth symptoms. *Eur J Cancer B Oral Oncol*, 31B (4), 253–7.

38 Shorthose K, Davies A (2005). Halitosis, in Davies A, Finlay I (eds) *Oral Care in Advanced Disease*, pp. 125–31. Oxford University Press, Oxford.

39 Davies AN, Brailsford SR, Beighton D (2006). Oral candidosis in patients with advanced cancer. *Oral Oncol*, 42(7), 698–702.

40 Leone CW, Oppenheim FG (2001). Physical and chemical aspects of saliva as indicators of risk for dental caries in humans. *J Dental Educ*, 65(10), 1054–62.

41 Ship JA (2004). Xerostomia: aetiology, diagnosis, management and clinical implications, in Edgar M, Dawes C, O'Mullane D (eds) *Saliva and Oral Health*, 3rd edn, pp. 50–70. British Dental Association, London.

42 Bagg J (2005). Bacterial infections, in Davies A, Finlay I (eds) *Oral Care in Advanced Disease*, pp. 73–86. Oxford University Press, Oxford.

43 Pankhurst CL, Dunne SM, Rogers JO (1996b). Restorative dentistry in the patient with dry mouth: part 2. Problems and solutions. *Dent Update*, 23(3), 110–14.

44 Rydholm M, Strang P (2002). Physical and psychosocial impact of xerostomia in palliative cancer care: a qualitative interview study. *Int J Palliat Nurs*, 8(7), 318–23.

45 Jellema AP, Slotman BJ, Doornaert P, Leemans CR, Langendijk JA (2007). Impact of radiation-induced xerostomia on quality of life after primary radiotherapy among patients with head and neck cancer. *Int J Radiat Oncol Biol Phys*, 69(3), 751–60.

46 Robbins LJ (1983). Dry mouth and delayed dissolution of sublingual nitroglycerin. *New Engl J Med*, 309(16), 985.

47 Davies AN, Vriens J (2005). Oral transmucosal fentanyl citrate and xerostomia. *J Pain Symptom Manage*, 30(6), 496–7.

48 Korsten MA, Rosman AS, Fishbein S, Shlein RD, Goldberg HE, Biener A (1991). Chronic xerostomia increases esophageal acid exposure and is associated with esophageal injury. *Am J Med*, 90(6), 701–6.

49 Wang SL, Zhao ZT, Li J, Zhu XZ, Dong H, Zhang YG (1998). Investigation of the clinical value of total saliva flow rates. *Arch Oral Biol*, 43(1), 39–43.

50 Thomson WM, Williams SM. Further testing of the xerostomia inventory (2000). *Oral Surg Oral Med Oral Pathol Oral Radiol Endod*, 89(1), 46–50.

51 Eisbruch A, Kim HM, Terrell JE, Marsh LH, Dawson LA, Ship JA (2001). Xerostomia and its predictors following parotid-sparing irradiation of head-and-neck cancer. *Int J Radiat Oncol Biol Phys*, 50(3), 695–704.

52 National Cancer Institute Common Terminology Criteria for Adverse Events (CTCAE). Available from National Cancer Institute (US National Institutes of Health) website: http://www.cancer.gov/

53 Meirovitz A, Murdoch-Kinch CA, Schipper M, Pan C, Eisbruch A (2006). Grading xerostomia by physicians or by patients after intensity-modulated radiotherapy of head-and-neck cancer. *Int J Radiat Oncol Biol Phys*, 66(2), 445–53.

54 Koukourakis MI, Danielidis V (2005). Preventing radiation induced xerostomia. *Cancer Treat Rev*, 31(7), 546–54.

55 Seikaly H, Jha N, McGaw T, Coulter L, Liu R, Oldring D (2001). Submandibular gland transfer: a new method of preventing radiation-induced xerostomia. *Laryngoscope*, 111(2), 347–52.

56 Jha N, Seikaly H, Harris J, et al. (2003). Prevention of radiation induced xerostomia by surgical transfer of submandibular salivary gland into the submental space. *Radiother Oncol*, 66(3), 283–9.

57 Seikaly H, Jha N, Harris J, et al. (2004). Long-term outcomes of submandibular gland transfer for prevention of postradiation xerostomia. *Arch Otolaryngol Head Neck Surg*, 130(8), 956–61.

58 Al-Qahtani K, Hier MP, Sultanum K, Black MJ (2006). The role of submandibular salivary gland transfer in preventing xerostomia in the chemoradiotherapy patient. *Oral Surg Oral Med Oral Pathol Oral Radiol Endod*, 101(6), 753–6.

59 Kam MK, Leung SF, Zee B, et al. (2007). Prospective randomized study of intensity-modulated radiotherapy on salivary gland function in early-stage nasopharyngeal carcinoma patients. *J Clin Oncol*, 25(31), 4873–9.

60 Eisbruch A (2007). Reducing xerostomia by IMRT: what may, and may not, be achieved. *J Clin Oncol*, 25(31), 4863–4.

61 Sasse A D, Clark LG, Sasse EC, Clark OA (2006). Amifostine reduces side effects and improves complete response rate during radiotherapy: results of a meta-analysis. *Int J Radiat Oncol Biol Phys*, 64(3), 784–91.

62 Schuchter L, Meropol NJ, Winer EP, Hensley ML, Somerfield MR (2003). Amifostine and chemoradiation therapy: ASCO responds. *Lancet Oncol*, 4(10), 593.

63 Warde P, O'Sullivan B, Aslanidis J, et al. (2002). A Phase III placebo-controlled trial of oral pilocarpine in patients undergoing radiotherapy for head-and-neck cancer. *Int J Radiat Oncol Biol Phys*, 54(1), 9–13.

64 Fisher J, Scott C, Scarantino CW, et al. (2003). Phase III quality-of-life study results: impact on patients' quality of life to reducing xerostomia after radiotherapy for head-and-neck cancer-RTOG 97-09. *Int J Radiat Oncol Biol Phys*, 56(3), 832–6.

65 Rode M, Smid L, Budihna M, Soba E, Rode M, Gaspersic D (1999). The effect of pilocarpine and biperiden on salivary secretion during and after radiotherapy in head and neck cancer patients. *Int J Radiat Oncol Biol Phys*, 45(2), 373–8.

66 Grotz KA, Wustenberg P, Kohnen R, et al. (2001). Prophylaxis of radiogenic sialadenitis and mucositis by coumarin/troxerutine in patients with head and neck cancer – a prospective, randomized, placebo-controlled, double-blind study. *Br J Oral Maxillofac Surg*, 39(1), 34–9.

67 Atkinson JC, Baum BJ (2001). Salivary enhancement: currrent status and future therapies. *J Dent Educ*, 65(10), 1096–101.

68 Bjornstrom M, Axell T, Birkhed D (1990). Comparison between saliva stimulants and saliva substitutes in patients with symptoms related to dry mouth. A multi-centre study. *Swed Dent J*, 14(4), 153–61.

69 Stewart CM, Jones AC, Bates RE, Sandow P, Pink F, Stillwell J (1998). Comparison between saliva stimulants and a saliva substitute in patients with xerostomia and hyposalivation. *Spec Care Dentist*, 18(4), 142–8.

70 Abelson DC, Barton J, Mandel ID (1989). Effect of sorbitol sweetened breath mints on salivary flow and plaque pH in xerostomic subjects. *J Clin Den*, 1(4), 102–5.

71 Davies AN (1997). The management of xerostomia: a review. *Eur J Cancer Care*, 6(3), 209–14.

72 Davies AN (2000). A comparison of artificial saliva and chewing gum in the management of xerostomia in patients with advanced cancer. *Palliat Med*, 14(3), 197–203.

73 Aagaard A, Godiksen S, Teglers PT, Schiodt M, Glenert U (1992). Comparison between new saliva stimulants in patients with dry mouth: a placebo-controlled double-blind crossover study. *J Oral Pathol Med*, 21(8), 376–80.

74 Spielman A, Ben-Aryeh H, Gutman D, Szargel R, Deutsch E (1981). Xerostomia - diagnosis and treatment. *Oral Surg Oral Med Oral Pathol*, 51(2), 144–7.

75 Senahayake F, Piggott K, Hamilton-Miller JM (1998). A pilot study of Salix SST (saliva-stimulating lozenges) in post-irradiation xerostomia. *Curr Med Res Opin*, 14(3), 155–9.

76 Newbrun E (1981). Xerostomia. *Oral Surg Oral Med Oral Pathol*, 52(3), 262.

77 Ferguson MM (1993). Pilocarpine and other cholinergic drugs in the management of salivary gland dysfunction. *Oral Surg Oral Med Oral Pathol*, 75(2), 186–91.

78 Fox PC, Atkinson JC, Macynski AA, et al. (1991). Pilocarpine treatment of salivary gland hypofunction and dry mouth (xerostomia). *Arch Intern Med*, 151(6), 1149–52.

79 Davies AN, Daniels C, Pugh R, Sharma K (1998). A comparison of artificial saliva and pilocarpine in the management of xerostomia in patients with advanced cancer. *Palliat Med*, 12(2), 105–11.

80 Johnson JT, Ferretti GA, Nethery WJ, et al. (1993). Oral pilocarpine for post-irradiation xerostomia in patients with head and neck cancer. *New Engl J Med*, 329(6), 390–5.

81 LeVeque FG, Montgomery M, Potter D, et al. (1993). A multicentre, randomized, double-blind, placebo-controlled, dose-titration study of oral pilocarpine for treatment of radiation-induced xerostomia in head and neck cancer patients. *J Clin Oncol*, 11(6), 1124–31.

82 Singhal S, Mehta J, Rattenbury H, Treleaven J, Powles R (1995). Oral pilocarpine hydrochloride for the treatment of refractory xerostomia associated with chronic graft-versus-host disease. *Blood*, 85(4), 1147–8.

83 Nagler RM, Nagler A (1999). Pilocarpine hydrochloride relieves xerostomia in chronic graft-versus-host disease: a sialometrical study. *Bone Marrow Transplant*, 23(10), 1007–11.

84 Davies AN, Singer J (1994). A comparison of artificial saliva and pilocarpine in radiation-induced xerostomia. *J Laryngol Otol*, 108(8), 663–5.

85 Davies AN, Shorthose K (2007). Parasympathomimetic drugs for the treatment of salivary gland dysfunction due to radiotherapy. Cochrane Database of Systematic Reviews, Issue 3. Art. No.: CD003782.

86 Joensuu H, Bostrom P, Makkonen T (1993). Pilocarpine and carbacholine in treatment of radiation-induced xerostomia. *Radiother Oncol*, 26(1), 33–7.

87 Everett HC (1975). The use of bethanechol chloride with tricyclic antidepressants. *Am J Psychiatry*, 132, 1202–4.

88 Epstein JB, Burchell JL, Emerton S, Le ND, Silverman S Jr (1994). A clinical trial of bethanechol in patients with xerostomia after radiation therapy. A pilot study. Oral Surg *Oral Med Oral Pathol*, 77(6), 610–14.

89 Gorsky M, Epstein JB, Parry J, Epstein MS, Le ND, Silverman S Jr (2004). The efficacy of pilocarpine and bethanechol upon saliva production in cancer patients with hyposalivation following radiation therapy. *Oral Surg Oral Med Oral Pathol Oral Radiol Endod*, 97(2), 190–5.

90 Petrone D, Condemi JJ, Fife R, Gluck O, Cohen S, Dalgin P (2002). A double-blind, randomized, placebo-controlled study of cevimeline in Sjögren's syndrome patients with xerostomia and keratoconjunctivitis sicca. *Arthritis Rheum*, 46(3), 748–54.

91 Chambers MS, Posner M, Jones CU, et al. (2007). Cevimeline for the treatment of postirradiation xerostomia in patients with head and neck cancer. *Int J Radiat Oncol Biol Phys*, 68(4), 1102–9.

92 Chambers MS, Jones CU, Biel MA (2007). Open-label, long-term safety study of cevimeline in the treatment of postirradiation xerostomia. *Int J Radiat Oncol Biol Phys*, 69(5), 1369–76.

93 Carpenter PA, Schubert MM, Flowers ME (2006). Cevimeline reduced mouth dryness and increased salivary flow in patients with xerostomia complicating chronic graft-versus-host disease. *Biol Blood Marrow Transplant*, 12(7), 792–4.

94 Wolpert E, Jung F, Middelhoff HD, Piegler T (1980). Zur Behandlung medikamentos bedingter Mundtrockenheit bei psychiatrischen Patienten – Eine Kontrollierte Vergleischsstudie. *Fortschritte der Neurologie, Psychiatrie und Ihrer Grenzgebiete*, 48(4), 224–33.

95 Teichman SL, Ferrick A, Kim SG, Matos JA, Waspe LE, Fisher JD (1987). Disopyramide-pyridostigmine interaction: selective reversal of anticholinergic symptoms with preservation of antiarrhythmic effect. *J Am Coll Cardiol*, 10(3), 633–41.

96 Blom M, Dawidson I, Angmar-Mansson B (1992). The effect of acupuncture on salivary flow rates in patients with xerostomia. *Oral Surg Oral Med Oral Pathol*, 73(3), 293–8.

97 Rydholm M, Strang P (1999). Acupuncture for patients in hospital-based home care suffering from xerostomia. *J Palliat Care*, 15(4), 20–3.

98 Blom M, Dawidson I, Fernberg JO, Johnson G, Angmar-Mansson B (1996). Acupuncture treatment of patients with radiation-induced xerostomia. *Eur J Cancer B Oral Oncol*, 32B(3), 182–90.

99 Johnstone PA, Peng YP, May BC, Inouye WS, Niemtzow RC (2001). Acupuncture for pilocarpine-resistant xerostomia following radiotherapy for head and neck malignancies. *Int J Radiat Oncol Biol Phys*, 50(2), 353–7.

100 Jedel E (2005). Acupuncture in xerostomia – a systematic review. J Oral Rehabil, 32(6), 392–6.

101 Johnstone PA, Niemtzow RC, Riffenburgh RH (2002). Acupuncture for xerostomia: clinical update. *Cancer*, 94(4), 1151–6.

102 Walsh B (2001). Control of infection in acupuncture. *Acupunct Med*, 19(2), 109–11.

103 Hamada T, Nakane T, Kimura T, et al. (1999). Treatment of xerostomia with the bile secretion-stimulating drug anethole trithione: a clinical trial. *Am J Med Sci*, 318, 146–51.

104 Bagheri H, Schmitt L, Berlan M, Montastrue JL (1997). A comparative study of the effects of yohimbine and anetholtrithione on salivary secretion in depressed patients treated with psychotropic drugs. *Eur J Clin Pharmacol*, 52, 339–42.

105 Fox PC, Cummins MJ, Cummins JM (2001). Use of orally administered anhydrous crystalline maltose for relief of dry mouth. *J Altern Complement Med*, 7(1), 33–43.

106 Grisius MM (2001). Salivary gland dysfunction: a review of systemic therapies. *Oral Surg Oral Med Oral Pathol Oral Radiol Endod*, 92(2), 156–62.

107 Sugano S, Takeyama I, Ogino S, Kenmochi M, Kaneko T (1996). Effectiveness of formula ophiopogoins in the treatment of xerostomia and pharyngoxerosis. *Acta Otolaryngol*, Suppl 522, 124–9.

108 Haila S, Koskinen A, Tenovuo J (2005). Effects of homeopathic treatment on salivary flow rate and subjective symptoms in patients with oral dryness: a randomized trial. *Homeopathy*, 94, 175–81.

109 Weiss WW Jr, Brenman HS, Katz P, Bennett JA (1986). Use of an electronic stimulator for the treatment of dry mouth. *J Oral Maxillofac Surg*, 44(11), 845–50.

110 Strietzel FP, Martin-Granizo R, Fedele S, et al. (2006). Electrostimulating device in the management of xerostomia. *Oral Dis*, 13(2), 206–13.

111 Wong RK, Jones GW, Sagar SM, Babjak A-F, Whelan T (2003). A phase I-II study in the use of acupuncture-like transcutaneous nerve stimulation in the treatment of radiation-induced xerostomia in head-and-neck cancer patients treated with radical radiotherapy. *Int J Radiat Oncol Biol Phys*, 57(2), 472–80.

112 Duxbury AJ, Thakker NS, Wastell DG (1989). A double-blind cross-over trial of a mucin-containing artificial saliva. *Br Dent J*, 166, 115–20.

113 Wiesenfeld D, Stewart AM, Mason DK (1983). A critical assessment of oral lubricants in patients with xerostomia. *Br Dent J*, 155, 155–7.

114 Olsson H, Axell T (1991). Objective and subjective efficacy of saliva substitutes containing mucin and carboxymethylcellulose. *Scand J Dent Res*, 99, 316–19.

115 Epstein JB, Stevenson-Moore P (1992). A clinical comparative trial of saliva substitutes in radiation-induced salivary gland hypofunction. *Spec Care Dentist*, 12(1), 21–3.

116 Wynn RL, Meiller TF (2000). Artificial saliva products and drugs to treat xerostomia. *Gen Dent*, 48(6), 630–6.

117 Vissink A, 's-Gravenmade EJ, Panders AK, et al. (1983). A clinical comparison between commercially available mucin- and CMC-containing saliva substitutes. *Int J Oral Surg*, 12(4), 232–8.

118 Visch LL, 's-Gravenmade EJ, Schaub RM, Van Putten WL, Vissink A (1986). A double-blind crossover trial of CMC- and mucin-containing saliva substitutes. *Int J Oral Maxillofac Surg*, 15(4), 395–400.

119 Epstein JB, Emerton S, Le ND, Stevenson-Moore P (1999). A double-blind crossover trial of Oral Balance gel and Biotene toothpaste versus placebo in patients with xerostomia following radiation therapy. *Oral Oncol*, 35(2), 132–7.

120 Shahdad SA, Taylor C, Barclay SC, Steen IN, Preshaw PM (2005). A double-blind, crossover study of Biotene Oralbalance and BioXtra systems as salivary substitutes in patients with post-radiotherapy xerostomia. *Eur J Cancer Care*, 14(4), 319–26.

121 Tenovuo J (2002). Clinical applications of antimicrobial host proteins lactoperoxidase, lysozyme and lactoferrin in xerostomia: efficacy and safety. *Oral Dis*, 8(1), 23–9.

122 Andersson G, Johansson G, Attstrom R, Edwardsson S, Glantz PO, Larsson K (1995). Comparison of the effect of the linseed extract Salinum and a methyl cellulose preparation on the symptoms of dry mouth. *Gerodontology*, 12(1), 12–17.

123 Rhodus NL, Bereuter J (2000). Clinical evaluation of a commercially available oral moisturizer in relieving signs and symptoms of xerostomia in postirradiation head and neck cancer patients and patients with Sjogren's syndrome. *J Otolaryngol*, 29(1), 28–34.

124 Vissink A, Gravenmade EJ, Panders AK, et al. (1984). Artificial saliva reservoirs. *J Prosthet Dent*, 52(5), 710–15.

125 Vissink A, Huisman MC, Gravenmade EJ (1986). Construction of an artificial saliva reservoir in an existing maxillary denture. *J Prosthet Dent*, 56(1), 70–4.

126 Robinson PG, Pankhurst CL, Garrett EJ (2005). Randomized-controlled trial: effect of a reservoir biteguard on quality of life in xerostomia. *J Oral Pathol Med*, 34(4), 193–7.

127 Frost PM, Shirlaw PJ, Walter JD, Challacombe SJ (2002). Patient preferences in a preliminary study comparing an intra-oral lubricating device with the usual dry mouth lubricating methods. *Br Dent J*, 193(7), 403–8.

128 Herod EL (1994). The use of milk as a saliva substitute. *J Public Health Dent*, 54, 184–9.

129 Kusler DL, Rambur BA (1992). Treatment for radiation-induced xerostomia. An innovative remedy. *Cancer Nurs*, 15, 191–5.

130 Walizer EM, Ephraim PM (1996). Double-blind cross-over controlled clinical trial of vegetable oil versus Xerolube for xerostomia: an expanded study abstract. *ORL Head Neck Nurs*, 14, 11–12.

131 Greenspan D (1990). Management of salivary dysfunction. *NCI Monogr*, 9, 159–61.

132 Furumoto EK, Barker GJ, Carter-Hanson C, Barker BF (1998). Subjective and clinical evaluation of oral lubricants in xerostomic patients. *Spec Care Dent*, 18, 113–18.

133 Klestov AC, Webb J, Latt D, et al. (1981). Treatment of xerostomia: a double-blind trial of 108 patients with Sjogren's syndrome. *Oral Surg Oral Med Oral Pathol*, 51(6), 594–9.

134 Van Drimmelen J, Rollins HF (1969). Evaluation of a commonly used oral hygiene agent. *Nurs Res*, 18(4), 327–32.

135 Sweeney P (2005). Oral hygiene, in Davies A, Finlay I (eds) *Oral Care in Advanced Disease*, pp. 21–35. Oxford University Press, Oxford.

Chapter 22

Taste disturbance

Carla Ripamonti and Fabio Fulfaro

Introduction

The sensation of taste is mediated by the taste buds. There are nearly 10 000 taste buds, situated within the mucosa of the tongue, soft palate, uvula, pharynx, upper third of the oesophagus, epiglottis, larynx, lips, and cheeks[1,2].

The taste buds are connected to the oral cavity via the taste pores[1]. A 'gatekeeper' protein regulates the passage of saliva/tastants from the oral cavity, through the taste pore, and into the taste bud. The taste buds consist of about 50 cells, including specialized gustatory cells. Gustatory cells have a microvillus (containing the taste receptor), which projects into the taste pore; gustatory cells also have a synapse, which connects to sensory nerve fibres. The gustatory cells are continuously being replaced (gustatory cells survive for ~10 days).

Each taste bud is innervated by about 50 nerve fibres, whilst each nerve fibre receives input from about five taste buds[1]. Taste information is transmitted via the V, VII, IX, and X cranial nerves to the nucleus of the tractus solitaris in the medulla, then onwards to the ventral posterior medial nucleus of the thalamus, and then onwards to the post-central gyrus in the parietal lobe.

The four main taste qualities discernable by humans are bitter, salt, sour, and sweet. However, other taste qualities are also discernible by humans, such as umami (glutamate-related taste quality)[1]. Contrary to popular belief, the four main taste qualities are detectable in all areas of the tongue, and not just in specific areas of the tongue[1].

Genetic variation in taste is present within the population. Thus, people can be classified as 'non-tasters', 'tasters', or 'supertasters' according to their ability to recognize the bitterness of 6-*n*-propylthiouracil: 'non-tasters' cannot recognize the bitterness; 'tasters' can recognize the bitterness; 'supertasters' experience the most intense bitterness[3].

It should be noted that taste refers to the specific perception of taste qualities (bitter, salt, sour, and sugar), whilst flavour refers to the composite perceptions of taste, smell, and oral somatosensory sensations (touch, temperature, and nociception)[4].

Definitions

Taste disturbance occurs as a result of a reduction in taste sensation (hypogeusia), an absence of taste sensation (ageusia), or a distortion of normal taste sensation (dysgeusia)[5].

Epidemiology

The prevalence of taste disturbance has been reported to be 31–35% in mixed oncology patients[6,7], and to be 44–50% in advanced oncology patients[8,9]. Taste disturbance is relatively common in patients with cancers of the head and neck region[10], and extremely common in patients that have received radiotherapy to the head and neck region[11].

Aetiology

There are a variety of different causes of taste disturbance in the general population[2]. Increasing age may represent an important variable, because healthy elderly individuals can have significant alterations in taste-perception thresholds[12]. Similarly, there are a variety of different causes of taste disturbance in the cancer population (Box 22.1).

Box 22.1 – Aetiology of taste disturbance in patients with cancer

- ◆ **Cancer - related**
  - Specific effect: damage of taste buds/cranial nerves (V, VII, IX, X)/central nervous system
  - Non-specific effect
- ◆ **Cancer treatment - related**
  - Local surgery
  - Local radiotherapy
  - Systemic chemotherapy
- ◆ **Oral problems**
  - Salivary gland dysfunction
  - Poor oral hygiene
  - Oral infections
  - Other oral pathology
  - Dental prosthesis ('denture')
- ◆ **Neurological problems**
  - Damage of cranial nerves (V, VII, IX, X)
  - Damage of central nervous system
- ◆ **Metabolic problems**
  - Malnutrition
  - Zinc deficiency
  - Renal dysfunction
  - Liver dysfunction
  - Endocrine dysfunction
- ◆ **Miscellaneous**
  - Ageing
  - Menopause
  - Drug treatment
  - Smoking
  - Other chronic diseases

Radiotherapy

Amongst the antineoplastic therapies, radiotherapy is the one most clearly linked to taste disturbance. Many patients have taste problems prior to head and neck radiotherapy, but almost all
patients develop taste problems during head and neck radiotherapy[10,13]. Taste disturbance
develops soon after the commencement of treatment (initial effect at ~1 week), and progresses
during the early stage of treatment (maximum effect: ~3–4 weeks)[14].

In a recent study, patients reported a variety of taste alterations following radiotherapy, including absence of taste (16%), bitter taste (8%), salty taste (5%), sour taste (4%), sweet taste (5%),
metallic taste (10%), and other assorted tastes (e.g. 'pepper', 'greasy', 'soapy', 'powdery', 'chemical')[15]. In a previous study, some patients reported a heightened taste sensation following
radiotherapy[16].

In some cases, improvement in taste disturbance occurs within a few weeks or months of
treatment. Nevertheless, in many cases, taste problems persist for a long time following treatment. For example, Maes et al. reported that 50% of patients had subjective taste disturbance
12 months post radiotherapy[10]. Similarly, Mossman reported that some patients had objective
taste disturbance 7 years post radiotherapy[17].

Taste disturbance is the result of damage to the taste buds and/or salivary gland dysfunction. However, other factors may be relevant in some patients, such as the development of oral
infection[18]. It is likely that the contribution of these factors varies from one individual to
another. Thus, salivary gland dysfunction may be the most important factor in those patients that
have persistent problems. (Salivary gland dysfunction is a long-term complication of head and
neck radiotherapy).

Chemotherapy

The antineoplastic drugs that have been associated with taste changes include bleomycin, carbo-
platin, cisplatin, cyclophsophamide, doxorubicin, 5-fluorouracil, gemcitabine, levamisole, and
methotrexate[19]. Bernhardson et al. reported variable taste changes in a heterogeneous group of
patients receiving chemotherapy[20]; the taste changes were temporary in nature, and all had
settled within 3.5 months of the end of treatment[20]. Cisplatin is associated with the development of a metallic taste, which may last from a few hours to 3 weeks following a dose of the
drug[19].

Drug therapy

A variety of different drugs have been reported to cause taste disturbance[2]. However, certain
classes of drug seem to be particularly problematic, including anti-inflammatory agents and
antimicrobial agents[21]. Some drugs cause taste disturbance *per se*, whilst others cause it through
indirect mechanisms, e.g. induction of salivary gland dysfunction.

Zinc deficiency

Zinc depletion has been linked to impaired taste function in pregnant women, in the elderly, in
patients with cancer[22], and in patients with other chronic illnesses (e.g. renal impairment)[23].
Furthermore, drugs with sulphydryl groups, which chelate zinc, are associated with taste
disturbance (e.g. D-penicillamine)[24].

The specific role of zinc in the control of taste is unknown[14]. Zinc is the co-factor for alkaline
phosphatase, the most abundant enzyme in the taste bud membrane. Furthermore, zinc (and
other metals) controls the conformation of the 'gatekeeper' protein that regulates the passage of
tastants from the oral cavity, through the taste bud pore, and into the taste bud.

Clinical features

Taste disturbance can lead to other physical, psychological, and social problems, which, in turn, can lead to a further deterioration in quality of life[25]. Box 22.2 displays quotations from patients with taste disturbance, which highlight some of these associated problems[26].

Patients may complain of a single taste problem (e.g. ageusia for all foods), or a combination of taste problems (e.g. hypogeusia for some foods, dysgeusia for other foods). For example, in a study involving patients with advanced cancer and taste disturbance, 40% reported ageusia, 31% reported hypogeusia, and 53% reported dysgeusia[27]. Patients with dysgeusia may report a variety of different sensations, but invariably report that food tastes unpleasant[28].

Table 28.3 depicts the severity of taste problems in a group of patients with advanced cancer[29]. It can be seen that the majority (70%) of patients reported that their taste disturbance was 'moderate', 'severe', or 'very severe'. Similarly, Table 28.4 shows the distress caused by taste problems in the same group of patients with advanced cancer[29]. It can be seen that the majority (51%) of patients reported that their taste disturbance caused significant distress. Other studies have reported very similar results[8,27].

Impairment of taste may be associated with anorexia[30], decreased nutritional intake[25], and weight loss[22,25]. It appears that the more severe the taste disturbance, the greater the impact on these other factors[25]. Impairment of taste may affect other aspects of gastrointestinal function, i.e. reduce salivary gland secretion and reduce gastrointestinal motility[5].

Assessment

It is uncommon for patients to report taste disturbance[5]. The reasons why patients do not report taste disturbance are unknown. However, patients may not report a symptom if: (1) they perceive the symptom to be inevitable; (2) they perceive there is no treatment for the symptom; (3) they sense that healthcare professionals perceive the symptom to be unimportant; and/or (4) other symptoms predominate[31]. Thus, it is important that patients are specifically asked about taste disturbance.

Box 22.2 Quotations from patients with taste disturbance [26]

◆ **Quote A:**
"Sweet food had a bad taste, strong food was burning and tingling on the tongue. Fluids with carbonic acid felt like hydrochloric acid".

◆ **Quote B:**
"We were to celebrate my birthday and I had helped to prepare salmon and looked forward to have dinner with the family. The taste alteration was incredible, the food tasted of absolutely nothing or possibly of wheat flower; I was disappointed and depressed and felt sorry for myself, I couldn't feel or share happiness with my family during that occasion".

◆ **Quote C:**
"I wanted to surprise my family with a nice meal, with my speciality which is salty herring. Normally, I am very proud of it but I totally failed with the seasoning as I did not feel the taste, I used far too much salt, the meal was uneatable. I was so embarrassed".

The assessment of taste disturbance involves taking a history, performing an examination, and undertaking appropriate investigations[32]. However, it is usually not necessary to undertake an objective assessment of the taste disturbance (i.e. measure taste acuity). The assessment of oral problems is discussed in detail in Chapter 3.

Taste acuity may be assessed using the standard three-stimulus drop technique, which measures the detection and recognition thresholds for the four main taste qualities (bitter, salt, sour, and sweet)[33]. The detection threshold is the lowest concentration of solute that the subject distinguishes as being different from water, whereas the recognition threshold is the lowest concentration of solute that the subject recognizes correctly.

Management

The management of taste disturbance involves: (1) treatment of the underlying cause; (2) dietary therapy; (3) zinc therapy; and/or (4) other therapies.

Treatment of the underlying cause

In some cases, it may be possible to treat the underlying cause of the taste disturbance, e.g. salivary gland dysfunction. Indeed, studies have shown that saliva stimulants improve both the xerostomia, and the associated taste disturbance[34]. (Saliva substitutes improve the xerostomia, but not the associated taste disturbance[34]). Nevertheless, in many cases, it is not possible to identify and/or treat the underlying cause of the taste disturbance.

Dietary therapy

Dietary therapy involves: (1) utilization of foods that taste 'good'; (2) avoidance of foods that taste 'bad'; (3) enhancing the taste of the food (using salt, sugar, and other flavourings); and (4) addressing the presentation, smell, consistency, and temperature of the food[35,36]. Ideally, a dietician should review all patients with taste disturbance, since dietary therapy requires an individualized approach[37].

Zinc therapy

The most studied treatment in patients with taste disturbance is zinc therapy. Studies in patients with radiotherapy-related taste disturbance have produced conflicting results (Table 22.1). Thus, two small studies in patients with established taste disturbance suggest a possible therapeutic role for oral zinc supplements[13,38]. Similarly, two small studies in patients undergoing radiotherapy suggest an additional prophylactic role for oral zinc supplements[39, 40]. However, the recent large North Central Cancer Treatment Group (NCCTG) study reported neither a significant prophylactic effect, nor a significant therapeutic effect, for oral zinc supplements[15].

Studies in other patient groups have also produced conflicting results. For example, some large studies involving patients with idiopathic/mixed-aetiology taste disturbance have reported a negative effect[41,42]. In contrast, some smaller studies involving patients with renal disease have reported a positive effect (i.e. objective improvement)[23,43]. Thus, it may be that zinc is effective for some, but not all, causes of taste disturbance. It should be noted that there appear to have been no studies in cancer patients with taste disturbance secondary to causes other than radiotherapy.

Oral zinc supplements are generally well tolerated, although they can cause dyspepsia and abdominal pain. Thus, it would seem reasonable to offer patients with taste disturbance a trial of an oral zinc supplement (in the absence of other treatment options).

Table 22.1 Studies of zinc administration in patients with cancer

Study	Design	Regimen	Outcomes
Mossman, 1978 [13]	Case series (n = 7; patients with taste disturbance post head and neck radiotherapy)	Variable 25 or 100 mg/day zinc for 2–6 months	Improvement in objective taste disturbance.
Silverman and Thompson, 1984 [38]	Case series (n = 30; patients with taste disturbance post head and neck radiotherapy)	Variable 100–150 mg/day zinc for at least 1 month	Improvement in subjective taste disturbance (37% patients).
Silverman et al., 1983 [39]	Randomised controlled trials vs placebo (n = 19; patients pre head & neck radiotherapy)	18 mg qds zinc for duration of radiotherapy	No difference in objective taste disturbance during radiotherapy between groups. Earlier recovery of subjective taste disturbance in treatment group (64% vs 22% patients at 3 weeks post treatment).
Ripamonti et al., 1998 [40]	Randomised controlled trials vs placebo (n = 18; patients with taste disturbance during head & neck radiotherapy)	45 mg tds zinc sulphate from onset of subjective taste disturbance until 1 month post radiotherapy	Less objective taste disturbance during radiotherapy in treatment group. Earlier recovery of objective taste disturbance in treatment group
Hakyard et al., 2007 [15]	Randomised controlled trials vs placebo (n = 169; patients pre head and neck radiotherapy)	45 mg tds zinc sulphate from onset of radiotherapy (≤ 7 days) until 1 month post radiotherapy	No difference in subjective taste disturbance during radiotherapy between groups. No difference in recovery of subjective taste disturbance between groups

Other treatments

Other treatments that have been used to treat taste disturbance include copper[44], nickel[45], corticosteroids[35], and various complementary therapies[46]. However, the evidence for their efficacy/tolerability is very limited.

References

1 Ganong WF (2003). *Review of medical physiology*, 21st edn, pp. 191–4. Lange Medical Books, New York.

2 Schiffman SS (1983). Taste and smell in disease (first of two parts). *New Engl J Med* 1983, 308(21), 1275–9.

3 Bartoshuk LM (2000). Comparing sensory experiences across individuals: recent psychophysical advances illuminate genetic variation in taste perception. *Chem Senses*, 25(4), 447–60.

4 Duffy VB, Fast K, Lucchina LA, Bartoshuk LM (2002). Oral sensation and cancer, in Berger AM, Portenoy RK, Weissman DE (eds) *Principles and Practice of Palliative Care and Supportive Oncology*, 2nd edn, pp. 178–93. Lippincott Williams & Wilkins, Philadelphia.

5   De Conno F, Sbanotto A, Ripamonti C, Ventafridda V (2003). Mouth care, in Doyle D, Hanks G, Cherny N, Calman K (eds) *Oxford Textbook of Palliative Medicine*, 3rd edn, pp. 673–87. Oxford University Press, Oxford.

6   Portenoy RK, Thaler HT, Kornblith AB, et al. (1994). Symptom prevalence, characteristics and distress in a cancer population. *Qual Life Res*, 3(3), 183–9.

7   Chang VT, Hwang SS, Feuerman M, Kasimis BS, Thaler HT (2000). The Memorial Symptom Assessment Scale Short Form (MSAS-SF). *Cancer*, 89(5), 1162–71.

8   Tranmer JE, Heyland D, Dudgeon D, Groll D, Squires-Graham M, Coulson K (2003). Measuring the symptom experience of seriously ill cancer and noncancer hospitalized patients near the end of life with the Memorial Symptom Assessment Scale. *J Pain Symptom Manage*, 25(5), 420–9.

9   Shorthose K, Davies A (2003). Symptom prevalence in palliative care. *Palliat Med*, 17(8), 723–4.

10 Maes A, Huygh I, Weltens C et al. (2002). De Gustibus: time scale of loss and recovery of tastes caused by radiotherapy. *Radiother Oncol*, 63(2), 195–201.

11 Ruo Redda MG, Allis S (2006). Radiotherapy-induced taste impairment. *Cancer* Treat Rev, 32(7), 541–7.

12 Ng K, Woo J, Kwan M, et al. (2004). Effect of age and disease on taste perception. *J Pain Symptom Manage*, 28(1), 28–34.

13 Mossman KL, Henkin RI (1978). Radiation-induced changes in taste acuity in cancer patients. *Int J Radiat Oncol Biol Phys*, 4(7–8), 663–70.

14 Ripamonti C, Fulfaro F (1998). Taste alterations in cancer patients. *J Pain Symptom Manage*, 16(6), 349–51.

15 Halyard MY, Jatoi A, Sloan JA, et al. (2007). Does zinc sulfate prevent therapy-induced taste alterations in head and neck cancer patients? Results of phase III double-blind, placebo-controlled trial from the North Central Cancer Treatment Group (N01C4). *Int J Radiat Oncol Biol Phys*, 67(5), 1318–22.

16 Bonanni G, Perazzi F (1965). Il comportamento della sensibilita' gustativa in pazienti sottoposti a trattamento radiologico con alte energie per tumori del cavo orale. *Nunt Radiol*, 31(4), 383–97.

17 Mossman KL, Shatzman AR, Chencharick JD (1982). Long-term effects of radiotherapy on taste and salivary function in man. *Int J Radiat Oncol Biol Phys*, 8(6), 991–7.

18 Fernando IN, Patel T, Billingham L, et al. (1995). The effect of head and neck irradiation on taste dysfunction: a prospective study. *Clin Oncol (R Coll Radiol)*, 7(3), 173–8.

19 Wickham RS, Rehwaldt M, Kefer C, et al. (1999). Taste changes experienced by patients receiving chemotherapy. *Oncol Nurs Forum*, 26(4), 697–706.

20 Bernhardson B-M, Tishelman C, Rutqvist LE (2007). Chemosensory changes experienced by patients undergoing cancer chemotherapy: a qualitative interview study. *J Pain Symptom Manage*, 34(4), 403–12.

21 Schiffman SS, Zervakis J, Westall HL, et al. (2000). Effect of antimicrobial and anti-inflammatory medications on the sense of taste. *Physiol Behav*, 69(4–5), 413–24.

22 DeWys WD, Walters K (1975). Abnormalities of taste sensation in cancer patients. *Cancer*, 36(5), 1888–96.

23 Atkin-Thor E, Goddard BW, O'Nion J, Stephen RL, Kolff WJ (1978). Hypogeusia and zinc depletion in chronic dialysis patients. *Am J Clin Nutr*, 31(10), 1948–51.

24 Willoughby JM (1983). Drug-induced abnormalities of taste sensation. Adverse *Drug React Bull*, 100, 368–71.

25 Hutton JL, Baracos VE, Wismer WV (2007). Chemosensory dysfunction is a primary factor in the evolution of declining nutritional status and quality of life in patients with advanced cancer. *J Pain Symptom Manage*, 33(2), 156–65

26 Rydholm M, Strang P (2002). Physical and psychosocial impact of xerostomia in palliative cancer care: a qualitative interview study. *Int J Palliat Nurs*, 8(7), 318–23.

27 Davies AN, Kaur K (1998). Taste problems in patients with advanced cancer. *Palliat Med*, 12(2), 482–3.

28 Shapiro SL (1974). Abnormalities of taste. *Eye Ear Nose Throat Mon*, 53(7), 293–6.

29 Davies AN (2000). An investigation into the relationship between salivary gland hypofunction and oral health problems in patients with advanced cancer [Dissertation]. King's College: University of London.

30 Stubbs L (1989). Taste changes in cancer patients. *Nurs Times*, 85(3), 49–50.

31 Shorthose K, Davies AN (2003). Symptom prevalence in palliative care. *Palliat Med*, 17(8), 73–4.

32 Birnbaum W, Dunne SM (2000). *Oral diagnosis: the clinician's guide.* Wright, Oxford.

33 Henkin RI, Schechter PJ, Hoye R, Mattern CF (1971). Idiopathic hypogeusia with dysgeusia, hyposmia and dysosmia. A new syndrome. *J Am Med Assoc*, 217(4), 434–40.

34 Davies AN, Singer J (1994). A comparison of artificial saliva and pilocarpine in radiation-induced xerostomia. *J Laryngol Otol*, 108(8), 663–5.

35 Twycross RG, Lack SA (1986). *Control of alimentary symptoms in far advanced cancer.* Churchill Livingstone, Edinburgh.

36 Komurcu S, Nelson KA, Walsh D (2001). The gastrointestinal symptoms of advanced cancer. *Support Care Cancer*, 9(1), 32–9.

37 Davidson I, Richardson R (2003). Dietary and nutritional aspects of palliative medicine, in Doyle D, Hanks G, Cherny N, Calman K (eds) *Oxford Textbook of Palliative Medicine*, 3rd edn, pp. 546–52. Oxford University Press, Oxford.

38 Silverman S Jr, Thompson JS (1984). Serum zinc and copper in oral/oropharyngeal carcinoma. A study of seventy-five patients. *Oral Surg Oral Med Oral Pathol*, 57(1), 34–6.

39 Silverman JE, Weber CW, Silverman S Jr, Coulthard SL, Manning MR (1983). Zinc supplementation and taste in head and neck cancer patients undergoing radiation therapy. *J Oral Med*, 38(1), 14–16.

40 Ripamonti C, Zecca E, Brunelli C, et al. (1998). A randomized, controlled clinical trial to evaluate the effects of zinc sulfate on cancer patients with taste alterations caused by head and neck irradiation. *Cancer*, 82(10), 1938–45.

41 Henkin RI, Schecter PJ, Friedewald WT, Demets DL, Raff M (1976). A double blind study of the effects of zinc sulfate on taste and smell dysfunction. *Am J Med Sci*, 272(3), 285–99.

42 Sakai F, Yoshida S, Endo S, Tomita H (2002). Double-blind, placebo-controlled trial of zinc picolinate for taste disorders. *Acta Otolaryngol Suppl (Stockh)*, (546), 129–33.

43 Mahajan SK, Prasad AS, Lambujon J, Abbasi AA, Briggs WA, McDonald FD (1980). Improvement of uremic hypogeusia by zinc: a double-blind study. *Am J Clin Nutr*, 33(7), 1517–21.

44 Henkin RI, Keiser HR, Jafee IA, Sternlieb I, Scheinberg IH (1967). Decreased taste sensitivity after D-penicillamine reversed by copper administration. *Lancet*, 2(7529), 1268–71.

45 Henkin RI, Bradley DF (1970). Hypogeusia corrected by Ni++ and Zn++. *Life Sci II*, 9(12), 701–9.

46 Peregrin T (2006). Improving taste sensation in patients who have undergone chemotherapy or radiation therapy. *J Am Diet Assoc*, 106(10), 1536–40.

Chapter 23

Halitosis

Stephen Porter

Definition

Halitosis has been defined as 'offensive odours from the mouth or hollow cavities such as the nose, sinuses, and pharynx'[1]. Other terms used to describe this condition include oral malodour, *foetor oris* ('stench of the mouth'), *foetor ex ore* ('stench from the mouth'), and 'bad breath'[2].

Epidemiology

Halitosis is a problem that everyone has from time to time, but that some people have on a more regular basis[3]. The prevalence of chronic objective halitosis is reported to be 2.4–30% in the general population[4]. It should be noted that the lower figure represents the prevalence of detectable oral odour, whilst the higher figure represents the prevalence of 'objectionable' oral odour. The prevalence of objective halitosis is unreported in the oncology population. Nevertheless, halitosis is a significant problem for certain groups of cancer patients (e.g. head and neck cancer patients), and a potential problem for all individual cancer patients.

Aetiology

Oral causes

Oral malodour upon awakening ('morning breath' or 'morning halitosis') affects all individuals from time to time, being worse if the bedroom is dry and warm and/or they have any nasal obstruction[5]. Certain foods, tobacco, and alcohol predictably cause alteration in the smell of the breath[6], although such breath changes may not be considered to be notably abnormal or unpleasant within different cultures.

Long-term oral malodour is almost always the consequence of oral disease (Table 23.1)[7]. Accumulation of food debris in the mouth and bacterial plaque on the teeth and tongue (due to poor oral hygiene), and the resultant gingival and periodontal inflammation are the usual sources of oral malodour[8]. All types of plaque-related gingivitis and periodontitis can give rise to halitosis, but acute necrotizing ulcerative gingivitis (Vincent's disease or 'trench mouth') and aggressive forms of periodontitis (e.g. as arising in chronic neutropenic states) can give rise to particularly unpleasant breath odour[9]. Long-standing xerostomia alone, or as a result of increasing the severity of gingivitis, may also give rise to halitosis[10,11]. It is also reported that denture wearing predisposes to oral malodour[11,12].

Halitosis arsing from the mouth is due to microbial putrefaction of food debris, epithelial cells, saliva, and blood. The implicated oral microbes are Gram-negative bacteria and include *Prevotella (Bacteroides) melaninogenica, Treponema denticola, Porphyromonas gingivalis, Porphyromonas endodontalis, Prevotella intermedius, Bacteroides loescheii, Enterobacteriacceae, Tannerella forsythensis*

Table 23.1 Causes of halitosis[5]

Category	Example
Volatile foodstuffs	Garlic
	Onions
Oral disease	Food impaction
	Poor oral hygiene
	Xerostomia
	Periodontal disease
	Pericoronitis
	Dry socket
	Oral ulceration
	Malignancy
Respiratory disease	Sinusitis
	Tonsillitis
	Bronchiectasis
	Lung abscess
	Foreign body
	Malignancy
Gastrointestinal disease	Pharyngo-oesophageal diverticulum
	Gastric *Helicobacter pylori* infection
	Gastro-oesophageal reflux disease
	Gastric outflow obstruction
	Gastro-intestinal obstruction
	Aorto-enteric anastomosis
Hepatic disease	Hepatic failure (foetor hepaticus)
Renal disease	Renal failure
Haematological disease	Leukaemia
Endocrine disease	Diabetic ketoacidosis
	(Menstruation (menstruation breath))
Metabolic disease	Trimethylaminuria ('Fish odour syndrome')
	Hypermethioninaemia
Drugs	Alcohol
	Tobacco
	Solvent abuse
	Nitrates
	Phenothiazines
	Amphetamines
	Chloral hydrate
	Disulfiram
	Paraldehyde

(*Bacteroides forsythus*), *Centipeda periodontii*, *Eikenella corrodens*, *Fusobacterium nucleatum vincentii*, *Fusobacterium nucleatum nucleatum*, *Fusobacterium nucleatum polymorphum*, and *Fusobacterium periodontium*[9,13]. However, there is no obvious association between halitosis and any specific bacterial infection, and oral malodour probably reflects complex interactions between several oral bacterial species.

The microbial events giving rise to halitosis occur in the gingival crevices, periodontal pockets, and also the back of the dorsum of the tongue (where the papillary surface provides an environment for the entrapment of both oral debris and bacteria)[14]. Patients who are unable to clean their mouths (or move their tongues) are liable to accumulation of plaque at the aforesaid sites[15,16]. The agents that give rise to oral malodour include volatile sulphur compounds (VSCs), diamines, and short-chain fatty acids (Table 23.2)[5].

In cancer care, oral malodour is likely to be most common in patients with head and neck malignancy affecting the mouth or upper airways, and arising as a consequence of tissue necrosis, nasal obstruction, and/or poor oral hygiene. Leukaemias may, occasionally, give rise to oral malodour as a result of enhanced gingival inflammation and/or neutropenic ulceration (which can be rather necrotic)[17]. Radiotherapy- and chemotherapy-induced mucositis can give rise to oral malodour as patients may not be able to maintain good oral hygiene. In addition, the ulceration and necrosis of mucositis may itself give rise to an unpleasant smell. Radiotherapy-induced xerostomia can cause oral malodour due to foodstuffs adhering to the oral surfaces, and an increased liability to plaque-related gingivitis.

Systemic causes

Respiratory diseases are probably the most common group of systemic causes of oral malodour. Upper respiratory tract infections, tonsillitis, and tonsoliths commonly cause bad breath, although pulmonary disease such as tuberculosis, bronchiectasis, lung abscess, and malignancy are causes of particularly unpleasant breath odour. Other recognized systemic causes of altered breath odour are indicated in Table 23.1[5]. A recent report suggested an association between dimethyl sulphide in oral breath and the systemic causes of halitosis[18].

There is a group of individuals who complain, often with great conviction, of oral malodour and yet have no detectable halitosis. This symptom is, often, considered to be delusional or a reflection of monosymptomatic hypochondriasis (self-oral malodour or halitophobia). Affected individuals, often, wrongly interpret the actions of others as an indication that their breath is offensive, and can adopt a variety of behaviours to minimize their perceived problem (e.g. covering the mouth when talking, avoiding social interactions)[19].

Table 23.2 Odiferous agents arising from the mouth[5]

Category	Compound
Volatile sulphur compounds (VSCs)	Methyl mercaptan
	Hydrogen sulphide
	Dimethyl sulphide
Diamines	Putrescine
	Cadaverine
Short chain fatty acids	Butyric acid
	Valeric acid
	Propionic acid

Clinical features

Halitosis may seem a minor problem, but it can be a significant cause of morbidity/impairment of quality of life.

The person may not be aware that they have halitosis, because they have also developed an olfactory disturbance[20], or because they have developed tolerance to the malodour (habituation)[21]. Even if the person is aware that they have halitosis, it is unusual for them to complain about the halitosis. It should be noted that some people present with taste disturbance ('bad taste'), whilst others present with symptoms relating to the underlying cause of the halitosis[20].

Halitosis can have profound psychological and social effects[22]. The person may be embarrassed/depressed by the malodour, and so avoid contact with other people (e.g. family, friends). Similarly, other people may find it difficult to tolerate the malodour, and so avoid contact with the person. Moreover, healthcare professionals may limit their interactions with the person[23].

Investigation

The diagnosis of clinically significant halitosis is straightforward, as the smell is usually apparent during routine clinical examination. A formal assessment of oral malodour may involve a variety of subjective methods (i.e. assessment of odour intensity or quality) and, less commonly, objective methods (i.e. detection of odiferous agents or bacteria)[24].

The organolpetic method involves assessing the intensity of the odour; it does not require formal training, and can be incorporated into routine clinical practice. The organolpetic method entails smelling/comparing the exhaled air of the mouth and nose, and attributing a grade to the intensity of the malodour (organolpetic score) (Table 23.3)[25]. Odour detectable from the mouth, but not from the nose, is likely to be of oral or pharyngeal origin[24]. Odour from the nose alone is likely to be coming from the nose or sinuses. A systemic cause of the malodour is likely in the rare instances when the odour from the nose and mouth are of similar intensity. The hedonic method involves assessing the quality of the odour; it does require formal training, and is not indicated in routine clinical practice (but may be relevant in translational research)[26,27].

The objective measurement of the breath components has little application in routine clinical practice. Volatile sulphur compounds in oral breath can be estimated using sulphide monitors, but as halitosis usually involves a combination of odiferous agents, the results may not truly reflect the source and/or severity of any oral odours[5]. An optical 'bio-sniffer' for the detection of methyl mercaptan has been developed, but it remains unclear if this has any value in clinical practice[28]. Gas chromatography of oral breath is considered the gold standard investigation, but this is a research tool rather than a clinical tool. The bacteria that give rise to oral malodour

Table 23.3 Organoleptic scoring scale[25]

Category	Description
0: Absence of odour	Odour cannot be detected
1: Questionable odour	Odour is detectable, although the examiner could not recognize it as malodour
2: Slight malodour	Odour is deemed to exceed the threshold of malodour recognition
3: Moderate malodour	Malodour is definitely detected
4: Strong malodour	Strong malodour is detected, but can be tolerated by examiner
5: Severe malodour	Overwhelming malodour is detected and cannot be tolerated by examiner (examiner instinctively averts the nose)

can be detected via a number of different techniques (e.g. benzoyl-DL-arginine-naphthylamide (BANA) test, dark-field microscopy, real-time polymerase chain reaction (PCR)), although at present such investigations have no practical application in the care of patients with oral malodour[29,30].

Treatment

The majority of patients with halitosis will have some or complete resolution of symptoms by following certain simple oral procedures. As most oral malodour is the consequence of plaque-related gingival and periodontal disease the mainstay of therapy is to remove as much plaque as possible[31]. Effective teeth cleaning, including brushing and interdental flossing, will help to reduce halitosis[9,32]. If oral malodour persists, the tongue may be the source of odour, and so tongue cleaning may be indicated. Tongue cleaning can reduce levels of VSCs in breath, but this may be of only transient benefit[33,34]. Chewing gum only seems to cause transient reduction in oral malodour[35], although gum containing magnolia bark extract may lessen the oral bacteria associated with halitosis[36].

A range of mouthwashes have been suggested for the treatment of oral malodour, and these act either by reducing the bacterial load or the associated odoriferous compounds[5]. Unfortunately, there are few randomized controlled trials of the effectiveness of these mouthwashes. Chlorhexidine gluconate produces a decline in the number of VSC-producing bacteria[37], and can be more effective than oral hygiene alone at reducing oral malodour[38]. A combined chlorhexidine/zinc mouthwash has been reported to be effective for halitosis[39]. Similarly, a mouthwash of chlorhexidine/cetylpyridinium chloride/zinc lactate also reduces oral malodour[40]. However, patients may be reluctant to use chlorhexidine long term as it has an unpleasant taste, can give rise to a burning sensation of the oral mucosa, and can cause (reversible) staining of the teeth.

Triclosan has a direct anti-bacterial effect and anti-VSC action, and when used in toothpastes and mouthrinses may reduce oral malodour. The anti-VSC action of triclosan seems to depend upon the solubizing agent with which it is delivered[41]. Thus, a formulation of triclosan/co-polymer/sodium fluoride (Colgate Total®) seems to be particularly effective in reducing oral malodour[42–44].

A two-phase oil–water rinse (Dentyl$_{pH}$®) can reduce oral malodour for several hours[45,46]. Other mouth rinses that can also reduce oral malodour for several hours include cetylpyridinium chloride[47], chlorine dioxide[48,49] and zinc chloride[37,50]. Application of 0.454% stabilized stannous fluoride sodium hexametaphosphate dentifrice has recently been found to reduce halitosis[51], whilst the finding that a metronidazole mouth rinse may be of benefit has never been confirmed[52].

A number of novel methods for reducing halitosis have been proposed, including the use of glycosylation inhibitors (e.g. D-galactosamine)[53], probiotic bacteria that replace bacteria causative of oral malodour (e.g. *Streptococcus salivarius*)[54,55], light exposure that directly inhibits VSC-producing bacteria[56], and lethal photosensitization (of relevant bacteria)[57]. Green tea has also been suggested as a means of transiently reducing halitosis[58].

Patients with oral malodour secondary to systemic disease should have a reduction in breath smell following successful treatment of the underlying disease. Halitophobia remains difficult to resolve, since affected individuals usually have complex underlying psychological drivers. Furthermore, few of these patients are willing to follow the necessary line of therapy (i.e. psychological/psychiatric interventions)[5].

It should be noted that there are no proven methods of lessening the halitosis of patients with cancer, and so the aforementioned approaches should be employed/tailored to individual patients with cancer. For example, patients with oral mucositis may not tolerate normal oral hygiene care measures (e.g. teeth brushing, chlorhexidine mouthwashes). Nevertheless, even in these circumstances, rinsing the mouth with normal saline can remove oral debris, improve oral hygiene, and so lessen oral malodour.

References

1 Nachnani S, Clark GT (1997). Halitosis: a breath of fresh air. *Clin Infect Dis*, 25(Suppl 2), S218–9.

2 Spouge JD (1964). Halitosis, A review of its causes and treatment. *Dent Pract Dent Rec*, 14(8), 307–17.

3 Scully C, Porter S, Greenman J (1994). What to do about halitosis. *Br Med J*, 308(6923), 217–18.

4 Loesche WJ, Kazor C (2002). Microbiology and treatment of halitosis. *Periodontol 2000*, 28, 256–79.

5 Porter SR, Scully C (2006). Oral malodour (halitosis). *Brit Med J*, 333(7569), 632–5.

6 Parmar G, Sangwan P, Vashi P, Kulkarni P, Kumar S (2008). Effect of chewing a mixture of areca nut and tobacco on periodontal tissues and oral hygiene status. *J Oral Sci*, 50(1), 57–62.

7 Rio AC, Franchi-Teixeira AR, Nicola EM (2008). Relationship between the presence of tonsilloliths and halitosis in patients with chronic caseous tonsillitis. *Br Dent J*, 204(2), E4.

8 Tsai CC, Chou HH, Wu TL, et al. (2008). The levels of volatile sulfur compounds in mouth air from patients with chronic periodontitis. *J Periodontal Res*, 43(2), 186–93.

9 Morita M, Wang HL (2001). Association between oral malodor and adult periodontitis: a review. *J Clin Periodontol*, 28(9), 813–19.

10 Kleinberg I, Wolff MS, Codipilly DM (2002). Role of saliva in oral dryness, oral feel and oral malodour. *Int Dent J*, 52(Suppl 3), 236–40.

11 Nalcaci R, Baran I (2008). Factors associated with self-reported halitosis (SRH) and perceived taste disturbance (PTD) in elderly. *Arch Gerontol Geriatr*, 46(3), 307–16.

12 Aizawa F, Kishi M, Moriya T, Takahashi M, Inaba D, Yonemitsu M (2005). The analysis of characteristics of elderly people with high VSC level. *Oral Dis*, 11(Suppl 1), 80–2.

13 Awano S, Gohara, K, Kurihara E, Ansai T, Takehara T (2002). The relationship between the presence of periodontopathogenic bacteria in saliva and halitosis. *Int Dent J*, 52(Suppl 3), 212–16.

14 Haraszthy VI, Zambon JJ, Sreenivasan PK, et al. (2007). Identification of oral bacterial species associated with halitosis. *J Am Dent Assoc*, 138(8), 1113–20.

15 Yaegaki K, Sanada K (1992b). Biochemical and clinical factors influencing oral malodor in periodontal patients. *J Periodontol*, 63(9), 783–9.

16 Washio J, Sato T, Koseki T, Takahashi N (2005). Hydrogen sulfide-producing bacteria in tongue biofilm and their relationship with oral malodour. *J Med Microbiol*, 54(Pt 9), 889–95.

17 Nasim VS, Shetty YR, Hegde AM (2007). Dental health status in children with acute lymphoblastic leukemia. *J Clin Pediatr Dent*, 31(3), 210–13.

18 Tangerman A, Winkel EG (2007). Intra- and extra-oral halitosis: finding of a new form of extra-oral blood-borne halitosis caused by dimethyl sulphide. *J Clin Periodontol*, 34(9), 748–55.

19 Yaegaki K, Coil JM (1999). Clinical dilemmas posed by patients with psychosomatic halitosis. *Quintessence Int*, 30(5), 328–33.

20 Bosy A (1997). Oral malodor: philosophical and practical aspects. *J Can Dent Assoc*, 63(3), 196–201.

21 Rosenberg M, Kozlovsky A, Gelernter I, et al. (1995). Self-estimation of oral malodor. *J Dent Res*, 74(9), 1577–82.

22 McKeown L (2003). Social relations and breath odour. *Int J Dent Hyg*, 1(4), 213–17.

23 Shorthose K, Davies A (2005). Halitosis, in Davies A, Finlay I (eds) *Oral Care in Advanced Disease*, pp. 125–31. Oxford University Press, Oxford.

24 Rosenberg M, McCulloch CA (1992). Measurements of oral malodor: current methods and future prospects. *J Periodontol*, 63(9), 776–82.

25 Yaegaki K, Coil JM (2000). Examination, classification, and treatment of halitosis; clinical perspectives. *J Can Dent Assoc*, 66(5), 257–61.

26 Greenman J, Duffield J, Spencer P, et al. (2004). Study on the Organleptic Intensity Scale for measuring oral malodor. *J Dent Res*, 83(1), 81–5.

27 Nachnani S, Majerus G, Lenton P, Hodges J, Magallanes E (2005). Effects of training on odor judges scoring intensity. *Oral Dis*, 11(Suppl 1), 40–4.

28 Mitsubayashi K, Minamide T, Otsuka K, Kudo H, Saito H (2006). Optical bio-sniffer for methyl mercaptan in halitosis. *Anal Chim Acta*, 573–4, 75–80.

29 Kato H, Yoshida A, Awano S, Ansai T, Takehara T (2005). Quantitative detection of volatile sulfur compound-producing microoorganisms in oral specimens using real-time PCR. *Oral Dis*, 11(Suppl 1), 67–71.

30 Riggio MP, Lennon A, Rolph HJ, et al. (2008). Molecular identification of bacteria on tongue dorsum of subjects with and without halitosis. *Oral Dis*, 14(3), 251–8.

31 Van den Broek AM, Feenstra L, de Baat C (2008). A review of the current literature on the management of halitosis. *Oral Dis*, 14(1), 30–9.

32 Rosenberg M (1996). Clinical assessment of bad breath: current concepts. *J Am Dent Assoc*, 127(4), 475–82.

33 Outhouse TL, Al Alawi R, Fedorowicz Z, Keenan JV (2006). Tongue scraping for treating halitosis. *Cochrane Database Syst Rev*, (2), CD005519.

34 Haas AN, Silveira EM, Rosing CK (2007). Effect of tongue cleansing on morning oral malodour in periodontally healthy individuals. *Oral Health Prev Dent*, 5(2), 89–94.

35 Reingewirtz Y, Girault O, Reingewirtz N, Senger B, Tenenbaum H (1999). Mechanical effects and volatile sulfur compound-reducing effects of chewing gums: comparison between test and base gums and a control group. *Quintessence Int*, 30(5), 319–23.

36 Greenberg M, Urnezis P, Tian M (2007). Compressed mints and chewing gum containing magnolia bark extract are effective against bacteria responsible for oral malodor. *J Agric Food Chem*, 55(23), 9465–9.

37 Pratten J, Pasu M, Jackson G, Flanagan A, Wilson M (2003). Modelling oral malodour in a longitudinal study. *Arch Oral Biol*, 48(11), 737–43.

38 Quirynen M, Mongardini C, van Steenberghe D (1998). The effect of a 1-stage full-mouth disinfection on oral malodor and microbial colonization of the tongue in periodontitis. A pilot study. *J Periodontol*, 69(3), 374–82.

39 Thrane PS, Young A, Jonski G, Rolla G (2007). A new mouthrinse combining zinc and chlorhexidine in low concentrations provides superior efficacy against halitosis compared to existing formulations: a double-blind clinical study. *J Clin Dent*, 18(3), 82–6.

40 Winkel EG, Roldan S, Van Winkelhoff AJ, Herrera D, Sanz M (2003). Clinical effects of a new mouthrinse containing chlorhexidine, cetylpyridinium chloride and zinc-lactate on oral halitosis. A dual-center, double-blind placebo-controlled study. *J Clin Periodontol*, 30(4), 300–6.

41 Young A, Jonski G, Rolla G (2002). A study of triclosan and its solubilizers as inhibitors of oral malodour. *J Clin Periodontol*, 29(12), 1078–81.

42 Gaffar A, Nabi N, Kashuba B, et al. (1990). Antiplaque effects of dentifrices containing triclosan/copolymer/NaF system vs triclosan dentifrices without the copolymer. *Am J Dent*, (3 Spec No), S7–S14.

43 Hu D, Zhang YP, Petrone M, Volpe AR, Devizio W, Giniger M (2005). Clinical effectiveness of a triclosan/copolymer/sodium fluoride dentifrice in controlling oral malodor: a 3-week clinical trial. *Oral Dis*, 11(Suppl 1), 51–3.

44 Niles HP, Hunter C, Vazquez J, Williams MI, Cummins D (2005). The clinical comparison of a triclosan/copolymer/fluoride dentifrice vs a breath-freshening dentifrice in reducing breath odor overnight: a crossover study. *Oral Dis*, 11(Suppl 1), 54–6.

45 Yaegaki K, Sanada K (1992c). Effects of a two-phase oil-water mouthwash on halitosis. *Clin Prev Dent*, 14(1), 5–9.

46 Kozlovsky A, Goldberg S, Natour I, Rogatky-Gat A, Gerlernter I, Rosenberg M (1996). Efficacy of a 2-phase oil: water mouthrinse in controlling oral malodor, gingivitis, and plaque. *J Periodontol*, 67(6), 577–82.

47 Borden LC, Chaves ES, Bowman JP, Fath BM, Hollar GL (2002). The effect of four mouthrinses on oral malodor. *Compend Contin Educ Dent*, 23(6), 531–40.

48 Frascella J, Gilbert R, Fernandez P (1998). Odor reduction potential of a chlorine dioxide mouthrinse. *J Clin Dent*, 9(2), 39–42.

49 Frascella J, Gilbert RD, Fernandez P, Hendler J (2000). Efficacy of a chlorine dioxide-containing mouthrinse in oral malodor. *Compend Contin Educ Dent*, 21(3), 241–8.

50 Tonzetich J (1978). Oral malodour: an indicator of health status and oral cleanliness. *Int Dent J*, 28(3), 309–19.

51 Farrell S, Barker ML, Gerlach RW (2007). Overnight malodor effect with a 0.454% stablized stannous fluoride sodium hexametaphosphate dentifrice. *Compend Contin Educ Dent*, 28(12), 658–61.

52 Louis J, Moyer J, Angelini J, Kagan SH (1997). Metronidazole oral rinse helps to alleviate odor associated with oral lesions. *Oncol Nurs Forum*, 24(8), 1331.

53 Sterer N, Rosenberg M (2002). Effect of deglycosylation of salivary glycoproteins on oral malodour production. *Int Dent J*, 52(Suppl 3), 229–32.

54 Burton JP, Chilcott CN, Tagg JR (2005). The rationale and potential for the reduction of oral malodour using Streptococcus salivarius probiotics. *Oral Dis*, 11(Suppl 1), 29–31.

55 Burton JP, Chilcott CN, Moore CJ, Speiser G, Tagg JR (2006). A preliminary study of the effect of probiotic Streptococcus salivarius K12 on oral malodour parameters. *J Appl Microbiol*, 100(4), 754–64.

56 Sterer N, Feuerstein O (2005). Effect of visible light on malodour production by mixed oral microflora. *J Med Microbiol*, 54(Pt 12), 1225–9.

57 Krespi YP, Slatkine M, Marchenko M, Protic J (2005). Lethal photosensitization of oral pathogens via red-filtered halogen lamp. *Oral Dis*, 11(Suppl 1), 92–5.

58 Lodhia P, Yaegaki K, Khakbaznejad A, et al. (2008). Effect of green tea on volatile sulfur compounds in mouth air. *J Nutr Sci Vitaminol (Tokyo)*, 54(1), 89–94.

Chapter 24

Orofacial pain

Paul Farquhar Smith and Joel Epstein

Introduction

The International Association for the Study of Pain (IASP) have defined pain as 'an unpleasant sensory and emotional experience associated with actual or potential tissue damage or described in terms of such damage'[1,2]. The aforementioned definition endorses the concept that pain is subjective in nature, and that pain is not synonymous with nociception (i.e. 'the neural processes of encoding and processing noxious stimuli')[2].

Pain is common in patients with cancer, and extremely common in patients with advanced cancer[3]. Not surprisingly, orofacial pain is also common in patients with primary/secondary cancer involving the structures of the head and neck region. The cause of pain in patients with cancer is invariably physical in nature, but the experience of pain in this group of patients may be influenced by associated psychological, spiritual, and social factors (the concept of 'total pain')[3]. Pain dramatically impacts on the quality of life.

Anatomy and physiology

Sensation to most of the orofacial structures is supplied by the trigeminal nerve (cranial nerve V). The maxillary branch (V_2) innervates the roof of the mouth and parts of the nasopharynx via the superior alveolar nerves, and the greater and lesser palatine nerves (Figure 2.6). Sensation in the buccal cavity and the anterior two-thirds of the tongue is mediated by the mandibular division of the trigeminal nerve (V_3) via the buccal, inferior alveolar, and lingual nerves. The posterior-third of the tongue is supplied by the lingual branches of the glossopharyngeal nerve (cranial nerve IX), and partly by the internal branch of the superior laryngeal nerve of the vagus (cranial nerve X). Trigeminal primary afferents project from the periphery to the brainstem.

C and Aδ fibres exist as free nerve endings, and respond to painful stimulation (nociceptors). These peripheral fibres may undergo plastic changes following inflammation and nerve damage as a result of mediators released by tumour, tissue damage, immune cells, and the nerves themselves ('peripheral sensitization')[4,5]. Tissue injury may lead to release of nerve growth factors with impact on nerve-sprouting changing receptor fields and function, and to release of other mediators that affect the activity of peripheral nociceptors. These changes may lead to spontaneous pain, hyperaesthesia, and allodynia[6]. However, there may be significant differences in trigeminal nerve changes compared to other spinal nerves[7], including a lack of sympathetic involvement following trigeminal nerve injury[8].

Sensitization of nociceptors, and changes in receptor fields, may also occur in response to alterations in descending control mechanisms. Trigeminal nociceptors have a range of potential influences in the brainstem. Trigeminal afferents synapse with second order neurones in the trigeminal main sensory nucleus and the trigeminal spinal tract nucleus. The latter is divided into three subnuclei, with the subnucleus caudalis being the main relay for nociceptive information (evidenced by the fact most C and Aδ fibres synapse here in laminae I, II, and V)[4,6]. It is also the subnucleus caudalis that expresses receptors and mediators associated with spinal pain mechanisms such as N-methyl-D-aspartate (NMDA), and receptors for neurokinins/neuropeptide neurotransmitters such as substance P.

Second-order neurones behave as either nociceptive-specific neurones (NS; excited only by input from painful stimuli), or as wide-dynamic-range neurones (WDR: responding to noxious and non-noxious input). Second-order neurones in the trigeminal brainstem complex are sensitized following peripheral inflammation and damage[4]. The subnucleus caudalis can undergo central sensitization involving activation of NMDA receptors[9]. The NS and WDR neurones display decreased activation thresholds, and increased reaction to painful stimuli, as well as expansion of the peripheral receptive field[4]. They may also precipitate spontaneous pain.

Epidemiology

Orofacial pain may occur in patients with head and neck cancer, and also patients with other types of cancer (see below). Pain is reported to be a frequent presenting complaint in certain types of head and neck cancer (e.g. nasopharyngeal cancer[10]), but may occur in all types of head and neck cancer. However, the reported rates are extremely variable[10,11].

A retrospective examination of clinical notes found pain was a presenting complaint in only 19% of patients with oral cancer[12]. In another study of oral cancers, pain was often not a symptom associated with patients seeking medical advice[13]. However, in those with symptoms for over 6 months, nearly 60% complained of the presence of pain[13]. This implies pain is more common with advanced disease. Indeed, patients with squamous cell cancer of the mouth are more likely to have pain with increasing tumour stage[14], but not necessarily with increasing tumour size[15].

Tumours of the oral cavity were more likely to cause pain than tumours in the oropharyngeal space, based on pain-related elements of quality of life scores[16]. Similarly, at time of diagnosis, pain was more important in oral tumours rather than nasopharyngeal tumours[17], and pain was not a major presenting symptom in tumours of the larynx[17]. Pain may be the first indicator of recurrence of head and neck cancer[18,19]. Indeed, in a small series of patients with head and neck cancer recurrence, pain preceded the other diagnostic indicators of disease progression/recurrence[19].

Aetiology

Orofacial pain in patients with cancer may be due to:

♦ Direct effect of tumour

♦ Indirect effect of tumour

♦ Effect of cancer therapy (e.g. surgery, radiotherapy, chemotherapy)

♦ Concurrent problem (e.g. temporomandibular disorder pain, trigeminal neuralgia, burning mouth syndrome, dental pain).

Pain due to direct effect of tumour

The head and neck region is densely vascular and innervated, and so tumours may impinge and invade on these structures earlier than elsewhere in the body. Some nerves in the head and neck region are encased by bony structures, which may make them susceptible to compression due to direct tumour invasion and/or associated inflammation. Tumours close to the course of trigeminal nerve are particularly likely to precipitate pain (and neurological symptoms).

Systemic malignancies such as lymphoma and leukaemia may present with orofacial pain due to tissue infiltration, mucosal ulceration, or secondary infection (due to the primary disease). Lymphoma is the second most common malignancy of the head and neck region, and some case series of extranodal lymphoma report that over 50% patients present with pain[20]. Pain may also be the effect of a paraneoplastic syndrome (i.e. neuropathy).

Primary bone tumours (e.g. osteosarcoma, chondrosarcoma) are relatively rare, and can cause orofacial pain[21]. However, in a small case series of osteosarcoma of the jaw, none of the patients complained of pain (a situation markedly different to studies of osteosarcoma of the long bones) [22]. However, neurosensory disturbance in the distribution of the mandibular branch of the trigeminal nerve is more common. Multiple myeloma often presents with bony pain, yet pain may not be reported in multiple myeloma in the head and neck region[23]. However, these systemic malignancies can present with 'numb chin syndrome', which signifies neurosensory loss in the distribution of the inferior alveolar nerve (and branches).

Metastatic bone disease of the jaws is relatively uncommon, but may cause significant orofacial pain. A recent review of 673 cases of oral metastases showed that in 23% the primary malignancy had not been diagnosed, and in 25% the mouth was the first sites of metastatic spread[24]. Metastases presented in the jaw (mostly in mandible) with swelling, pain, and paraesthesia. In women, 40% of jaw metastasis originated from a primary breast cancer, but this cancer only accounted for only 25% of the soft-tissue oral metastases. Lung cancer was the most prevalent source of jaw spread (25% of cases), and soft oral-tissue involvement (31% of cases), in men.

Pain due to effect of cancer therapy

Treatment of cancer with surgery, radiotherapy, and/or chemotherapy causes both acute and chronic pain[25,26]. Pain has a major impact upon on quality of life, and reduction in activities of daily living in cancer survivors. For example, pain was a major reason why nearly 40% of patients were no longer working following treatment of head and neck cancer[27].

Surgery

Chronic pain following surgery has been well described, and several risk factors have been identified.[28] Examination of pain scores following surgery showed that higher scores were reported for oral cavity cancers compared to cancers at other sites in the head and neck[29].

In a large survey of surgically treated oral cancer patients moderate to severe pain was reported by approximately one-third of cases at review (≥6 months post surgery)[13]. The most frequent pain locations were the shoulder (31–38.5%), the neck (4.9–34.9%), the temporomandibular joint (4.9–20.1%), the oral cavity (4.2–18.7%), and the face/other regions (4.2–15.6%)[13]. Indeed, only 39.2% of patients were free of pain. Of note, analgesics and physiotherapy seem largely ineffective in the treating these chronic pains (which may imply neuropathic mechanisms). However, there was a tendency for symptoms to improve with time, with a smaller proportion of reviewed patients having persistent pain at 54–60 months post surgery (i.e. 14.9%)[13]. Nevertheless, long-term head and neck cancer survivors still suffer from significantly more pain than matched subjects, although they do have a tendency to return to normal general function[30,31].

Pain following neck dissection may consist of neuropathic as well as musculoskeletal pain[32]. Modified surgical techniques may be successful in reducing chronic pain, without adversely affecting treatment outcome. For example, modified/more limited neck dissection is associated with less functional problems, including less pain[33]. Damage to the accessory nerve has been implicated in the development of chronic pain following head and neck surgery[32,34]: neck dissection where the spinal accessory nerve is spared leads to less pain (and better shoulder function)[32]. Good post-operative pain control is essential to reduce acute pain, and may ameliorate the development of chronic pain. Interestingly, increased pain during and following cancer treatment is correlated with higher incidence of pain pre-treatment[13].

Other modalities

Clinically significant oral mucositis is a common complication of cancer treatment, especially in haematopoetic stem cell transplantation (HSCT) patients treated with chemotherapy ± total body irradiation (>50%), and in head and neck cancer patients receiving radiotherapy ± chemotherapy (>90%). Furthermore, oral mucositis is common in patients receiving chemotherapy for common epithelial cell cancers (up to 25%). The incidence varies according to the treatment protocol (i.e. drug, dosage, and frequency)[35]. Oral mucositis is discussed in detail in Chapter 15.

A follow-up study of head and neck cancer patients reported persistent oral mucosal discomfort 6–12 months following radiotherapy (probably related to neuropathy)[36]. Graft-versus-host disease (GVHD) following HSCT can cause mucosal ulceration and pain[37]. Oral involvement is more common in chronic GVHD. Indeed, 80% of patients with chronic oral GVHD avoid certain foods because of related oral pain[38].

Clinical features

Tissue destruction by invasive tumours (or metastases) induces inflammation and nerve damage, with attendant acute pain that may, in some cases, lead on to chronic pain.

Tumour involvement of the oral and surrounding tissues may lead to pain during speech, mastication, and deglutition[13]. For example, in patients with oral squamous cell carcinoma, pain is more likely to be triggered by oral function than to be spontaneous in nature[15].

Orofacial cancer pain may mimic pain due to other causes, which may lead to diagnostic challenges (e.g. dental pain, temporomandibular disorder, trigeminal neuralgia, burning mouth syndrome)[39]. The corollary is that these non-malignant pains may trigger anxiety of disease recurrence in patients with cancer (and so affect pain experience and pain behaviour).

Temporomandibular disorder pain

Temporomandibular disorder (TMD) pain is a relatively common non-malignant orofacial pain. Differences in diagnostic criteria make it difficult to quantify the extent of TMD pain, but suggestive symptoms occur in up to 10% of people[40]. Head and neck cancers can cause similar complaints of pain. For example, in one study seven (of 52) patients with nasopharyngeal cancer presented with symptoms described as similar to those associated with TMD[10]. The symptoms of TMD include temporomandibular joint sounds with movement, limited jaw movement, pain in the temporomandibular joint, and pain in the muscles of mastication. TMD-related pain is typically increased with chewing. TMD pain may be associated with neck pain and headache.

Trigeminal neuralgia

Idiopathic trigeminal neuralgia (TN) has an incidence of four in 100 000, with a mean presenting age of 50[41]. One theory of TN causation is nerve-root compression by vascular structures[41]. Hence, it is not surprising that neoplasm-induced compression of the trigeminal nerve may cause similar pain. Indeed, in a series of 2972 patients diagnosed with TN, nearly 10% of the pains were ultimately found to be caused by an underlying malignancy (mostly meningiomas and posterior fossa tumours)[42].

Usually, the pain is paroxysmal, classically described as 'lancinating' or shock-like, in the distribution of the mandibular or maxillary divisions of the trigeminal nerve, and often precipitated by a 'trigger' (i.e. an orofacial stimulus)[41]. Patients with underlying malignancy tend to be younger, and the diagnosis is often made at the time of development of a trigeminal neurological deficit[42]. (Abnormal neurology such as sensory deficits is not present in idiopathic TN.)

Carbamazepine is commonly effective for TN, and response to treatment strengthens the diagnosis. Other agents, including oxcarbazepine provide alternatives if carbamazepine is not well tolerated[43]. Patients with underlying malignancy may demonstrate a more limited/short term response to carbamazepine treatment.

Burning mouth syndrome

Burning mouth syndrome (BMS) is defined as a burning persisting pain that may involve multiple oral surfaces, most commonly the tongue, palate, and lips, with a bilateral distribution, without clinical findings of tissue abnormality and in the absence of underlying systemic disease.

BMS may occur in 3.7% of the general population, and its aetiology has variously been described as biological and psychological[44]. However, characterization of sensory testing abnormalities in patients supports a type of trigeminal neuropathy as the underlying mechanism [45] and, indeed, topical clonazepam may be effective in 40% or more of patients[44].

The burning sensation may be accompanied by taste changes and a complaint of dry mouth. As with other types of non-malignant orofacial pain, an atypical presentation (e.g. unilateral distribution), and refractoriness to treatment should raise the suspicion of an underlying malignant disease.

Oral mucositis

Oral mucositis usually develops in 5–7 days following chemotherapy treatment. With radiotherapy, the onset of mucosits typically occurs following 2 weeks of treatment, with the peak intensity of mucositis occurring at 5 weeks of treatment[46]. Pain is the major symptom of mucositis, and can affect oral function including the ability to swallow (adversely affecting nutrition), and the ability to undertake oral hygiene measures[47]. Oral mucositis is discussed in detail in Chapter 15.

Management

The initial management involves a rigorous assessment process, which should be similar in nature to that of other types of cancer pain, and should consist of taking a detailed history, performing a thorough examination, and the appropriate use of investigations[48]. The treatment of orofacial pain in cancer should be multidisciplinary, and multidimensional in nature: therapeutic strategies include treatment of the underlying cause, treatment of precipitating/aggravating factors, use of non-pharmacological methods, use of pharmacological methods, and use of anaesthetic/ neurosurgical techniques. The subsequent management involves a robust re-assessment, which should again be similar in nature to that of other types of cancer pain, and should review changes in the pain as well as the efficacy/tolerability of all interventions. It is important that the patient is followed up on a regular basis; the timing of follow up will be influenced by the severity of the pain and its interference with activities of daily living.

Oral hygiene is recommended as a non-specific general approach to treating oral pain, with or without antibacterial mouth washes to reduce microbial contamination. Certain non-pharmacological methods/'complementary' therapies are also now accepted as part of the treatment approach to cancer pain (e.g. acupuncture, transcutaneous electrical nerve stimulation – TENS)[49]. Nevertheless, the paucity of high-quality data demand further research to support their continued utilization[50]. However, the mainstay of orofacial cancer pain management is the use of pharmacological methods. The current pharmacological treatment of orofacial pain associated with cancer is essentially similar to that of other types of cancer pain (although the elucidation of underlying pathophysiological mechanisms of orofacial pain promises targeted treatments).

Historically, the management of cancer pain has been based upon the World Health Organization Cancer Pain Relief guidelines[51]. The guidelines cover all aspects of the management of cancer pain, although they focus on the pharmacological management of cancer pain; the guidelines promote five main principles with regard to the pharmacological management of pain: (1) 'By mouth' – drugs should be given orally (if possible); (2) 'By the clock' – drugs should be given regularly; (3) 'By the ladder' – drugs are given in a step-wise manner; (4) 'For the individual' – opioid drugs should be individually titrated; and (5) 'Attention to detail'. The cornerstone of the WHO Cancer Pain Relief guidelines is the 'three-step analgesic ladder' (Figure 24.1). Treatment starts at the lowest rung of the ladder with the use of non-opioid analgesics. Failure of non-opioid analgesics prompts the use of the second-step medications, namely opioids for mild-to-moderate pain ('weak' opioids), and if pain is still not controlled, then opioids for moderate-to-severe pain ('strong' opioids) are invoked.

At any stage of the ladder, so-called adjuvant medications may also be given (Box 24.1). Adjuvant analgesics ('co-analgesics') are agents whose primary function is not analgesia, but which provide pain relief in certain circumstances (e.g. antiepileptics for neuropathic pain)[52]. Adjuvant drugs are agents whose function is not analgesia, but which provide relief from the adverse effects of analgesic drugs, or the complications of the pain (e.g. laxatives for opioid-related constipation) [52]. It is important to anticipate the adverse effects of analgesic drugs, and to provide the patient with adjuvant drugs to manage these adverse effects. Thus, all patients prescribed opioid analgesics should be prescribed laxatives (and probably anti-emetics). The three-step ladder does not

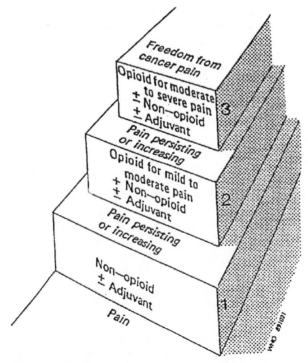

Fig. 24.1 World Health Organization three-step analgesic ladder[51].
Source: Reproduced with permission from World Health Organization (1996). Cancer Pain Relief, 2nd edn. World Health Organization, Geneva

Box 24.1 Categories of drugs used to treat cancer-related pain

Non-opioid analgesics

♦ Paracetamol/acetaminophen

♦ Non-steroidal anti-inflammatory drugs

♦ Other agents, e.g. dipyrone, nefopam

Opioids for mild-to-moderate pain ('weak') opioids, e.g. codeine, dihydrocodeine

Opioids for moderate-to-severe pain ('strong') opioids, e.g. morphine, oxycodone

Adjuvant analgesics*

♦ Antidepressants

♦ Anticonvulsants

♦ Corticosteroids

♦ Local anaesthetics

♦ Muscle relaxants

♦ Other agents, e.g. bisphosphonates, NMDA antagonists

Adjuvant drugs**

♦ Antiemetics

♦ Laxatives

♦ Other agents, e.g. hypnotics, psychostimulants

* Adjuvant analgesic = agents whose primary function is not analgesia, but which provide pain relief in certain circumstances

** Adjuvant drug = agents whose function is not analgesia, but which provide relief from the adverse effects of analgesic drugs (or the complications of the pain)

specifically include topical therapies, which have been shown to ameliorate oral pain, and which may decrease the requirement for systemic opioid use (e.g. local anaesthetics, coating agents).

A systematic review of evidence for the WHO ladder reported that 69–100% of patients achieved 'adequate' analgesia, although none of the included studies were randomized controlled trials (and many were methodologically questionable)[53]. A more recent systematic review reported that 45–100% of patients described their pain relief as 'adequate', although again the authors highlighted the lack of controlled studies[54]. Although both reviews acknowledged some merit in simple clinical protocols, they concluded there was insufficient evidence to support the use of the WHO ladder. There is little published data on the WHO ladder for (non-mucositis) orofacial pain.

Some experts have voiced additional concerns about the WHO ladder, due in part to its simplicity (which is at odds with the increasing knowledge of the complexity of cancer pain)[55], its inclusion of step 2/opioids for mild-to-moderate pain (which is contrary to the existing understanding of the pharmacology of opioid analgesics, and potentially exposes the patient to unnecessary/prolonged suffering)[56], and its relevance for patients with chronic cancer pain (e.g. cancer survivors)[57]. Indeed, although recent reviews and recommendation still advocate the WHO ladder[58], other contemporaneous guidelines for cancer pain treatment stress the importance of titration of short-acting opioids (and do not state that opioids for mild-to-moderate pain should be initially used)[59]. Morphine remains the mainstay of pain management, and has shown to be effective and well tolerated by most patients. However, some patients require the use of other opioids, due either to lack of efficacy of morphine and/or poor tolerability of morphine.

Interventional techniques (e.g. local anaesthetic nerve blocks, neurolytic nerve blocks) have been coined as the 'fourth step' of the WHO ladder[60], although they can be utilized at any stage of the patient's pain journey (either in conjunction with pharmacological therapy, or instead of pharmacological therapy). Invasive techniques have been used for head and neck pain of multiple aetiologies, although there are few published studies on their use in cancer-related head and neck pain[61]. However, selective interventions may be appropriate in certain instances of cancer-related head and neck pain[62,63].

References

1 Anonymous (1979). Pain terms: a list with definitions and notes on usage. Recommended by the IASP subcommittee on taxonomy. *Pain*, 6(3), 249–52.

2 Loeser JD, Treede RD (2008). The Kyoto protocol of IASP Basic Pain Terminology. *Pain*, 137(3), 473–7.

3 Twycross R (1994). *Pain relief in advanced cancer*. Churchill Livingstone, Edinburgh.

4 Sessle BJ (2005). Peripheral and central mechanisms of orofacial pain and their clinical correlates. *Minerva Anestesiol*, 71(4), 117–36.

5 Robinson PP, Boissonade FM, Loescher AR, et al. (2004). Peripheral mechanisms for the initiation of pain following trigeminal nerve injury. *J Orofac Pain*, 18(4), 287–92.

6 Benoliel R, Epstein J, Eliav E, Jurevic R, Elad S (2007). Orofacial pain in cancer: part 1 – mechanisms. *J Dent Res*, 86(6), 491–505.

7 Fried K, Bongenhielm U, Boissonade FM, Robinson PP (2001). Nerve injury-induced pain in the trigeminal system. *Neuroscientist*, 7(2), 155–65.

8 Bongenheilm U, Boissonade FM, Westermark A, Robinson PP, Fried K (1999). Sympathetic nerve sprouting fails to occur in the trigeminal ganglion after peripheral nerve injury in the rat. *Pain*, 82(3), 283–8.

9 Park SJ, Chiang CY, Hu JW, Sessle BJ (2001). Neuroplasticity induced by tooth pulp stimulation in trigeminal subnucleus oralis involves NMDA receptor mechanisms. *J Neurophysiol*, 85(5), 1836–46.

10 Epstein JB, Jones CK (1993). Presenting signs and symptoms of nasopharyngeal carcinoma. *Oral Surg Oral Med Oral Pathol*, 75(1), 32–6.

11 Su CY, Lui CC (1996). Perineural invasion of the trigeminal nerve in patients with nasopharyngeal carcinoma. Imaging and clinical correlations. *Cancer*, 78(10), 2063–9.

12 Cuffari L, Tesseroli de Siqueira JT, Nemr K, Rapaport A (2006). Pain complaint as the first symptom of oral cancer: a descriptive study. *Oral Surg Oral Med Oral Pathol Oral Radiol* Endod, 102(1), 56–61.

13 Gellrich NC, Schimming R, Schramm A, Schmalohr D, Bremerich A, Kugler J (2002). Pain, function, and psychologic outcome before, during, and after intraoral tumor resection. *J Oral Maxillofac Surg*, 60(7), 772–7.

14 Haya-Fernandez MC, Bagan JV, Murillo-Cortes J, Poveda-Roda R, Calabuig C (2004). The prevalence of oral leukoplakia in 138 patients with oral squamous cell carcinoma. *Oral Dis*, 10(6), 346–8.

15 Connelly ST, Schmidt BL (2004). Evaluation of pain in patients with oral squamous cell carcinoma. *J Pain*, 5(9), 505–10.

16 Borggreven PA, Verdonck-de Leeuw IM, Muller MJ, et al. (2007). Quality of life and functional status in patients with cancer of the oral cavity and oropharynx: pretreatment values of a prospective study. *Eur Arch Otorhinolaryngol*, 264(6), 651–7.

17 Hammerlid E, Bjordal K, Ahlner-Elmqvist M, et al. (2001). A prospective study of quality of life in head and neck cancer patients. Part I: at diagnosis. *Laryngoscope*, 111(4 Pt 1), 669–80.

18 Zakrzewska JM, Harrison SD (2008). Facial pain, in Jensen TS, Wilson PR, Rice AS (eds) *Chronic Pain*, 1st edn, pp. 481–504. Arnold, London.

19 Wong JK, Wood RE, McLean M (1998). Pain preceding recurrent head and neck cancer. *J Orofac Pain*, 12(1), 52–9.

20 Rosado MF, Morgensztern D, Peleg M, Lossos IS (2004). Primary diffuse large cell lymphoma of the mandible. *Leuk Lymphoma*, 45(5), 1049–53.

21 Bennett JH, Thomas G, Evans AW, Speight PM (2000). Osteosarcoma of the jaws: a 30-year retrospective review. *Oral Surg Oral Med Oral Pathol Oral Radiol Endod*, 90(3), 323–32.

22 Mardinger O, Givol N, Talmi YP, Taicher S (2001). Osteosarcoma of the jaw. The Chaim Sheba Medical Center experience. *Oral Surg Oral Med Oral Pathol Oral Radiol Endod*, 91(4), 445–51.

23 Witt C, Borges AC, Klein K, Neumann HJ (1997). Radiographic manifestations of multiple myeloma in the mandible: a retrospective study of 77 patients. *J Oral Maxillofac Surg*, 55(5), 450–3.

24 Hirshberg A, Shnaiderman-Shapiro A, Kaplan I, Berger R (2007). Metastatic tumours to the oral cavity - pathogenesis and analysis of 673 cases. *Oral Oncol*, 44(8), 473–52.

25 Marchettini P, Formaglio F, Lacerenza M (20010. Iatrogenic painful neuropathic complications of surgery in cancer. *Acta Anaesthesiol Scand*, 45(9), 1090–4.

26 Farquhar-Smith WP (2008). Pain in cancer survivors, in Sykes N, Bennett MI, Yuan C-S (eds) *Cancer Pain*, 2nd edn, pp. 399–410. Hodder Arnold, London.

27 Buckwalter AE, Karnell LH, Smith RB, Christensen AJ, Funk GF (2007). Patient-reported factors associated with discontinuing employment following head and neck cancer treatment. *Arch Otolaryngol Head Neck Surg*, 133(5), 464–70.

28 Perkins FM, Kehlet H (2000). Chronic pain as an outcome of surgery. A review of predictive factors. *Anesthesiology*, 93(4), 1123–33.

29 Terrell JE, Nanavati K, Esclamado RM, Bradford CR, Wolf GT (1999). Health impact of head and neck cancer. *Otolaryngol Head Neck Surg*, 120(6), 852–9.

30 Hammerlid E, Silander E, Hornestam L, Sullivan M (2001). Health-related quality of life three years after diagnosis of head and neck cancer – a longitudinal study. *Head Neck*, 23(2), 113–25.

31 Hammerlid E, Taft C (2001). Health-related quality of life in long-term head and neck cancer survivors: a comparison with general population norms. *Br J Cancer*, 84(2), 149–56.

32 Inoue H, Nibu K, Saito M, et al. (2006). Quality of life after neck dissection. *Arch Otolaryngol Head Neck Surg*, 132(6), 662–6.

33 Samant S, Robbins KT (2003). Evolution of neck dissection for improved functional outcome. *World J Surg*, 27(7), 805–10.

34 Terrell JE, Welsh DE, Bradford CR, et al. (2000). Pain, quality of life, and spinal accessory nerve status after neck dissection. *Laryngoscope*, 110(4), 620–6.

35 Volpato LE, Silva TC, Oliveira TM, Sakai VT, Machado MA (2007). Radiation therapy and chemotherapy-induced oral mucositis. *Braz J Otorhinolaryngol*, 73(4), 562–8.

36 Epstein JB, Stewart KH (1993). Radiation therapy and pain in patients with head and neck cancer. *Eur J Cancer B Oral Oncol*, 29B(3), 191–9.

37 Woo SB, Lee SJ, Schubert MM (1997). Graft-vs.-host disease. *Crit Rev Oral Biol Med*, 8(2), 201–16.

38 Treister NS, Cook EF Jr, Antin J, Lee SJ, Soiffer R, Woo SB (2008). Clinical evaluation of oral chronic graft-versus-host disease. *Biol Blood Marrow Transplant*, 14(1), 110–15.

39 Epstein JB, Elad S, Eliav E, Jurevic R, Benoliel R (2007). Orofacial pain in cancer: part II -clinical perspectives and management. *J Dent Res*, 86(6), 506–18.

40 Poveda RR, Bagan JV, Diaz Fernandez JM, Hernandez BS, Jimenez SY (2007). Review of temporomandibular joint pathology. Part I: classification, epidemiology and risk factors. *Med Oral Patol Oral Cir Bucal*, 12(4), E292–98.

41 Bagheri SC, Farhidvash F, Perciaccante VJ (2004). Diagnosis and treatment of patients with trigeminal neuralgia. *J Am Dent Assoc*, 135(12), 1713–17.

42 Cheng TM, Cascino TL, Onofrio BM (1993). Comprehensive study of diagnosis and treatment of trigeminal neuralgia secondary to tumors. *Neurology*, 43(11), 2298–302.

43 Jorns TP, Zakrzewska JM (2007). Evidence-based approach to the medical management of trigeminal neuralgia. *Br J Neurosurg*, 21(3), 253–61.

44 Minguez Serra MP, Salort LC, Silvestre Donat FJ (2007). Pharmacological treatment of burning mouth syndrome: A review and update. *Med Oral Patol Oral Cir Bucal*, 12(4), E299–304.

45 Forssell H, Jaaskelainen S, Tenovuo O, Hinkka S (2002). Sensory dysfunction in burning mouth syndrome. *Pain*, 99(1-2), 41–7.

46 Epstein JB, Emerton S, Kolbinson DA, et al. (1999). Quality of life and oral function following radiotherapy for head and neck cancer. *Head Neck*, 21(1), 1–11.

47 Trotti A, Bellm LA, Epstein JB, et al. (2003). Mucositis incidence, severity and associated outcomes in patients with head and neck cancer receiving radiotherapy with or without chemotherapy: a systematic literature review. *Radiother Oncol*, 66(3), 253–62.

48 Foley KM (2004). Acute and chronic cancer pain syndromes, in Doyle D, Hanks G, Cherny N, Calman K (eds) *Oxford Textbook of Palliative Medicine*, 3rd edn, pp. 298–316. Oxford University Press, Oxford.

49 Filshie J, Rubens CN (2006). Complementary and alternative medicine. *Anesthesiol Clin*, 24(1), 81–111, viii.

50 Bardia A, Barton DL, Prokop LJ, Bauer BA, Moynihan TJ (2006). Efficacy of complementary and alternative medicine therapies in relieving cancer pain: a systematic review. *J Clin Oncol*, 24(34), 5457–64.

51 World Health Organization (1996). *Cancer Pain Relief*, 2nd edn. World Health Organization, Geneva.

52 Lussier D, Portenoy RK (2004). Adjuvant analgesics in pain management, in Doyle D, Hanks G, Cherny N, Calman K (eds). *Oxford Textbook of Palliative Medicine*, 3rd edn, pp. 349–78. Oxford University Press, Oxford.

53 Jadad AR, Browman GP (1995). The WHO analgesic ladder for cancer pain management. Stepping up the quality of its evaluation. *J Am Med Assoc*, 274(23), 1870–73.

54 Azevedo Sao Leao Ferreira K, Kimura M, Jacobsen Teixeira M (2006). The WHO analgesic ladder for cancer pain control, twenty years of use. How much pain relief does one get from using it? *Support Care Cancer*, 14(11), 1086–93.

55 Laird B, Colvin L, Fallon M (2008). Management of cancer pain: basic principles and neuropathic cancer pain. *Eur J Cancer*, 44(8), 1078–82.

56 Burton AW, Hamid B (2007). Current challenges in cancer pain management: does the WHO ladder approach still have relevance? *Expert Rev Anticancer Ther*, 7(11), 1501–2.

57 Burton AW, Fanciullo GJ, Beasley RD, Fisch MJ (2007). Chronic pain in the cancer survivor: a new frontier. *Pain Med*, 8(2), 189–98.

58 Fallon M, Hanks G, Cherny N (2006). Principles of control of cancer pain. *Br Med J*, 332(7548), 1022–4.

59 Swarm R, Anghelescu DL, Benedetti C, et al. (2007). Adult cancer pain. *J Natl Compr Canc Netw*, 5(8), 726–51.

60 Miguel R (2000). Interventional treatment of cancer pain: the fourth step in the World Health Organization analgesic ladder? *Cancer Control*, 7(2), 149–56.

61 Rosenberg M, Phero JC (2003). Regional anesthesia and invasive techniques to manage head and neck pain. *Otolaryngol Clin North Am*, 36(6), 1201–19.

62 Varghese BT, Koshy RC (2001). Endoscopic transnasal neurolytic sphenopalatine ganglion block for head and neck cancer pain. *J Laryngol Otol*, 115(5), 385–7.

63 Varghese BT, Koshy RC, Sebastian P, Joseph E (2002). Combined sphenopalatine ganglion and mandibular nerve, neurolytic block for pain due to advanced head and neck cancer. *Palliat Med*, 16(5), 447–8.

Chapter 25

Miscellaneous oral problems

Andrew Davies

Sialorrhoea

Sialorrhoea has been defined as 'an excessive secretion of saliva'. Sialorrhoea is not synonymous with drooling (see below), although patients with sialorrhoea may also experience drooling.

Sialorrhoea is relatively uncommon in patients with cancer (as compared to salivary gland hypofunction). Nevertheless, sialorrhoea is an issue for a number of patients with cancer.

Box 25.1 depicts the more important causes of sialorrhoea in the general population[1,2]. Other specific causes of sialorrhoea in the cancer population include paraneoplastic encephalitis[3], and chemotherapy (e.g. 5-fluorouracil, irinotecan)[4,5].

Sialorrhoea is an unpleasant symptom, which may be associated with physical, psychological, and social complications[1]. The most important physical complication is aspiration, which may result in laryngitis, bronchitis, and/or pneumonia (and may present with a hoarse voice, 'choking' sensation, and/or persistent cough). Sialorrhoea may result in sleep disturbance, and so lead to daytime somnolence/fatigue. Sialorrhoea may also result in bloating/flatulence as a result of repeated associated swallowing of air (with saliva).

The management of sialorrhoea involves treatment of the cause of the problem, and/or symptomatic management. The symptomatic management of sialorrhoea is similar to the symptomatic management of drooling (see below).

Drooling

Drooling has been defined as 'abnormal spillage of saliva from the mouth on to the lips, chin and clothing'[6]. As discussed above, drooling is not synonymous with sialorrhoea. Indeed, many patients with drooling have salivary gland hypofunction rather than sialorrhoea[7].

Drooling is relatively uncommon in patients with cancer as compared to patients with other chronic diseases (e.g. Parkinson's disease, motor neurone disease)[7]. Nevertheless, drooling is an issue for a number of patients with specific cancers (e.g. head and neck cancer, oesophageal cancer, brain tumours). Drooling is usually not related to sialorrhoea, but is related to difficulty in retaining saliva within the mouth (secondary to facial weakness/deformity) and/or removing saliva from the mouth (secondary to dysphagia).

Drooling is an unpleasant symptom, which may be associated with physical, psychological, and social complications[7,8]. The physical complications include maceration of the perioral skin, secondary infection of the perioral skin, and generalized malodour. Moreover, leakage of saliva may result in problems similar to salivary gland hypofunction (e.g. difficulty chewing, difficulty swallowing). The psychological complications include low self-esteem and depression. The social complications include social isolation and financial repercussions (i.e. increased laundry costs and increased clothing costs).

Box 25.1 Causes of sialorrhoea in the general population[1,2]

Hyperhydration
Nausea (& vomiting)
Drug-induced

- Parasympathomimetic drugs (i.e. choline esters, cholinesterase inhibitors)
- Sympathomimetic drugs
- Other drugs (e.g. lithium, antipsychotics, benzodiazepines, cocaine, amphetamine, ketamine, digoxin, reserpine)

Chemical-induced

- Organophosphate pesticides
- Mercury
- Selenium

Oropharyngeal mucosal irritation
Poorly fitting dentures
Nasal mucosal irritation
Oesophageal inflammation
Oesophageal obstruction
Rabies
Pre-eclampsia
Wilson's disease
Idiopathic paroxysmal sialorrhoea

A number of strategies have been employed to control drooling in the general population (see Table 25.1)[9–15]. Strategies that have been reported to control drooling in patients with cancer include drugs (see below)[16–22], botulinum toxin A[23], parasympathetic nerve ablation[24], and salivary gland duct relocation[25]. The choice of treatment depends on a number of factors, including the patient's performance status, the patient's prognosis, the distress caused by the drooling, and (particularly) the patient's choice of treatment.

Table 25.1 Interventions for the management of drooling in general population

	Intervention
Non pharmacological methods	Behavioural therapy[9]
	Intra oral appliances[10]
Pharmacological methods	Drugs[11]
	Botulinum toxin A[12]
Radiotherapy	Salivary gland radiotherapy[13]
Surgery	Parasympathetic nerve ablation[14]
	Salivary gland duct ligation[14]
	Salivary gland duct relocation[14]
	Salivary gland excision[14]
Complementary therapies	Acupuncture[15]

Table 25.2 Drug regimens used to manage drooling in patients with cancer

Drug	Route	Dose
Atropine	Sublingual	0.5mg q.d.s[16]
Glycopyrronium bromide	Oral PEG Nebulized	0.2–0.4mg t.d.s[17] 0.2mg q.d.s[18] 0.6–1.0mg t.d.s[19] 0.2mg q.d.s[18]
Hyoscine hydrobromide (scopolamine)	Transdermal Nebulized	0.02mg/hr[20] 0.8mg b.d–t.d.s[21] 0.4mg q.d.s[22]

Drugs are the mainstay of treatment in patients with drooling[11]. The drug regimens that have been reported to control drooling in patients with cancer are depicted in Table 25.2[16–22]. Nevertheless, other drug regimens are often used in clinical practice. The principles of drug use are: (1) start at a low dose; (2) titrate the dose in small increments; (3) titrate the dose upwards if symptoms persist; and (4) titrate the dose downwards if side effects develop. It is particularly important not to substitute the problem of drooling with a more troublesome problem of salivary gland hypofunction.

Tenacious saliva

Tenacious (thick) saliva is a common complaint in patients with head and neck cancer, particularly in patients that have received head and neck radiotherapy. However, this problem may occur in other groups of patients with cancer, and it is usually secondary to salivary gland dysfunction, although it is sometimes secondary to dehydration. The thick saliva accumulates in the oropharynx, where it causes discomfort, may cause a choking sensation, and can lead to nausea and vomiting.

The strategies used to manage tenacious saliva include treatment of any salivary gland dysfunction (see Chapter 21), treatment of any dehydration (and encouragement of drinking), oral rinsing (e.g. soda water, sodium bicarbonate), humidification, and dietary manipulation (e.g. avoidance of milk, avoidance of caffeine)[26]. Other strategies have been reported to be effective in patients with non-malignant diseases, include drinking of fruit juices (e.g. dark grape, pineapple)[27], and treatment with beta-blockers (e.g. propranolol 10 mg bd, metoprolol 25 mg bd)[28].

Haemorrhage

Intraoral haemorrhage is a relatively common problem in patients with cancer, and may be related to the cancer, treatment for the cancer, a concomitant problem, treatment for the concomitant problem, or a combination of these reasons (Table 25.3). It should be noted that the presence of blood in the oral cavity does not necessarily mean that the source of the blood is within the oral cavity. Extraoral (loco-regional) haemorrhage is also a relatively common problem in patients with head and neck cancer[29,30].

In most instances, haemorrhage is of little clinical significance (although it may be distressing to the patient and their carers)[31]. For example, many patients with oral mucositis develop a degree of intraoral haemorrhage, which is of no particular consequence, and which is of limited duration. However, in some cases, haemorrhage can be a major source of morbidity. For example, chronic bleeding can lead to anaemia with all of the associated problems (e.g. fatigue, dyspnoea).

Table 25.3 Causes of haemorrhage

Category	Comment
Local causes	
Cancer	Oral haemorrhage may originate from the tumour, or the adjacent tissues.
Cancer treatment	Oral haemorrhage is a complication of both traditional cancer treatments (e.g. head and neck radiotherapy, systemic chemotherapy), and new cancer treatments (e.g. biological therapies).
Oral trauma	Causes include (vigorous) oral hygiene, and dental surgery.
Oral infection	Causes include periodontal disease, and HSV infection.
Other oral conditions	Causes include vascular anomalies, and blistering disorders.
Systemic causes	
Thrombocytopaenia	Thrombocytopaenia is usually secondary to either bone marrow infiltration (e.g. leukaemia, solid tumour), or bone marrow suppression (e.g. chemotherapy, radiotherapy).
Platelet dysfunction	Platelet dysfunction is usually secondary to drug treatment (e.g. aspirin, non-steroidal anti-inflammatory drugs).
Coagulation factor deficiencies	Causes include malabsorption, and liver disease/dysfunction.
Anticoagulant therapy	Anticoagulants may cause bleeding per se, or aggravate bleeding due to other causes.
Disseminated intravascular coagulation (DIC)	DIC is a recognized complication of cancer.
Systemic vascular conditions	Causes include hereditary haemorrhagic telangiectasia, and vitamin C deficiency ('scurvy').

Box 25.2 Non-specific methods for treating haemorrhage

- Local pressure[33,34]
- Ice chips/packs[33,34]
- Topical vasoconstrictor agents (e.g. adrenaline[31,34], cocaine[31,34])
- Topical haemostatic agent (e.g. thrombin[31], thromboplastin[32], fibrin sealants[33], cyanoacrylate products[31], sucralfate[35], gelatin[34])
- Topical antifibrinolytic agents (e.g. aminocaproic acid[31], tranexamic acid[33])
- Haemostatic dressings (e.g. alginate[34], collagen[34], collagen/oxidised regenerated cellulose[34], fibrin[32], gelatin[34])
- Cautery (e.g. silver nitrate[34])
- Systemic antifibrinolytic agents (e.g. aminocaproic acid[36], tranexamic acid[37]

Similarly, in some cases, haemorrhage can be the cause of mortality. Indeed, haemorrhage is an important cause of death in patients with head and neck cancer (3–12%)[29,30].

The management of haemorrhage depends on a number of factors including the intensity of the bleeding, the cause of the bleeding, the availability of interventions, and (particularly) the patient's general condition/prognosis[32]. Thus, the management of patients with early cancer will tend to be more intensive than that of patients with advanced cancer. However, active treatment often offers better palliation than 'supportive care', and so active treatment should always be considered an option for management.

The management of haemorrhage is highly individualized, and may involve some or all of the following strategies: (1) resuscitation of the patient (when appropriate); (2) non-specific treatments to stop the bleeding (Box 25.2)[33–37]; (3) assessment of the cause of the bleeding (e.g. full blood count, coagulation screen, endoscopy, angiography); (4) specific treatments to stop the bleeding/prevent further bleeding (Box 25.3)[38–48]; and (5) avoidance of aggravating factors (e.g. modification of oral hygiene measures, modification of dietary intake)[33].

As discussed above, haemorrhage is an important cause of death in patients with head and neck cancer (e.g. carotid artery rupture). Patients at risk of a major bleed should be identified, and the management strategy determined (i.e. active treatment or supportive care). Major bleeds are invariably preceded by minor ('herald') bleeds. Active management involves surgical/interventional radiological techniques to manage the haemorrhage (Box 25.3). Ideally, patients should be treated proactively rather than reactively (i.e. patients should be treated prior to a major bleed). Supportive management involves pharmacological interventions to manage the associated distress (e.g. midazolam). The following discussion relates to the supportive management of a major bleed.

In most cases, a subcutaneous injection of 10 mg of midazolam will adequately sedate the patient[49]. However, some patients require further/larger doses of midazolam (e.g. patients on long-term benzodiazepine therapy). It is recommended that a pre-filled syringe of midazolam be kept in close proximity to the patient[49]. Such pre-filled syringes should be changed on a weekly basis[50]. Similarly, it is recommended that other relevant items are also kept in close proximity to the patient (i.e. pressure dressings, coloured blankets)[49].

It is generally appropriate to warn patients at high risk about the possibility of such a problem occurring. Indeed, in many cases, the patient will already have considered the issue, and may be 'thinking the worst'. (In such cases, an open and honest conversation may actually help to relieve some of the psychological distress associated with these issues). Moreover, it is generally appropriate to warn the

---

Box 25.3 Specific methods for treating haemorrhage

- Radiotherapy[38]
- Surgery (e.g. excision of bleeding tissue[32], ligation of blood vessels[39,40], reconstruction of blood vessels[40]
- Interventional radiology (e.g. transcutaneous arterial embolization[41,42], insertion of endovascular stent[43,44])
- Blood products (e.g. platelets for thrombocytopenia[45], fresh frozen plasma/cryoprecipitate/ cryosupernatant for multiple coagulation factor deficiencies[46])
- Specific interventions (e.g. vitamin K ± coagulation factors to reverse warfarin anticoagulation[47], protamine to reverse unfractionated heparin anticoagulation[48]

carers of patients at high risk about the possibility of such a problem occurring. Nevertheless, in some circumstances, such conversations may, in fact, do more harm than good.

References

1 Boyce HW, Bakheet MR (2005). Sialorrhea. A review of a vexing, often unrecognized sign of oropharyngeal and esophageal disease. *J Clin Gastroenterol*, 39(2), 89–97.

2 Schubert MM, Izutsu KT (1987). Iatrogenic causes of salivary gland dysfunction. *J Dent Res*, 66 (Spec Iss), 680–8.

3 Tonomura Y, Kataoka H, Hara Y, et al. (2007). Clinical analysis of paraneoplastic encephalitis associated with ovarian teratoma. *J Neurooncol*, 84(3), 287–92.

4 Laufman LR, Brenckman WD, Stydnicki KA, et al. (1989). Clinical experience with leucovorin and 5-fluorouracil. *Cancer*, 63(6), 1031–5.

5 Dodds HM, Bishop JF, Rivory LP (1999). More about: irinotecan-related cholinergic syndrome induced by coadministration of Oxaliplatin. *J Natl Cancer Inst*, 91(1), 91–2.

6 Brodsky L (1993). Drooling in children, in Arvedson JC, Brodsky L (eds) *Pediatric Swallowing and Feeding: Assessment and Management*. Singular Publishing Group, San Diego.

7 Meningaud J-P, Pitak-Arnnop P, Chikhani L, Bertrand J-C (2006). Drooling of saliva: a review of the etiology and management options. *Oral Surg Oral Med Oral Pathol Oral Radiol Endod*, 101(1), 48–57.

8 Kilpatrick NM, Johnson H, Reddihough D (2000). Sialorrhea: a multidisciplinary approach to the management of drooling children. *J Disab Oral Health*, 1(1), 3–9.

9 Van der Burg JJ, Didden R, Jongerius PH, Rotteveel JJ (2007). Behavioral treatment of drooling. A methodological critique of the literature with clinical guidelines and suggestions for future research. *Behav Modif*, 31(5), 573–94.

10 Moulding MB, Koroluk LD (1991). An intraoral prosthesis to control drooling in a patient with amyotrophic lateral sclerosis. *Spec Care Dentist*, 11(5): 200–2.

11 Jongerius PH, van Tiel P, van Limbeek J, Gabreels FJ, Rotteveel JJ (2003). A systematic review for evidence of efficacy of anticholinergic drugs to treat drooling. *Arch Dis Child*, 88(10), 911–14.

12 Benson J, Daugherty KK (2007). Botulinum toxin A in the treatment of sialorrhea. *Ann Pharmacother*, 41(1), 79–85.

13 Borg M, Hirst F (1998). The role of radiation therapy in the management of sialorrhea. *Int J Radiat Oncol Biol Phys*, 41(5), 1113–19.

14 Goode RL, Smith RA (1970). The surgical management of sialorrhea. *Laryngoscope*, 80(7), 1078–89.

15 Wong V, Sun JG, Wong W (2001). Traditional Chinese medicine (tongue acupuncture) in children with drooling problems. *Pediatr Neurol*, 25(1), 47–54.

16 De Simone GG, Eisenchlas JH, Junin M, Pereyra F, Brizuela R (2006). Atropine drops for drooling: a randomized controlled trial. *Palliat Med*, 20(7), 665–71.

17 Olsen AK, Sjogren P (1999). Oral glycopyrrolate alleviates drooling in a patient with tongue cancer. *J Pain Symptom Manage*, 18(4), 300–2.

18 Rashid H, Long JD, Wadleigh RG (1997). Management of secretions in esophageal cancer patients with glycopyrrolate. *Ann Oncol*, 8(2), 198–9.

19 Lucas V (1998). Use of enteral glycopyrrolate in the management of drooling. *Palliat Med*, 12(3), 207–8.

20 Tassinari D, Poggi B, Fantini M, Tamburini E, Sartori S (2005). Treating sialorrhea with transdermal scopolamine. Exploiting a side effect to treat an uncommon symptom in cancer patients. *Support Care Cancer*, 13(7), 559–61.

21 Zeppetella G (1999). Nebulized scopolamine in the management of oral dribbling: three case reports. *J Pain Symptom Manage*, 17(4), 293–5.

22 Doyle J, Walker P, Bruera E (2000). Nebulized scopolamine. *J Pain Symptom Manage*, 19(5), 327–8.

23 Laskawi R, Ellies M (2007). The role of botulinum toxin in the management of head and neck cancer patients. *Curr Opin Otolaryngol Head Neck Surg*, 15(2), 112–16.

24 Parisier SC, Blitzer A, Binder WJ, Friedman WF, Marovitz WF (1978). Tympanic neurectomy and chorda tympanectomy for the control of drooling. *Arch Otolaryngol*, 104(5), 273–7.

25 Cohen IK, Holmes EC, Edgerton MT (1971). Parotid duct transplantation for correction of drooling in patients with cancer of the head and neck. *Surg Gynecol Obstet*, 133(4), 663–5.

26 British Columbia Cancer Agency website: http://www.bccancer.bc.ca/

27 Anonymous (2000). *Practical management of motor neurone disease: speech pathology*, 3rd edn. Bethlehem Hospital Inc, Caulfield.

28 Newall AR, Orser R, Hunt M (1996). The control of oral secretions in bulbar ALS/MND. *J Neurol Sci*, 139 (Suppl), 43–4.

29 Forbes K (1997). Palliative care in patients with cancer of the head and neck. *Clin Otolaryngol Allied Sci*, 22(2), 117–22.

30 Shedd DP, Carl A, Shedd C (1980). Problems of terminal head and neck cancer patients. *Head Neck Surg*, 2(6), 476–82.

31 National Cancer Institute website: http://www.cancer.gov/cancertopics/pdq/supportivecare/oralcomplications/HealthProfessional

32 Perreira J, Phan T (2004). Management of bleeding in patients with advanced cancer. *Oncologist*, 9(5), 561–70.

33 Sadler GR, Stoudt A, Fullerton JT, Oberle-Edwards LK, Nguyen Q, Epstein JB (2003). Managing the oral sequelae of cancer therapy. *Medsurg Nurs*, 12(1), 28–36.

34 Seaman S (2006). Management of malignant fungating wounds in advanced cancer. *Semin Oncol Nurs*, 22(3), 185–93.

35 Regnard CF (1991). Control of bleeding in advanced cancer. *Lancet*, 337(8747), 974.

36 Dean A, Tuffin P (1997). Fibrinolytic inhibitors for cancer-associated bleeding problems. *J Pain Symptom Manage*, 13(1), 20–4.

37 Seto AH, Dunlap DS (1996). Tranexamic acid in oncology. *Ann Pharmacother*, 30(7-8), 868–70.

38 Hoskin PJ (2004). Radiotherapy in symptom management, in Doyle D, Hanks G, Cherny N, Calman K (eds) *Oxford Textbook of Palliative Medicine*, 3rd edn, pp. 239–55. Oxford University Press, Oxford.

39 Witz M, Korzets Z, Shnaker A, Lehmann JM, Ophir D (2002). Delayed carotid artery rupture in advanced cervical cancer: a dilemma in emergency management. *Eur Arch Otorhinolaryngol*, 259(1), 37–9.

40 Upile T, Triaridis S, Kirkland P, et al. (2005). The management of carotid artery rupture. *Eur Arch Otorhinolaryngol*, 262(7), 555–60.

41 Sesterhenn AM, Iwinska-Zelder J, Dalchow CV, Bien S, Werner JA (2006). Acute haemorrhage in patients with advanced head and neck cancer: value of endovascular therapy as palliative treatment option. *J Laryngol Otol*, 120(2), 117–24.

42 Chou WC, Lu CH, Lin G, et al. (2007). Transcutaneous arterial embolization to control massive tumor bleeding in head and neck cancer: 63 patients' experiences from a single medical center. *Support Care Cancer*, 15(10), 1185–90.

43 Warren FM, Cohen JL, Nesbit GM, Barnwell SL, Wax MK, Andersen PE (2002). Management of carotid ,blowout' with endovascular stent grafts. *Laryngoscope*, 112(3), 428–33.

44 Desuter G, Hammer F, Gardiner Q, et al. (2005). Carotid stenting for impending carotid blowout: suitable supportive care for head and neck cancer patients? *Palliat Med*, 19(5), 427–9.

45 British Committee for Standards in Haematology (2003). Guidelines for the use of platelet transfusions. *Br J Haem* 122(1), 10–23.

46 British Committee for Standards in Haematology (2004). Guidelines for the use of fresh-frozen plasma, cryoprecipitate and cryosupernatant. *Br J Haem*, 126(1), 11–28.

47 Baglin TP, Keeling DM, Watson HG (2006). Guidelines on oral anticoagulation (warfarin): third edition – 2005 update. *Br J Haem*, 132(3), 277–85.

48 Baglin T, Barrowcliffe TW, Cohen A, Greaves M (2006). Guidelines on the use and monitoring of heparin. *Br J Haem*, 133(1), 19–34.

49 Lovel T (2000). Palliative care and head and neck cancer. *Br J Oral Maxillofac Surg*, 38(4), 253–4.

50 Gagnon B, Mancini I, Pereira J, Bruera E (1998). Palliative management of bleeding events in advanced cancer patients. *J Palliat Care*, 14(4), 50–4.

Chapter 26

Oral care in paediatric cancer patients

Alessandra Majorana and Fulvio Porta

Introduction

Childhood cancers account for ~2% of the total number of cancer cases registered worldwide. Data collected from cooperative paediatric clinical trial groups suggests that the overall incidence of childhood cancer increased by 4.1% in the period 1973–88, and thereafter increased by 1% per year. However, caution must be used in interpreting these data, which may be the result of factors such as better reporting of cancer, and random variation in the occurrence of cancer. In the USA, the probability of developing cancer by the age of 20 is 1 in 300–333 for children born in 1999 (male children: 1 in 300; female children: 1 in 333)[1].

The types of cancer that occur in the paediatric population are very different from those that occur in the adult population. The most frequent neoplasms are acute lymphocytic leukaemia, acute myeloid leukaemia, central nervous system (CNS) tumours (e.g. medulloblastoma, brain-stem glioma), neuroblastoma, Non-Hodgkin's lymphoma, Hodgkin's disease, Wilm's tumour, rhabdomyosarcoma, retinoblastoma, osteosarcoma, and Ewing's sarcoma (Figure 26.1)[2]. A detailed discussion of these conditions is beyond the scope of this chapter, and readers are encouraged to consult an appropriate paediatric oncology textbook[3,4].

Significant advances have been achieved in the treatment of most paediatric cancers in terms of overall survival[1]. Indeed, the chance of being cured from a paediatric cancer is ~70% overall. The best results have been achieved in children affected by acute lymphocytic leukaemia, lymphomas, and sarcomas. The improvements in survival are related not only to improvements in anti-cancer therapies, but also to improvements in supportive care (i.e. management of the life-threatening complications of cancer/anti-cancer therapies). Nevertheless, cancer is the most common cause of death from disease in childhood.

The treatment schedules for children often differ from those of adults, since the biology of childhood tumours is different from those of adult tumours. For example, the schedule for the treatment of acute lymphocytic leukaemia involves a sequential combination of drugs at low to intermediate dosages, and consists of an induction phase, a consolidation phase and a maintenance phase (of about 18 months). Haematopoietic stem cell transplantation (HSCT) may be indicated in patients with relapsed acute lymphocytic leukaemia, high-risk acute myeloid leukaemia, stage IV rhabdomyosarcoma, and stage IV neuroblastoma.

Oral complications are common consequences for paediatric patients undergoing systemic chemotherapy, head and neck radiotherapy, and HSCT. Indeed, children and adolescents develop more acute/long-term oral side effects than adults (overall incidence: 30–100%)[5]. Oral complications are a significant cause of morbidity, and a potential cause of mortality. The more common oral side effects are discussed in the following section (and in relevant chapters within the book).

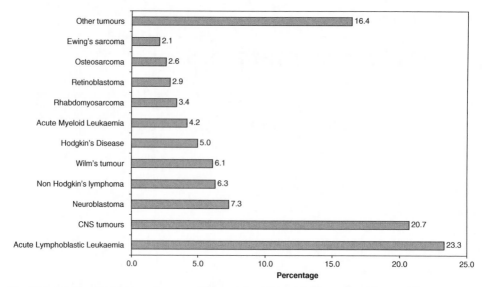

Fig. 26.1 Relative distribution of cancer diagnoses in children younger than 15 years.[2]
Source: Reproduced from Gurney JG, Severson RK, Davis S, Robinson LL (1995). Incidence of cancer in children in the United States. Sex-, Race-, and 1-year age-specific rates by histologic type. Cancer, 75: 2186

Oral complications

Early complications

Oral mucositis

Cancer therapy-induced mucositis occurs in 40–80% of children, and is highest in patients undergoing myeloablative chemotherapy and/or whole body radiotherapy prior to HSCT[5–10]. The overall risk of mucositis is greater in children and adolescents compared with in adults, due to the high incidence of haematological malignancies, the use of more intensive treatment protocols, and the higher mitotic index of the epithelial basal cells.

Oral mucositis is one of the most debilitating complications of cancer therapy in children. The clinical features are similar to those seen in adults (see Chapter 15). Children initially describe (when possible) a burning or tingling sensation, followed by an intolerance to food. Drooling may occur in children that cannot swallow normally. The severity of mucositis in childhood is clearly related to the use of narcotic analgesics, use of total parenteral nutrition, use of antibiotics, development of life-threatening infections, 100-day mortality statistic, and higher cost of care[5–8,11–15]. Oral mucositis tends to resolve more quickly in children than in adults.

The management of oral mucositis is mostly palliative/supportive, since in most cases there is no effective measure for preventing oral mucositis. The management is similar to that used in adults (see Chapter 15). The use of topical local anaesthetics should be supervised in children, to avoid the risk of swallowing with consequent loss of the gag reflex.

Oral infections

Children are at risk for all types of oral infections, due to compromise of the immune system and the mucosal barrier[5–7].

Fungal infections – candidosis, aspergillosis, mucormycosis[16–19] Oral fungal infections often develop in children undergoing systemic chemotherapy (especially during severe immuno-suppression), and head and neck radiotherapy. Prevention of fungal colonization and control of local infection are of critical importance in avoiding systemic fungal infections. Oral fungal infections are discussed, in detail, in Chapter 18.

Bacterial infections Bacterial infections most commonly involve the gingival tissues, although potentially any mucosal surface is at risk. Oral mucosal infections may cause fevers, and can result in systemic bacteraemia. Infection can also be associated with exfoliation of primary teeth and eruption of permanent teeth. Oral bacterial infections are discussed, in detail, in Chapter 19.

Viral infections[20,21] Herpes simplex virus (HSV) causes most of the oral infections in children with cancer. The clinical features of HSV infection are oral/extra-oral ulcers with associated erythema and crusting. It is not unusual to see the sudden emergence of widespread herpetic stomatitis in children with cancer. Oral viral infections are discussed, in detail, in Chapter 20.

Salivary gland dysfunction

Salivary gland dysfunction may be related to toxicity from systemic chemotherapy, head and neck radiotherapy, and HSCT[5,6,22]. Chemotherapy-induced salivary gland dysfunction is generally transient, usually resolving 48 h following treatment. Radiotherapy-induced salivary gland dysfunction is generally permanent. However, despite the damage caused by radiation to the acini of the salivary glands, some paediatric patients do achieve an improvement in salivary gland function 2–12 months following radiotherapy.

The clinical features of salivary gland dysfunction are similar to those seen in adults (see Chapter 21). In paediatric patients, decreased salivary flow leads to modified oral bacteria, favouring the development of dental caries (e.g. *Streptococcus mutans*, *Lactobacillus spp*) and opportunistic infections.

The management of salivary gland dysfunction is primarily symptomatic, and is similar to that used in adults (see Chapter 21). In order to reduce the risk of aggressive dental decay, intensive oral hygiene/care, use of topical fluorides, use of fissure sealants, and adoption of a sugar-free diet should be encouraged in children with salivary glands dysfunction.

Taste disturbance

Cancer therapy is a frequent cause of loss of taste discrimination, and/or altered sense of taste. [5–7,23] However, children usually recover their sense of taste 1–3 months after the cancer therapy has ended.

These sequelae may cause significant distress to the patient, reduce their nutritional intake, and interfere with their physiological growth. It should be noted that nutritional intake may also be affected by other common therapy-related problems such as anorexia, nausea and vomiting, and oral mucositis/stomatitis.

Current management protocols focus on improving the appearance, smell, and texture of the food. It is recommended choosing foods typically preferred by children and adolescents (i.e. snacks or liquid nutritional supplements). Zinc supplements have been reported to be effective in helping the recovery of the sense of taste in some instances.

Taste disturbance is discussed, in detail, in Chapter 22.

Oral haemorrhage

The incidence of oral bleeding ranges from 6% to 42% in children undergoing cancer therapy. The most common risk factors are thrombocytopaenia, coagulopathies, mucosal infections, mucosal trauma, mobile primary teeth, orthodontic appliances, and poor oral hygiene. Spontaneous bleeding is rare with a platelet count of $\geq$50 000/mm^3, and the incidence and severity of oral bleeding are decreased if the platelet counts can be maintained above 20 000/mm^3. Oral haemorrhage can vary from minor gingival oozing to major mucosal bleeding; oral bleeding can be clinically problematic if there is severe thrombocytopaenia in the presence of mucosal breakdown or infection. The management of oral haemorrhage is similar to that used in adults (see Chapter 25).

Long-term complications

Dental developmental abnormalities

Chemotherapy/radiotherapy administered during odontogenesis may cause various dental anomalies[5–7,24,25–29]. These sequelae are related to the child's age at the beginning of cancer therapy (the risk is greater when the cancer therapy starts prior to age 5), the stage of tooth development, and the type of treatment protocol. Children with mixed dentition that undergo cancer therapy have a higher incidence of dental anomalies, probably due to the rapid/major odontogenic changes that occur during this period.

Dental abnormalities caused by radiation are limited to the irradiated area. High-dose radiotherapy during the very early phases of tooth development may destroy the cells of the tooth germ, and lead to complete dental agenesis (Figures 26.2 and 26.3). Less drastic complications like microdontia (i.e. small teeth), enamel hypoplasia and defective calcification, and stunted or tapering roots (Figure 26.4) occur with lower dose radiotherapy, or when radiotherapy starts at a later stage of dental development. Radiotherapy-related changes/damage occur simultaneously in the pulp, periodontal ligament, and adjacent bone.

Chemotherapy may damage the developing odontogenic cells causing disturbances in dental development such as microdontia, crown hypoplasia, enlarged pulp chamber, and root anomalies (i.e. conical roots, short V-shaped roots, etc; Figure 26.5). Chemotherapeutic agents usually cause localized dental defects, with the changes occurring mostly in the lower incisors and premolars. Complete dental agenesis is rare, although it may result when intensive and repetitive chemotherapy is used. Chemotherapy is also associated with an increase of enamel hypoplasia and white

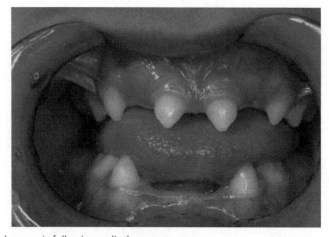

Fig. 26.2 Dental agenesis following radiotherapy.

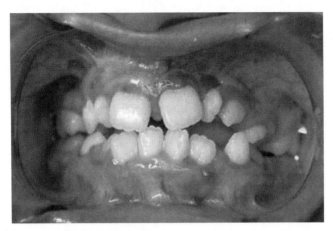

Fig. 26.3 Dental agenesis following radiotherapy.

spot lesions, caused by interference to ameloblasts during dental crown formation (Figure 26.6, see colour plate section).

In children undergoing cancer therapy, the eruption of teeth can be delayed, whilst the frequency of impacted maxillary canines also appears to be increased. Shortened root length can result in shortened alveolar processes, leading to a decreased vertical dimension of the mandible and the lower-third of the face. Additionally, damage to jaw-growth centres by treatment regimens can lead to decreased size (and mobility) of the jaw bones (Figure 26.7)[30].

Dental caries

Children with cancer are at high risk of dental caries as a result of multiple factors[5–7,24,31–34]. Damage to the salivary glands by radiotherapy and chemotherapeutic agents results in reduced salivary flow, which causes oral environment changes that favour caries-related microflora. Cancer therapy-induced enamel defects increase the risk of dental caries (see previous section). Other factors associated with the development of dental caries include poor oral hygiene, carbohydrate-rich diet, sucrose-rich paediatric medications, nausea and vomiting (causing acid erosion), prolonged hospitalization, and psychological factors.

Dental caries is discussed, in detail, in Chapter 19.

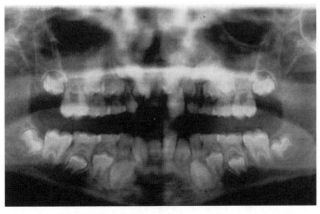

Fig. 26.4 Orthopantogram showing shortened roots.

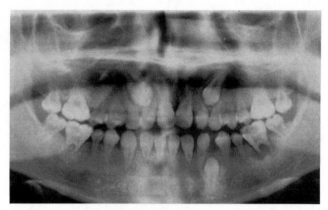

Fig. 26.5 Orthopantogram showing V-shaped roots.

Trismus

High doses of radiotherapy to the head and neck may cause fibrosis of the masticator muscles, which may lead to the development of trismus[5,35]. In order to prevent/ameliorate this condition, daily oral stretching exercises are recommended during and following radiotherapy (for 3–6 months).

Trismus is discussed in detail in Chapter 11.

Oral graft-versus-host disease (GVHD)

The frequency of GVHD is usually lower in paediatric patients who undergo HSCT than in adult patients. The oral cavity can be involved with both acute and chronic forms of the disease. The clinical features are similar to those seen in adults (see Chapter 14)[5–7,36].

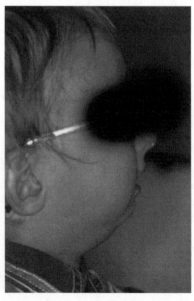

Fig. 26.7 Impaired jaw development following radiotherapy.

Oral GVHD usually presents as part of multi-system involvement, but in numerous patients it is the first or only manifestation of the condition. The management is similar to that used in adults (see Chapter 15).

Second tumours

One of the most serious oral complications facing long-term survivors of HSCT is secondary oral malignancy, such as oral squamous cell carcinoma and Non-Hodgkin's lymphoma[5–7,36]. GVHD appears to be a significant risk factor for this complication. Secondary oral malignancies may also occur in other patients that have received systemic chemotherapy and head and neck radiotherapy[37].

Role of paediatric dental professionals

Oral health care providers play an essential role in the management of paediatric patients undergoing cancer therapy. Paediatric dentists and dental hygienists should support the oncology team by providing basic oral/dental care, implementing oral hygiene measures, delivering emergency dental treatment, and assisting in managing oral complications from cancer therapy. The ultimate goals of the dental care team's coordinated efforts are to reduce the incidence and severity of oral complications, improve patient comfort during cancer treatment, improve patient outcomes from cancer treatment, and help to reduce the overall cost of care[5–7,38–42].

A pre-cancer therapy evaluation is the essential first step (see Chapter 5). The dental team should identify and eliminate all active or potential sources of oral infection. Thus, stabilization of oral infection prior to treatment can reduce the incidence and severity of oral and/or systemic complications. In particular, dental caries should, whenever possible, be treated prior to cancer therapy; while permanent restorations are the best option, temporary materials can stabilize the teeth in the short term. Incipient dental caries may be reversed with the use of topical fluorides, remineralizing solutions, and fissure sealants. In addition, the dental team should identify and eliminate all active or potential sources of oral trauma.

It is important that there is ongoing discussion with the child's oncologist/physician in order to coordinate the timing of oral care. Routine dental treatment should be completed, and initial healing of wounds should be established, prior to commencing the cancer treatment. Routine dental treatment should not be undertaken when the patient is immunosuppressed. The oral healthcare team has a key role in highlighting to patients and their parents the significance of oral health, and in supporting patients and their parents to undertake the necessary oral hygiene measures (see the following).

It is important that patients maintain an appropriate level of oral hygiene during cancer treatment. Parents should understand the oral hygiene protocol, and the effectiveness of the techniques advocated. Moreover, parents should ensure their children adhere to the oral hygiene protocol (and join them in adopting a non-cariogenic diet). Strategies to remove dental plaque from the teeth and gums are critically important in reducing the risk of oral complication such as local infection and haemorrhage. Children should be encouraged to use extra-soft nylon toothbrushes to limit the risk of trauma to gingival and other soft tissue. Brushing should always be supervised by either the parents or professional staff. Dental floss, dental toothpicks, and water-irrigation devices should be used carefully (if at all) to avoid tissue trauma.

Fluoridated toothpaste, fluoride varnish, and neutral fluoride rinses or gels are recommended for high-caries-risk patients during all phases of the cancer treatment. The routine use of topical antibacterial rinses remains controversial. However, chlorhexidine should be used in cases where mechanical dental plaque removal is not possible, or where significant gingival inflammation/ infection is present. Non-prescription mouthwashes containing alcohol and flavouring agents should be avoided whenever possible in children with mucositis/stomatitis, since these agents can cause burning and stinging.

Frequent follow-up dental visits, with the application of prevention protocols, may decrease or eliminate the need for invasive dental procedures in children with cancer. Furthermore, follow-up will ensure the earlier recognition/management of the other late effects of treatment. Once the patient has recovered sufficiently, and is immunologically stable, restorative dentistry can start, and orthodontic care can be resumed (at least 2 years for orthodontic care).

References

1 Surveillance, Epidemiology and End Results (National Cancer Institute) website: http://seer.cancer.gov/

2 Gurney JG, Severson RK, Davis S, Robinson LL (1995). Incidence of cancer in children in the United States. Sex-, Race-, and 1-year age-specific rates by histologic type. *Cancer*, 75: 2186.

3 Pizzo PA, Poplack DG (2005). *Principles and practice of pediatric oncology*, 5th edn. Lippincott Williams & Wilkin, Philadelphia.

4 Pinkerton C, Plowman N, Pieters R (2004). *Paediatric oncology*, 3rd edn. Hodder Arnold, London.

5 Hong CH, da Fonseca M (2008). Considerations in the Pediatric Population with Cancer. *Dent Clin N Am*, 52 (1), 155–181.

6 Belfield PM, Dwyer AA (2004). Oral complications of childhood cancer and its treatment: current best practice. *Eur J Cancer*. 40(7), 1035–41.

7 Majorana A, Schubert MM, Porta F, Ugazio AG, Sapelli PL (2000). Oral complications of pediatric hematopoietic cell transplantation: diagnosis and management. *Support Care Cancer*, 8(5), 353–65.

8 Cheng KK, Chang AM, Yuen MP (2004). Prevention of oral mucositis in paediatric patients treated with chemotherapy; a randomised crossover trial comparing two protocols of oral care. *Eur J Cancer*, 40(8), 1208–16.

9 Gandemer V, Le Deley MC, Dollfus C, et al (2007). Multicenter randomized trial of chewing gum for preventing oral mucositis in children receiving chemotherapy. *J Pediatr Hematol Oncol*, 29 (2), 86–94.

10 Peterson DE (2006). New strategies for management of oral mucositis in cancer patients. *J Support Oncol*, 4 (2 Suppl 1), 9–13.

11 Oliveira Lula EC, Oliveira Lula CE, Alves CM, Lopes FF, Pereira AL (2007). Chemotherapy-induced oral complications in leukemic patients. *Int J Pediatr Otorhinolaryngol*, 71(11),1681–5.

12 Scully C, Sonis S, Diz PD (2006). Oral mucositis. *Oral Dis*, 12(3), 229–41.

13 D'Hondt L, Lonchay C, Marc A, Canon JL (2006). Oral mucositis induced by anticancer treatments: physiopathology and treatments. *Therapeutics and Clinical Risk Management*, 2 (2), 159–68.

14 Redding SW (2005). Cancer therapy-related oral mucositis. *Dent Educ*, 69(8), 919–29.

15 Epstein JB, Schubert MM (2004). Managing pain in mucositis. *Semin Oncol Nurs*, 20(1), 30–7.

16 Gozdasoglu S, Ertem M, Buyukkececi Z, et al. (1999). Fungal colonization and infection in children with acute leukemia and lymphoma during induction therapy. *Med Pediatr Oncol*, 32(5), 344–8.

17 Gonzalez Gravina H, Gonzalez de Moran E, Zambrano O, et al. (2007). Oral candidiasis in children and adolescents with cancer. Identification of Candida spp. *Med Oral Patol Oral Cir Bucal*, 12(6), E419–23.

18 Alberth M, Majoros L, Kovalecz G, et al. (2006). Significance of oral Candida infections in children with cancer. *Pathol Oncol Res*, 12(4), 237–41.

19 Grigull L, Beier R, Schrauder A, et al. (2003). Invasive fungal infections are responsible for one-fifth of the infectious deaths in children with ALL. *Mycoses*, 46(11–12), 441–6.

20 Sepulveda E, Brethauer U, Rojas J, Fernandez E, Le Fort P (2005). Oral ulcers in children under chemotherapy: clinical characteristics and their relation with Herpes Simplex Virus type 1 and Candida albicans. *Med Oral Patol Oral Cir Bucal*, 10(Suppl 1), E1–8.

21 Carrega G, Castagnola E, Canessa A, et al. (1994). Herpes simplex virus and oral mucositis in children with cancer. *Support Care Cancer*, 2(4), 266–9.

22 Bagesund M, Winiarski J, Dahllof G (2000). Subjective xerostomia in long-term surviving children and adolescents after pediatric bone marrow transplantation. *Transplantation*, 69(5):822–6.

23 Skolin I, Wahlin YB, Broman DA, Koivisto Hursti UK, Vikstrom LM, Hernell O (2006). Altered food intake and taste perception in children with cancer after start of chemotherapy: perspectives of children, parents and nurses. *Support Care Cancer*, 14(4):369–78.

24 Alberth M, Kovalecz G, Nemes J, Math J, Kiss C, Marton IJ (2004). Oral health of long-term childhood cancer survivors. *Pediatr Blood Cancer*, 43(1), 88–90.

25 Vaughan MD, Rowland CC, Tong X, et al. (2005). Dental abnormalities after pediatric bone marrow transplantation. *Bone Marrow Transplant*, 36(8), 725–9.

26 Minicucci EM, Lopes LF, Crocci AJ (2003). Dental abnormalities in children after chemotherapy treatment for acute lymphoid leukaemia. *Leuk Res*, 27(1), 45–50.

27 Estilo CL, Huryn JM, Kraus DH, et al. (2003). Effects of therapy on dentofacial development in long-term survivors of head and neck rhabdomyosarcoma: the Memorial Sloan-Kettering Cancer Center experience. *J Pediatr Hematol Oncol*, 25(3), 215–22.

28 Cetiner S, Alpaslan C (2004). Long-term effects of cancer therapy on dental development: a case report. *J Clin Pediatr Dent*, 28(4), 351–3.

29 Zarina RS, Nik-Hussein NN (2005). Dental abnormalities of a long-term survivor of a childhood hematological malignancy: literature review and report of a case. *J Clin Pediatr Dent*, 29(2), 167–74.

30 Dahllof G (1998). Craniofacial growth in children treated for malignant diseases. *Acta Odontol Scand*, 56(6), 378–82.

31 Wogelius P, Dahllof G, Gorst-Rasmussen A, Sorensen HT, Rosthoj S, Poulsen S (2008). A population-based observational study of dental caries among survivors of childhood cancer. *Pediatr Blood Cancer*, 50(6), 1221–6.

32 Avsar A, Elli M, Darka O, Pinarli G (2007). Long-term effects of chemotherapy on caries formation, dental development, and salivary factors in childhood cancer survivors. *Oral Surg Oral Med Oral Pathol Oral Radiol Endod*, 104(6), 781–9.

33 Cubukcu CE, Gunes AM (2008). Caries experience of leukemic children during intensive course of chemotherapy. *J Clin Pediatric Dent*, 32(2), 155–8.

34 Dahllof G, Bagesund M, Ringden O (1997). Impact of conditioning regimens on salivary function, caries-associated microorganisms and dental caries in children after bone marrow transplantation. A 4-year longitudinal study. *Bone Marrow Transplant*, 20(6), 479–83.

35 Dijkstra PU, Kalk WW, Roodenburg JL (2004). Trismus in head and neck oncology: a systematic review. *Oral Oncol*, 40(9), 879–89.

36 Treister NS, Woo SB, O'Holleran EW, Lehmann LE, Parsons SK, Guinan EC (2005). Oral chronic graft-versus-host disease in pediatric patients after hematopoietic stem cell transplantation. *Biol Blood Marrow Transplant*, 11(9), 721–31.

37 National Cancer Institute website: http://www.cancer.gov/

38 American Academy of Pediatric Dentistry website: http://www.aapd.org/media/Policies_Guidelines/G_Chemo.pdf

39 Meraw SJ, Reeve CM (1998). Dental considerations and treatment of the oncology patient receiving radiation therapy. *J Am Dent Assoc*, 129(2), 201–5.

40 Glenny AM, Gibson F, Auld E et al. (2004). A survey of current practice with regard to oral care for children being treated for cancer. *Eur J Cancer*, 40(8), 1217–24.

41 da Fonseca MA (2003). Dental care of the pediatric cancer patient. *Pediatr Dent*, 26(1), 53–7.

42 Yamagata K, Onizawa K, Yoshida K, et al. (2006). Dental management of pediatric patients undergoing hematopoietic stem cell transplant. *Pediatr Hematol Oncol*, 23(7), 541–8.

Chapter 27

Oral supportive care and the geriatric oncology patient

Ira R. Parker, Joanne E. Mortimer, and Joel Epstein

Introduction

Cancer is the leading cause of death for Americans under the age of 85, and ranks second only to cardiovascular disease for those 85 years of age and older (Figure 1.1; Tables 27.1 and 27.2) [1,2]. It is anticipated that by 2018 cancer will surpass cardiovascular disease incidence rates in all age groups. The U.S. population over the age of 65 is increasing significantly and is expected to reach 21% of the overall population by 2030. The population age cohort 80 years and older are increasing at the highest rate. Although the elderly presently represent 12% of the total U.S. population, 60% of all cancer diagnoses, and 71% of all cancer deaths, occur in populations 65 years of age or older. Worldwide data demonstrate that incidence rates of common cancers increase as individual populations age.

The natural history of some malignancies are unique in the elderly (e.g. haematologic malignancies tend to be more aggressive). Although geriatric populations are not well represented in therapeutic clinical trials[3,4], elderly cancer patients tend to have worse treatment outcomes than younger individuals[5–8]. Age-related disease co-morbidities and age-specific psychosocial stressors often complicate cancer management. Furthermore, 'access to care' issues often compromise the delivery of quality cancer care to senior populations (e.g. public policy, healthcare financing/provider reimbursement, education/training of providers).

The ability to provide adequate cancer-related oral supportive care to senior adult cancer patients is impacted by: (1) the 'normal ageing' processes of the oral complex; (2) the increased prevalence of medical co-morbidities; (3) frailty and reduced 'physiological reserve'; (4) the increased likelihood of functional and psychosocial stressors; and (5) limited public policy, public health, provider training and age-focused research agendas.

The aim of this chapter is to examine the pertinent issues associated with the delivery of oral supportive care to elder adults impacted by cancer, utilizing the patient-centred philosophies and healthcare-delivery models of two recognized dental/medical disciplines (i.e. Geriatric Dentistry, Geriatric Oncology). It should be noted that a minimal amount of research has been conducted focusing on the interrelationship between provision of oral supportive care and geriatric-specific cancer-care management[9,10].

Geriatric dentistry/geriatric oncology

Geriatric Dentistry is the discipline of dental medicine that focuses on disease factors and patient/provider treatment decision-making processes that are unique to ageing populations. The preservation of oral wellness in healthy community-dwelling elder populations, and the control of disease and the optimization of oral quality-of-life for frail senior adult populations (e.g. cognitively/physically impaired groups, assisted living/nursing home groups) are the underlying objectives of the discipline.

Table 27.1 2005 age-adjusted incidence and mortality rates for breast, colon/rectum, and prostate cancers (per 100 000)[1]

Tumour type	Age range			
	50–64 yr	≥65 yr	65–74 yr	≥75 yr
Breast				
Incidence	275.267	406.956	399.215	415.426
Mortality	46.377	105.215	79.381	133.484
Colon/rectum				
Incidence (Female)	62.165	217.531	163.537	276.611
Mortality (Female)	16.900	87.669	49.439	129.501
Incidence (Male)	86.232	283.008	212.297	360.381
Mortality (Male)	25.545	126.075	80.430	176.021
Prostate				
Incidence	296.910	805.507	855.067	751.277
Mortality	10.021	182.480	69.138	306.500

The development of Geriatric Dentistry closely mirrors the evolution of Geriatric Medicine (but significantly less in magnitude and overall impact). Geriatric Dentistry is firmly grounded in the philosophy of delivery of 'rational dental care'. Ettinger's decision-making and delivery model utilizes both the 'dentist's resources' (e.g. technical capability, equipment availability) and the 'patient's resources'[11]. A patient's resources include his/her life expectancy, medical history, medication profile, mental status, dexterity/functionality/mobility, financial resources, and the level of commitment from the patient and his/her caregivers.

Table 27.2 2005 age-adjusted incidence and mortality rates for oral cavity/pharynx, and larynx cancers (per 100 000)[1]

Tumour type	Age range			
	50–64 yr	≥65 yr	65–74 yr	≥75 yr
Oral cavity and pharynx				
Incidence (Female)	11.104	24.509	21.695	27.589
Mortality (Female)	2.186	7.563	5.230	10.116
Incidence (Male)	37.562	55.083	50.701	59.877
Mortality (Male)	8.394	17.455	15.379	19.727
Larynx				
Incidence (Female)	2.682	5.199	6.051	4.267
Mortality (Female)	0.868	2.496	2.390	2.612
Incidence (Male)	12.599	29.322	28.167	30.585
Mortality (Male)	3.899	12.216	10.773	13.795

Geriatric Oncology is a relatively young discipline within the specialty of Haematology/ Oncology. Geriatric Oncology's philosophy integrates an understanding of the biology of ageing, with a comprehensive geriatric assessment and the delivery of patient-centred care. The discipline spans the entire cancer-care management continuum (i.e. from prevention/early detection through cancer disease treatment to palliative/end-of-life care or cancer survivorship). The emphasis is on the individual cancer patient's quality-of-life and overall functionality.

A fundamental clinical tool is the Comprehensive Geriatric Assessment (CGA). The CGA's dual utility is: (1) to provide a methodology for evaluating the patient's overall health status; and (2) to provide the practitioner with a framework to better assess/stage a patient's life expectancy and capacity to endure stress[12]. The basic elements of the CGA are: (1) functional status; (2) co-morbidity; (3) cognitive function; (4) nutritional status; (5) psychological state/social support; (6) social condition/economic condition; and (7) medication review[13–15].

For most solid tumours, cancer treatments provide the same efficacy in the older population as in the younger age group[16]. However, normal tissue toxicities appear to be more common, and more severe, in ageing populations[17]. The ability to distinguish physiological age from chronological age utilizing the CGA is critical in the development of a patient-specific cancer-treatment plan that will balance the benefits of therapy with the potential side effects of that intervention.

Oral supportive care

The primary goal of oral supportive care is to prevent or minimize short-term and long-term 'orally related' morbidities that are associated with locally or systemically targeted cancer interventions. The maintenance of a well-functioning oropharyngeal apparatus throughout a cancer patient's treatment regimen is an essential factor in the patient's overall health status and quality of life.

Long-standing cancer treatments such as surgery, radiotherapy, and chemotherapy have been substantially investigated with regard to oral complications and the need for oral supportive care. Newer cancer interventions potentially also have substantial levels of oral morbidity as a byproduct. These include such interventions as molecularly targeted therapies, chemotherapy combined with radiotherapy, haematopoietic stem cell transplantation, and the use of pharmaceuticals such as bisphosphonates.

Age-related changes affect the composition and function of various tissues and organs in the oral cavity (see following sections). The impact of these age-related variations upon cancer-care oral morbidity has not been extensively investigated. Nevertheless, it is thought that normal ageing, and reduced physiologic reserve, contribute to an increase in incidence and/or severity of treatment-related morbidities.

The low level of oral supportive care research (relating to age-related tissue changes) may be a byproduct of: (1) an insufficient quantity of clinical investigators participating in the field of study; and (2) a limited number of clinical interventions, devices, and pharmaceuticals that might be targeted for 'age-focused' research. The historical exclusion of older (and medically compromised) subjects in clinical trials has also contributed to this paucity of investigation. Hence, a concerted, multidisciplinary research effort is needed to determine the relationship between the 'ageing process' and oral/head and neck complications.

Oral mucositis

There is presently no scientific literature qualifying or quantifying the differences in incidence, pathobiology, severity, or treatment outcomes comparing elderly and non-elderly cancer-patient populations.

Osteonecrosis (post-radiation and bisphosphonate-related)

There are no significant age-related bone alterations in the maxilla, whereas mandibular bone sustains a number of changes. Mandibular bone becomes less cellular, less vascular, more dense, and more brittle throughout the ageing process. The number of osteocytes decreases, and glycoprotein levels increase, in the lacunae. There are distinct changes in the collagen matrix, as well as the formation of diffuse calcifications. How these age-related changes impact on the incidence of post-radiation osteonecrosis (PRON) has been assessed by Lye and his group[18]; 'age' was the only significant variable associated with the development of PRON following dental extractions in their study of 40 subjects who had previously received radiotherapy for nasopharyngeal cancer. PRON is discussed in detail in Chapter 12. Osteonecrosis of the jaw is also a complication of the prolonged administration of intravenous bisphosphonates (bisphosphonate-related osteonecrosis – BRON). Data suggests that the risk of BRON is greater in at least some groups of older patients (e.g. patients with myeloma treated with intravenous bisphosphonates). BRON is discussed in detail in Chapter 16.

Salivary gland dysfunction

Age-related changes in the salivary glands include reduction of acinar cells, decreased vascularity, increased fibrosis, increased adiposity, a decline in the rate of protein synthesis, and the development of structurally deviant proteins[19]. Nevertheless, it has been established that both resting and stimulated whole salivary rates do not differ markedly between older and younger age cohorts. However, many elderly persons are prescribed anti-cholinergic medications that promote hyposalivation, resulting in a large prevalence of 'dry mouth' in geriatric populations[20]. The subsequent reduction in flow significantly compromises the functional capacity of the oral cavity. Salivary gland dysfunction is discussed in detail in Chapter 21.

Taste disturbance

Studies have demonstrated that gustatory thresholds for salt and bitter tastes are heightened as a population increases in age (whereas those for sweet and sour perceptions are not)[21]. Taste disturbance is discussed in detail in Chapter 22.

Dysphagia

Swallowing transit time increases 25–50% in ageing populations[22]. This increased transit time is worsened by cancer-treatment-related hyposalivation, thickening of the saliva, and muscle fibrosis. Swallowing dysfunction will adversely affect nutritional intake, and may increase the risk of aspiration pneumonia[23].

Barriers to oral supportive care

The elderly, as a segment of the overall population, are at considerable risk with regard to fully accessing and utilizing those cancer-related oral supportive care services that may be available to them. The barriers may best be illustrated by recognizing them as 'personal/individual issues' and 'societal/institutional barriers'.

Personal/individual issues

Personal/individual issues are represented by such factors as: (1) the individual's physiological, functional, cognitive[24], and psychosocial levels; (2) the ability to perform those tasks that are required to maintain their oral health quality of life; and (3) the individual's support system (which provides guidance, assistance, encouragement, and reinforcement). Thus, frailty, fatigue, movement disorders, cognitive impairment, sensory deficiencies, and depression can all compromise the abilities of an elderly cancer patient.

When a potential barrier to patient-conducted oral supportive care is identified, a strategy must be developed to better empower the patient in his/her health-promotion tasks. Examples of healthcare provider-initiated interventions include constructing custom handles for toothbrushes and fluoride trays (Figure 6.1); promoting patient utilization of cue cards, calendar reminders, and recording forms (for those who are cognitively impaired); providing enhanced provider-based oversight for at-risk patients; and identifying/recruiting/training a caregiver (formal or informal) to assist the cancer patient in the conduct of oral supportive care.

Societal/institutional barriers

Examples of societal/institutional barriers that potentially may compromise an elderly patient's access to cancer-related oral supportive care are: (1) limitations in commercial dental insurance and governmental programmes with regard to oral supportive care service-related procedural coverage (and provider compensation); (2) an inadequate pool of appropriately trained healthcare providers in oral supportive care clinical competencies; and (3) oncologic institutional under-utilization of oral supportive care expertise and services (as well as a constrained allocation of resources for cancer-related oral supportive services).

In the USA, non-working and/or retired citizens older than 65 generally do not have dental insurance coverage because: (1) former employers customarily do not include dental care as a component of their retiree healthcare package; (2) the Medicare Program (Title 18), the federal healthcare initiative that targets all US citizens that are disabled or 65 years old and older, does not reimburse patients or healthcare providers for dental procedures; and (3) the Medicaid Program (Title 19), a federal-state healthcare initiative targeting low-income citizens, does not mandate the inclusion of adults for dental coverage in its programme requirements (resulting in very few states offering dental reimbursement). Moreover, those states that do compensate for adult dental services generally do so at reimbursement levels that are not conducive for healthcare-provider participation, particularly for more complex treatments such as those required by patients receiving cancer therapy.

There is limited coverage for oral supportive care procedures through the Medicare Program. Pre-cancer treatment dental examinations are covered in some cases, as well as medical and surgical procedures involving the oral cavity (e.g. management of oral infection, pre-radiotherapy tooth extractions). However, dental restorative and prosthodontic procedures, dental prophylaxes and periodontal procedures, periodic oral surveillance examinations, and the construction of radiotherapy-necessitated fluoride trays for 'tooth preserving care' are all examples of services that are not covered by Medicare (and must be directly paid by the patient). As Medicare coverage for specific healthcare procedures/interventions is based upon proven, scientifically based evidence, it is essential that quality cancer-related oral supportive care research be conducted in a timely manner (and legislative advocacy efforts be expanded). An Institute of Medicine report, and other reviews of the literature, have concluded that there is sufficient evidence-based proof to support the reimbursement of targeted oral care prior to head and neck radiotherapy, and chemotherapy in leukaemia patients[25,26].

There are also apparent 'access to care' barriers associated with dental professional training. All US schools of dental medicine provide didactic education in 'medically necessary dental healthcare' concepts. However, the probability of an undergraduate dental student having the opportunity to clinically observe or manage a cancer patient requiring oral supportive care is very low. Graduate dental programs are also not mandated to incorporate cancer-related oral supportive care into their training curriculae. Furthermore, although there has been a substantial National Institutes of Health/American Dental Association effort on the national level, continuing dental education providers have demonstrated limited interest in developing or facilitating offerings focusing on the dental professional's role in the cancer-related oral supportive care treatment paradigm[27]. These dental trainee curricula/continuing dental education programme deficiencies contribute to the reality of a nominally prepared US dental workforce to address the oral supportive care needs of cancer patients.

The overall cancer-care delivery system also plays an important role with regard to a patient's ability to access appropriate oral supportive care. Epstein and his group surveyed comprehensive cancer centres in the USA and Canada to assess each facility's oral supportive care policies and delivery mechanisms. Forty-four percent of responding US National Cancer Institute-designated cancer centres reported having no formal dental/oral supportive care service. Thus, oral supportive care was usually delivered by cancer-centre staff, or occasionally by community-based dentists. Canadian cancer centres reported a general lack of documented standards of care, and limited institutional support for dental staff with regard to oral supportive care. The majority of Canadian centres managed cancer-related oral care needs by referring their patients to their own dentist, or to another community-based dentist[28,29]. Barker et al surveyed an international cohort of experts in the discipline of cancer supportive care. Integrated dental services were reported available in only 25% of the relevant institutions. The majority of those patients needing oral supportive care were again referred to community-based dental professionals[30].

Increasing numbers of cancer patients are being admitted to US nursing homes, and ~11% of admissions to US nursing facilities had a cancer diagnosis in 2002. These patients present unique clinical management challenges for the nursing and medical staff[31]. There is no epidemiological evidence to date qualifying or quantifying the oral disease burden and/or oral supportive care treatment needs of nursing home residents that are actively being treated for cancer. However, there has been a large volume of research focusing on the delivery and quality of overall dental care in nursing home settings. The data suggests that the oral health status of residents (and the delivery of dental healthcare services in nursing facilities) may be considered suboptimal, due to factors such as patients' limited capacities to provide self-care, healthcare provider attitudes and behaviours, healthcare provider training and competencies, nursing manpower constraints, and reimbursement issues[32]. The expected increase in number of cancer patients/survivors residing in nursing facilities will only compound an already unsatisfactory situation.

Summary

Worldwide increases in geriatric population cohorts will substantially impact the profile of healthcare and its delivery, including comprehensive cancer care and its oral supportive care component. The expected growing demand for oral supportive care services will necessitate a heightened awareness of the pertinent issues, as well as targeted efforts from clinicians, researchers, public health specialists, cancer centre administrators, policy makers and advocates to overcome existing barriers to care.

There are ample opportunities for geriatric oral supportive care research, specifically focussing on determining the relationships between cancer treatment, patient comorbidities, oral tissue aging processes, and cancer treatment-related oral complications. Clinical competency, workforce, and access-to-care issues must also be addressed through improved healthcare professional training, and the upgrading of patient insurance coverage for oral supportive care services.

   The provision of high quality oral supportive care is an essential component of a comprehensive approach to the geriatric cancer patient. As cancer care delivery systems are impacted by the influx of thousands and thousands of healthy and medically-compromised senior adults, improved treatment protocols and delivery methodologies must be adopted to better serve this expanding patient population.

References

1   Surveillance Epidemiology and End Results website: http://seer.gov/

2   National Cancer Institute website: http://cancer.gov/

3   Kemeny MM, Peterson BL, Kornblith AB, et al. (2003). Barriers to clinical trial participation by older women with breast cancer. *J Clin Oncol*, 21(12), 2268–75.

4   Wyld L, Reed MW (2003). The need for targeted research into breast cancer in the elderly. *Br J Surg*, 90(4), 388–99.

5   Rao AV, Seo PH, Cohen HJ (2004). Geriatric assessment and comorbidity. *Semin Oncol*, 31(2), 149–59.

6   Satariano WA, Silliman RA (2003). Comorbidity: implications for research and practice in geriatric oncology. *Crit Rev Oncol Hematol*, 48(2), 239–48.

7   Extermann M (200). Measurement and impact of comorbidity in older cancer patients. *Crit Rev Oncol Hematol*, 35(3), 181–200.

8   Janssen-Heijnen ML, Houterman S, Lemmens VE, Louwman MW, Maas HA, Coebergh JW (2005). Prognostic impact of increasing age and co-morbidity in cancer patients: a population-based approach. *Crit Rev Oncol Hematol*, 55(3), 231–40.

9   Epstein JB, Lunn R, Le ND, Stevenson-Moore P, Gorsky M (2005). Patients with oropharyngeal cancer: a comparison of adults living independently and patients living in long-term care facilities. *Spec Care Dentist*, 25(2), 124–30.

10 Ingram SS, Seo PH, Sloane R, et al. (2005). The association between oral health and general health and quality of life in older male cancer patients. *J Am Geriatr Soc*, 53(9), 1504–9.

11 Ettinger RL (1984). Clinical decision making in the dental treatment of the elderly. *Gerodontology*, 3(2), 157–65.

12 Hamermann D (1999). Toward an understanding of frailty. *Ann Intern Med*, 130(11), 945–50.

13 Balducci L (2006). Management of cancer in the elderly. *Oncology (Williston Park)*, 20(2), 135–43.

14 Hurria A, Lachs MS, Cohen HJ, Muss HB, Kornblith AB (2006). Geriatric assessment for oncologists: rationale and future directions. *Crit Rev Oncol Hematol*, 59(3), 211–17.

15 Extermann M, Aapro M, Bernabei R, et al. (2005). Use of comprehensive geriatric assessment in older cancer patients: recommendations from the task force on CGA of the International Society of Geriatric Oncology (SIOG). *Crit Rev Oncol Hematol*, 55(3), 241–52.

16 Jiang P, Choi M, Smith D, Heilbrun L, Gadgeel SM (2006). Characteristics and outcomes of cancer patients ≥80 years treated with chemotherapy at a comprehensive cancer center. *J Clin Oncol*, 24(18S), 8548.

17 Repetto L (2003). Greater risks of chemotherapy toxicity in elderly patients with cancer. *J Support Oncol*, 1(4 Suppl 2), 18–24.

18 Lye KW, Wee J, Gao F, Neo PS, Soong YL, Poon CY (2007). The effect of prior radiation therapy for treatment of nasopharyngeal cancer on wound healing following extractions: incidence of complications and risk factors. *Int J Oral Maxillofac Surg*, 36(4), 315–20.

19 Ferguson DB (1987). *The aging mouth*. Karger AG, Basel.

20 Turner MD, Ship JA (2007). Dry mouth and its effects on the oral health of elderly people. *J Am Dent Assoc*, 138(Suppl), 15S–20S.

21 Weiffenbach JM, Baum BJ, Burghauser R (1982). Taste thresholds: quality specific variation with human aging. *J. Gerontol*, 37(3), 372–7.

22 Sonies BC, Stone M, Shawker T (1984). Speech and swallowing in the elderly. *Gerodontology*, 3(2), 115–23.

23 Palmer JL, Metheny NA (2008). Preventing aspiration in older adults with dysphagia. *Am J Nurs*, 108(2), 40–8.

24 Extermann M (2005). Older patients, cognitive impairment, and cancer: an increasingly frequent triad. *J Natl Compr Canc Netw*, 3(4), 593–6.

25 Field MJ, Lawrence RL, Zwanziger L (2000). *Extending Medicare coverage for preventive and other services*. National Academy Press, Washington DC.

26 Patton LL, White BA, Field MJ (2001). Extending Medicare coverage to medically necessary dental care. *J Am Dent Assoc*, 132(9), 1294–9.

27 Silverman S Jr (2005). Controlling oral and pharyngeal cancer. Can dental professionals make a difference? *J Am Dent Assoc*, 136(5), 576–8.

28 Epstein JB, Parker IR, Epstein MS, Gupta A, Kutis S, Witkowski DM (2007). A survey of National Cancer Institute-designated comprehensive cancer centers' oral health supportive care practices and resources in the USA. *Support Care Cancer*, 15(4), 357–62.

29 Epstein JB, Parker IR, Epstein MS, Stevenson-Moore P (2004). Cancer-related oral health care services and resources: a survey of oral and dental care in Canadian cancer centres. *J Can Dent Assoc*, 70(5), 302–4.

30 Barker GJ, Epstein JB, Williams KB, Gorsky M, Raber-Durlacher JE (2005). Current practice and knowledge of oral care for cancer patients: a survey of supportive health care providers. *Support Care Cancer*, 13(1), 32–41.

31 Rodin MB (2008). Cancer patients admitted to nursing homes: what do we know? *J Am Med Dir Assoc*, 9(3), 149–56.

32 Kiyak HA, Grayston MN, Crinean CL (1993). Oral health problems and needs of nursing home residents. *Community Dent Oral Epidemiol*, 21(1), 49–52.

Chapter 28

Oral care in advanced cancer patients

Andrew Davies

Introduction

Advanced cancer is defined as 'cancer that has spread to other places in the body and usually cannot be cured or controlled with treatment'[1]. In the United Kingdom, many patients with advanced cancer receive specialist palliative care, and indeed most patients receiving specialist palliative care have advanced cancer (e.g. ~93% home-care patients/inpatients in 2006) [National Council for Palliative Care (UK), personal communication]. The basis of this chapter is information derived from the somewhat limited palliative care literature on oral problems/oral care[2].

Epidemiology

Oral symptoms are common in patients with advanced cancer (Table 28.1)[3–8]. Most patients have at least one symptom, and many patients have several symptoms. Oral symptoms are also common relative to other symptoms in patients with advanced cancer[7,8]. Indeed, xerostomia (dry mouth) is consistently ranked as one of the five most common symptoms in this group of patients[7–10].

Investigators have found disparities between the recorded prevalence of certain oral symptoms and the true prevalence of these oral symptoms in patients with advanced cancer[11]. These disparities probably relate to service-related factors (e.g. inadequate oral assessment procedures), professional-related factors (e.g. perception that these symptoms are unimportant), and patient-related factors (e.g. perception that other symptoms are more important)[12]. It should be noted that the figures in Table 28.1 are based on studies where patients were specifically asked about the presence of oral symptoms, rather than studies where patients were expected to spontaneously report the presence of oral symptoms.

Oral infections are also common in patients with advanced cancer. A number of studies have assessed oral candidosis in this group of patients (Table 28.2)[3,4,13–17], and there appears to be an association between the presence of oral candidosis and poor performance status[16,17]. In contrast, few studies have assessed other oral infections in this group of patients. Nevertheless, dental caries has been reported in 20–35% patients[4,5], and gingivitis in 36% patients[3]. Oral herpes simplex virus infections are also relatively common in patients with advanced cancer[18].

Denture-related problems are again common in patients with advanced cancer. The reported prevalence of subjective problems is 45–86%[3–5], and of objective problems is 57–83% in edentulous patients with advanced cancer[3–5]. Most problems relate to poor fitting of the dentures (e.g. oral discomfort, oral ulceration, food getting stuck under denture). Denture-related fungal infections are also common in patients with advanced cancer (i.e. denture stomatitis, angular cheilitis). The reported prevalence of isolated denture stomatitis is 22%, of isolated angular cheilitis is 4%, and of combined denture stomatitis and angular cheilitis is 22% in edentulous patients with advanced cancer[7].

Table 28.1 Prevalence of oral symptoms in patients with advanced cancer

Study	Population type/size	Prevalence oral symptoms					
		Xerostomia (dry mouth)	Oral discomfort	Taste disturbance	Difficulty chewing	Difficulty swallowing	Difficulty speaking
Gordon et al., 1985 [3]	Hospice inpatients (n = 31)	62%	55%	31%	52%	No data	59%
Aldred et al., 1991 [4]	Hospice inpatients (n = 20)	58%	42%	26%	No data	37%	No data
Jobbins et al., 1992 [5]	Hospice inpatients (n = 197)	77%	33%	37%	No data	35%	No data
Oneschuk et al., 2000 [6]	'Advanced cancer' patients (n = 99)	88%	16%*	No data	No data	No data	No data
Davies, 2000 [7]	Hospital inpatients/outpatients (n = 120)	78%	46%	44%	23%	23%	31%
Tranmer et al., 2003 [8]	Hospital inpatients (n = 66)	82%	No data	50%	No data	24%	No data

* "Oral pain" rather than oral discomfort

Table 28.2 Prevalence of oral candidosis in patients with advanced cancer

Study	Population type/size	Prevalence oral candidosis
Boggs et al., 1961 [13]	Hospital inpatient (n = 90)	14%
Rodu et al., 1984 [14]	Hospital inpatient (n = 52)	8%
Gordon et al., 1985 [3]	Hospice inpatient (n = 31)	10%
Clarke et al., 1987 [15]	Hospice inpatient (n = 46)	83%
Aldred et al., 1991 [4]	Hospice inpatient (n = 20)	70%
Davies et al., 2001 [16]	Hospital support team patients (n = 120)	30%
Davies et al., 2008 [17]	Hospice day centre patients (n = 390)	13%

Aetiology

Oral problems in patients with advanced cancer may be related to: (1) a direct (anatomical) effect of the cancer; (2) an indirect (physiological) effect of the cancer; (3) an effect of the treatment of the cancer; (4) an effect of a coexisting disease; (5) an effect of the treatment of a coexisting disease; or (6) a combination of these factors[19].

The indirect effects of the cancer are a major underlying cause of the oral problems in this group of patients[19]. Thus, patients often develop physical problems (e.g. fatigue), which may impede their ability to undertake oral hygiene measures. Moreover, patients often develop psychological problems (e.g. depression) and/or cognitive problems (e.g. confusion), which may further affect their ability/desire to undertake oral hygiene measures.

It should be noted that many oral problems are related to the underlying presence of salivary gland dysfunction (e.g. xerostomia, taste disturbance, oral candidosis, dental caries).[20] Salivary gland dysfunction is extremely common in palliative care patients (Table 28.1), and is usually secondary to drug treatment in this group of patients[21,22]. Indeed, salivary gland dysfunction is a side effect of many of the drugs used in supportive care/palliative care (e.g. analgesics, antiemetics)[21,23]. Salivary gland dysfunction is discussed, in detail, in Chapter 21.

Clinical features

Oral problems are a significant direct cause of morbidity in palliative care patients. Table 28.3 shows the severity of oral symptoms, whilst Table 28.4 shows the distress caused by oral symptoms, in an advanced cancer population[7]. Moreover, oral problems can lead to a more generalised deterioration in a patient's physical state, and also in their psychological state[24]. Oral problems are also an indirect cause of mortality in palliative care patients (i.e. oral colonization/infection leading to systemic infection)[25,26].

Salivary gland dysfunction is one of the few oral problems to have been formally investigated in patients with advanced cancer[20–22,24,27]. Unsurprisingly, the data in patients with advanced cancer somewhat mirrors the data in the general population/other groups of patients[28].

Table 28.3 Severity of oral symptoms in patients with advanced cancer [7]

Symptom (n = 120)	'Slight'	'Moderate'	'Severe'	'Very severe'
Dry mouth (n = 93)	14%	37%	33%	16%
Mouth discomfort (n = 55)	40%	29%	22%	9%
Change in the way food tastes (n = 53)	30%	45%	19%	6%
Difficulty speaking (n = 37)	40%	30%	19%	11%
Difficulty swallowing (n = 28)	46%	29%	14%	11%
Difficulty chewing (n = 27)	41%	41%	11%	7%
Mouth sores (n = 17)	59%	35%	6%	0%

Thus, it has been reported that the severity of xerostomia is associated with the severity of oral discomfort, anorexia, taste disturbance, difficulty chewing, difficulty swallowing, and difficulty speaking in patients with advanced cancer[21]. Furthermore, xerostomia has been shown to be associated with the development of oral candidosis in this group of patients[16,17]. It has also been reported that the presence of an abnormally low unstimulated whole salivary flow rate (<0.1 ml/min) is associated with the presence of xerostomia, oral discomfort, difficulty swallowing, and difficulty speaking in patients with advanced cancer[22]. Salivary gland dysfunction is also associated with significant psychosocial morbidity in this group of patients (Box 28.1)[24].

Oral candidosis has also been formally investigated in patients with advanced cancer [13–17]. Oral candidosis is not a single entity, but a spectrum of very different clinical entities

Table 28.4 Distress caused by oral symptoms in patients with advanced cancer [7]

Symptom (n = 120)	'Not at all'	'A little bit'	'Somewhat'	'Quite a bit'	'Very much'
Dry mouth (n = 93)	16%	21%	23%	26%	14%
Mouth discomfort (n = 55)	16%	31%	18%	26%	9%
Change in the way food tastes (n = 53)	17%	32%	23%	21%	7%
Difficulty speaking (n = 37)	3%	32%	24%	22%	19%
Difficulty swallowing (n = 28)	11%	28%	36%	14%	11%
Difficulty chewing (n = 27)	11%	44%	15%	30%	0%
Mouth sores (n = 17)	18%	35%	18%	29%	0%

Box 28.1 Quotations from advanced cancer patients with salivary gland dysfunction [24]

- Quote A:
  "It's so dry and sticky, my mouth glues, sometimes I have difficulties even opening my mouth".

- Quote B:
  "Sweet food had a bad taste, strong food was burning and tingling on the tongue. Fluids with carbonic acid felt like hydrochloric acid".

- Quote C:
  "Eating takes a long time, I stayed there at the table for 30-45 minutes after everybody else. I had to sip before each swallowing, totally about 1 litre of water".

- Quote D
  "We were to celebrate my birthday and I had helped to prepare salmon and looked forward to have dinner with the family. The taste alteration was incredible, the food tasted of absolutely nothing or possibly of wheat flower; I was disappointed and depressed and felt sorry for myself, I couldn't feel or share happiness with my family during that occasion".

- Quote E:
  "I wanted to surprise my family with a nice meal, with my speciality which is salty herring. Normally, I am very proud of it but I totally failed with the seasoning as I did not feel the taste, I used far too much salt, the meal was uneatable. I was so embarrassed".

- Quote F:
  "I used to participate in choir singing, nowadays I can't sing at all because my voice is so weak, my vocal cords are so dry... so I won't participate at all, I avoid all these things and prefer staying at home. I feel sorry and depressed".

(e.g. pseudomembranous candidosis, erythematous candidosis, denture stomatitis, angular cheilitis)[29]. Patients with advanced cancer may exhibit any of the variants of oral candidosis, and frequently (25–31%) exhibit more than one variant of oral candidosis at the same time (Table 28.5)[16,17]. Oral candidosis is often extensive/multifocal in patients with advanced cancer, and also often a persistent/recurrent problem in this group of patients.

Assessment

The assessment of oral problems is essentially similar to the assessment of other medical problems. It involves taking a history, performing an examination, and the use of appropriate investigations[30]. Many of the oral assessment tools that are used in palliative care are not validated for use in this clinical setting (and indeed are not appropriate for use in this clinical setting)[31]. The assessment of oral problems is discussed, in detail, in Chapter 3.

A wide range of investigations are used in every day clinical practice[30], but only some of these investigations will be relevant in patients with advanced cancer (e.g. microbiological testing). The decision to perform an investigation will depend on the nature of the problem (important or not), the nature of the investigation (invasive or not), the likely outcome of the investigation (management altered or not), and the condition/prognosis of the patient[31].

Table 28.5 Prevalence of variants of oral candidosis in patients with advanced cancer [17]

Variants of oral candidosis	Number of subjects (n = 51)
Pseudomembranous	23
Denture stomatitis	6
Angular cheilitis	5
Erythematous	4
Pseudomernbranous + denture stomatitis	6
Pseudomembranous + angular cheilitis	1
Pseudomembranous + erythematous	1
Pseudomembranous + denture stomatitis + angular cheilitis	1
Pseudomembranous + denture stomatitis + erythematous	1
Denture stomatitis + angular cheilitis	2
Angular cheilitis + erythematous	1

Management

The successful management of oral problems involves adequate assessment, appropriate treatment, and adequate re-assessment. The aims of assessment are to determine the nature of the problem, and factors that may influence the choice of treatment. Inadequate assessment may result in the use of ineffective or inappropriate interventions. The aims of re-assessment are to determine the response to the treatment (i.e. efficacy of treatment, tolerability of treatment). Inadequate re-assessment may result in the continued use of ineffective or inappropriate interventions (and ongoing morbidity from the oral problem).

The treatment of oral problems may involve definitive management of the problem ('cure'), symptomatic management of the problem ('palliation'), management of the cause of the problem, and/or management of the complications of the problem. Whilst there may be a range of options for management in everyday practice, there may be fewer options for management in patients with advanced cancer. The decision to undertake a treatment depends on a number of factors, including the nature of the problem, the nature of the treatment, the availability of the treatment, the general health/condition of the patient, and, particularly, the wishes of the patient.

In some cases the most appropriate treatment for a patient with advanced cancer is the same treatment that would be given to a patient with early cancer (or even no cancer). Thus, intensive treatment of the oral problem often results in the foremost palliation of the oral problem. It is not justified to withhold treatment on the grounds that the patient has advanced cancer. However, it is justified to amend treatment (when appropriate) on the grounds that the patient has advanced cancer. For example, the standard treatment for a poorly fitting denture involves fabrication of a new denture. However, in patients with a poor performance status, an alternative treatment for a poorly fitting denture would involve re-lining of the old denture[32].

Multidisciplinary working

Oral care/problems should be the concern of all clinical members of the core palliative care multidisciplinary team (MDT). However, oral care is often delegated to the nursing staff, and performed by the junior nursing staff[33]. Studies suggest that most nurses receive minimal education about oral care during their training, and so require further/ongoing education about oral care in order to properly undertake this activity[34]. Similarly, most doctors receive minimal (if any) education about oral care during their training.

Dental professionals are important members of the extended palliative care MDT (i.e. dentists, dental hygienists)[35]. They have a number of key roles, including: (1) training of other members of the MDT; (2) management of specific oral problems (e.g. dental caries); and (3) management of complex oral problems (in combination with other members of the MDT). Many dental procedures can be performed in the home/hospice setting, although such 'domiciliary dentistry' requires specialized skills and appropriate equipment[32].

Other members of the MDT team will, of course, have a major role in the management of certain oral problems (e.g. speech and language therapists, dieticians).

Oral care in palliative care

Oral care in palliative care is frequently based on historical anecdote, rather than on available research evidence[36]. Hence, many patients continue to receive relatively ineffective treatments for their oral problems (e.g. ice cubes for xerostomia), whilst some patients continue to receive entirely inappropriate treatments for their oral problems (e.g. pineapple chunks for xerostomia)[37].

Nevertheless, evidence-based guidelines on the management of oral problems in patients with advanced cancer have been developed[2,18]. The evidence for these guidelines comes from studies involving different groups of patients, and increasingly from studies involving patients with advanced cancer (see below). These guidelines stress the particular importance of individualized care in this group of patients.

The management of salivary gland dysfunction has been the focus of several clinical trials in patients with advanced cancer. The results of relevant randomized controlled clinical trials involving saliva stimulants are shown in Table 28.6[38,39], whilst the results of relevant randomized controlled clinical trials involving saliva substitutes are shown in Table 28.7[38–40]. The management of salivary gland dysfunction is discussed, in detail, in Chapter 21.

The management of oral candidosis has also been the focus of several clinical trials in patients with advanced cancer. Studies suggest that azole (i.e. fluconazole, itraconazole) resistance is now common, whilst polyene (i.e. amphotericin, nystatin) resistance remains uncommon, amongst the yeasts colonizing the oral cavity of patients with advanced cancer[41,42]. It is thought that the reason for the increase in azole resistance is related to the increase in the use of azole drugs in the general population, and the associated increase in non-*Candida albicans* species colonizing the oral cavity of patients with advanced cancer (e.g. *C. glabrata*, *C. dubliniensis*)[43].

Oral care in the terminal phase

Oral care often takes prominence during the terminal phase of the illness. Indeed, oral care is a major component of so-called integrated care pathways ('care of the dying' pathways)[44].

Table 28.6 Randomized controlled trials of saliva stimulants in the palliative care setting

Study	Treatment	Effectiveness of treatment	Side effects of treatment	Other comments
Davies et al., 1998 [38]	Pilocarpine 5mg tds	Improvement in xerostomia ♦ 90% subjects	Side effects ♦ 84% subjects ♦ sweating, dizziness, lacrimation	RCT: mucin-based artificial saliva vs pilocarpine. 76% of patients wanted to continue with pilocarpine. Pilocarpine more effective than mucin-based artificial saliva.
Davies 2000 [39]	Chewing gum 1-2 pieces qds	Improvement in xerostomia ♦ 90 % subjects	Side effects ♦ 22% subjects ♦ irritation of mouth, nausea, unpleasant taste	RCT: mucin-based artificial saliva vs chewing gum. 86% of patients wanted to continue with chewing gum. Chewing gum as effective as mucin-based artificial saliva. (Patients preferred chewing gum).

However, the oral care protocols in these pathways are not evidence-based, and are reported to produce somewhat disappointing outcomes[45].

Certain authors recommend 1–2 hourly oral care patients in the terminal phase[46]. This is very obtrusive for patients (and families), and very time consuming for healthcare professionals. Some patients may require this frequency of care, although many patients require much less frequent care, to maintain oral comfort. Thus, the frequency of oral care should be determined on an individual basis rather than on the basis of a written protocol.

Oral care is often delegated to families in the terminal phases[47]. Some family members relish this task, whilst others find it difficult and/or distressing. It is important, if appropriate, that families are given the opportunity to provide oral care. Equally, it is important that families are not coerced into providing oral care. Furthermore, healthcare professionals must provide adequate instructions, and on going support and supervision, for families that do undertake this task.

One of the most common problems amongst unconscious patients is the presence of a desiccated oral mucosa. Family members (and healthcare professionals) often perceive this as a source of discomfort, although it is unlikely to be the case in an unconscious patient. Oral care protocols often recommend the regular application of water. However, this strategy is largely ineffective, since the water rapidly dissipates as a result of swallowing and/or evaporation. A more effective intervention involves the regular application of a suitable water-based moisturizing gel (e.g. KY® jelly, Oral Balance® gel).

The philosophy of care in the terminal phase should be the maintenance of patient comfort[48]. It is relatively easy to determine the merits of oral care in conscious patients. Thus, healthcare professionals should always ask patients about their experiences of oral care (i.e. whether the oral care makes them feel better, whether the oral care causes any problems). Nevertheless, it is much less easy to determine the merits of oral care in unconscious patients. However, if an intervention causes or appears to cause distress, then that intervention should be discontinued (irrespective of the perceived merits of the intervention).

Table 28.7 Randomized controlled trials of saliva substitutes in the palliative care setting

Study	Treatment	Effectiveness of treatment	Side effects of treatment	Other comments
Sweeney et al., 1997[40]	Mucin-based artificial saliva prn	Improvement in xerostomia ◆ 60% subjects	Side effects ◆ none reported	RCT: mucin-based artificial saliva vs 'placebo' spray. 93% of patients wanted to continue with artificial saliva.
Davies et al., 1998 [38]	Mucin-based artificial saliva qds	Improvement in xerostomia ◆ 73% subjects	Side effects ◆ 31% subjects ◆ nausea, diarrhoea, irritation of mouth	RCT: mucin-based artificial saliva vs pilocarpine. 64% of patients wanted to continue with artificial saliva.
Davies AN 2000 [39]	Mucin-based artificial saliva qds	Improvement in xerostomia ◆ 89 % subjects	Side effects ◆ 19% subjects ◆ nausea, unpleasant taste, irritation of mouth	RCT: mucin-based artificial saliva vs chewing gum. 74% of patients wanted to continue with artificial saliva.

References

1 National Cancer Institute (US National Institutes of Health) website: http://www.cancer.gov/

2 Davies A, Finlay I (2005). *Oral care in advanced disease.* Oxford University Press, Oxford.

3 Gordon SR, Berkey DB, Call RL (1985). Dental need among hospice patients in Colorado: a pilot study. *Gerodontics,* 1(3), 125–9.

4 Aldred MJ, Addy M, Bagg J, Finlay I (1991). Oral health in the terminally ill: a cross-sectional pilot survey. *Spec Care Dentist,* 11(2), 59–62.

5 Jobbins J, Bagg J, Finlay IG, Addy M, Newcombe RG (1992). Oral and dental disease in terminally ill cancer patients. *Br Med J,* 304(6842), 1612.

6 Oneschuk D, Hanson J, Bruera E (2000). A survey of mouth pain and dryness in patients with advanced cancer. *Support Care Cancer,* 8(5), 372–6.

7 Davies AN (2000). *An investigation into the relationship between salivary gland hypofunction and oral health problems in patients with advanced cancer [Dissertation].* King's College: University of London.

8 Tranmer JE, Heyland D, Dudgeon D, Groll D, Squires-Graham M, Coulson K (2003). Measuring the symptom experience of seriously ill cancer and noncancer hospitalized patients near the end of life with the Memorial Symptom Assessment Scale. *J Pain Symptom Manage* 25(5), 420–9.

9 Reuben DB, Mor V, Hiris J (1988). Clinical symptoms and length of survival in patients with terminal cancer. *Arch Intern Med,* 148(7), 1586–91.

10 Ventafridda V, De Conno F, Ripamonti C, Gamba A, Tamburini M (1990). Quality-of-life assessment during a palliative care programme. *Ann Oncol,* 1(6), 415–20.

11 Shah S, Davies AN (2001). Medical records vs. patient self-rating. *J Pain Symptom Manage,* 22(4), 805–6.

12 Shorthose K, Davies A (2003). Symptom prevalence in palliative care. *Palliat Med,* 17(8), 723–4.

13 Boggs DR, Williams AF, Howell A (1961). Thrush in malignant neoplastic disease. *Arch Intern Med,* 107, 354–60.

14 Rodu B, Griffin IL, Gockerman JP (1984). Oral candidosis in cancer patients. *Southern Med J,* 77(3), 312–14.

15 Clarke JMG, Wilson JA, von Haacke NP, Milne LJ (1987). Oral candidiasis in terminal illness. *Health Bull (Edinb),* 45(5), 268–71.

16 Davies AN, Brailsford SR, Beighton D (2006). Oral candidosis in patients with advanced cancer. *Oral Oncology,* 42(7), 698–702.

17 Davies AN, Brailsford SR, Beighton D, Shorthose K, Stevens VC (2008). Oral candidosis in community-based patients with advanced cancer. *J Pain Symptom Manage,* 35(5), 508–14.

18 Sweeney MP, Bagg J (2000). The mouth and palliative care. *Am J Hosp Palliat Care,* 17(2), 118–24.

19 Davies A (2005a). Introduction, in Davies A, Finlay I (eds) *Oral Care in Advanced Disease,* pp. 1–6. Oxford University Press, Oxford.

20 Sweeney MP, Bagg J, Baxter WP, Aitchison TC (1998). Oral disease in terminally ill cancer patients with xerostomia. *Oral Oncol,* 34(2), 123–6.

21 Davies AN, Broadley K, Beighton D (2001). Xerostomia in patients with advanced cancer. *J Pain Symptom Manage,* 22(4), 820–5.

22 Davies AN, Broadley K, Beighton D (2002). Salivary gland hypofunction in patients with advanced cancer. *Oral Oncol,* 38(7), 680–5.

23 Sreebny LM, Schwartz SS (1997). A reference guide to drugs and dry mouth, 2nd edn. *Gerodontology,* 14(1), 33–47.

24 Rydholm M, Strang P (2002). Physical and psychosocial impact of xerostomia in palliative cancer care: a qualitative interview study. *Int J Palliat Nurs,* 8(7), 318–23.

25 Meurman JH, Pyrhonen S, Teerenhovi L, Lindqvist C (1997). Oral sources of septicaemia in patients with malignancies. *Oral Oncol,* 33(6), 389–97.

26 Mandel ID (2004). Oral infections: impact on human health, well-being, and health-care costs. *Compend Contin Educ Dent*, 25(11), 881–90.

27 Chaushu G, Bercovici M, Dori S, et al. (2000). Salivary flow and its relation with oral symptoms in terminally ill patients. *Cancer*, 88(5), 984–7.

28 Sreebny LM (1996). Xerostomia: diagnosis, management and clinical complications, in Edgar WM, O'Mullane DM (eds) *Saliva and Oral Health*, 2nd edn, pp. 43–66. British Dental Association, London.

29 Axell T, Samaranayake LP, Reichart PA, Olsen I (1997). A proposal for reclassification of oral candidosis. *Oral Surg Oral Med Oral Pathol Oral Radiol Endod*, 84(2), 111–12.

30 Birnbaum W, Dunne SM (2000). *Oral diagnosis: the clinician's guide.* Wright, Oxford.

31 Davies A (2005b). Assessment, in Davies A, Finlay I (eds) *Oral Care in Advanced Disease*, pp.7–19. Oxford University Press, Oxford.

32 Walls A (2005). Domiciliary dental care, in Davies A, Finlay I (eds) *Oral Care in Advanced Disease*, pp. 37–45. Oxford University Press, Oxford.

33 Miller M, Kearney N (2001). Oral care for patients with cancer: a review of the literature. *Cancer Nurs*, 24(4), 241–53.

34 Southern H (2007). Oral care in cancer nursing: nurses' knowledge and education. *J Adv Nurs*, 57(6), 631–8.

35 Cummings I (1998). The interdisciplinary team, in Doyle D, Hanks G, Cherny NI, Calman K (eds) *Oxford Textbook of Palliative Medicine*, 2nd edn, pp. 21. Oxford University Press, Oxford.

36 Davies A (1998). Clinically proven treatments for xerostomia were ignored. *Br Med J*, 316(7139), 1247.

37 De Conno F, Sbanotto A, Ripamonti C, Ventafridda V (2004). Mouth care, in Doyle D, Hanks G, Cherny NI, Calman K (eds) *Oxford Textbook of Palliative Medicine*, 2nd edn, pp. 673–87. Oxford University Press, Oxford.

38 Davies AN, Daniels C, Pugh R, Sharma K (1998). A comparison of artificial saliva and pilocarpine in the management of xerostomia in patients with advanced cancer. *Palliat Med*, 12(2), 105–11.

39 Davies AN (2000). A comparison of artificial saliva and chewing gum in the management of xerostomia in patients with advanced cancer. *Palliat Med*, 14(3), 197–203.

40 Sweeney MP, Bagg J, Baxter WP, Aitchison TC (1997). Clinical trial of a mucin-containing oral spray for treatment of xerostomia in hospice patients. *Palliat Med*, 11(3), 225–32.

41 Davies A, Brailsford S, Broadley K, Beighton D (2002). Resistance amongst yeasts isolated from the oral cavities of patients with advanced cancer. *Palliat Med*, 16(6), 527–31.

42 Bagg J, Sweeney MP, Lewis MA, et al. (2003). High prevalence of non-albicans yeasts and detection of antifungal resistance in the oral flora of patients with advanced cancer. *Palliat Med*, 17(6), 477–81.

43 Finlay I, Davies A (2005). Fungal infections, in Davies A, Finlay I (eds) *Oral Care in Advanced Disease*, pp. 55–71. Oxford University Press, Oxford.

44 Ellershaw J, Ward C (2003). Care of the dying patient: the last hours or days of life. *Br Med J*, 326(7379), 30–4.

45 Fowell A, Finlay I, Johnstone R, Minto L (2002). An integrated care pathway for the last two days of life: Wales-wide benchmarking in palliative care. *Int J Palliat Nurs*, 8(12), 566–73.

46 Anonymous (1996). *Managing oral care problems throughout the cancer illness trajectory*, pp. 9. The Macmillan Practice Development Unit, London.

47 Goodman M (2003). Symptom control in care of the dying. Section 3, in Ellershaw J, Wilkinson S (eds) *Care of the Dying. A Pathway to Excellence*, pp. 55–7. Oxford University Press, Oxford.

48 Sweeney P (2005). Oral hygiene, in Davies A, Finlay I (eds) *Oral Care in Advanced Disease*, pp. 21–35. Oxford University Press, Oxford.

Chapter 29

Quality of life and health economics

Jennifer Beaumont, David Cella, and Joshua Epstein

What is quality of life?

Quality of life (QoL) is a subjective concept that encompasses all of life's circumstances, including personal resources, environmental and social conditions, health and its impact on daily function, emotional well-being, and overall satisfaction with life[1].

Health-related quality of life (HRQoL) 'refers to the extent to which one's usual or expected physical, emotional, and social well-being are affected by a medical condition or its treatment'[2]. HRQoL consists of those aspects of QoL – physical, emotional, and social – which can be directly or indirectly related to one's health.

Quality of life is an inherently subjective concept, and so it is imperative to obtain information from the patient. Thus, even when objective measures are available for the given condition, the patient's perspective is necessary to obtain a full understanding of a condition. For example, clinician ratings of oral mucositis are highly dependent on the examiner's ability to assess the severity of the ulceration[3], and may not allow for immediate detection of changes in the condition. Indeed, in a recent phase III study of palifermin, patients reported onset, peak, and resolution of oral pain 1–3 days earlier than clinician-observed changes in oral mucositis[4].

How do you measure health-related quality of life?

Many instruments exist to measure QoL. Administration of these measures can include interview, self-administration of paper questionnaires, computer-assisted telephone interviews, Internet-based questionnaires, and computer-adaptive test administration. The choice of instrument (and method of administration) depends on the population under study, and the specific outcomes of interest.

Generic health-related quality of life tools

Generic measures ask questions that are applicable to everyone, irrespective of the presence or absence of particular health conditions. Generic measures allow for the comparison of HRQoL status across disease groups, and they enable comparison of individuals and groups to the general population.

One of the most widely used general HRQoL measures is the Medical Outcomes Study 36-item Short Form Health Survey (SF-36)[5]. The SF-36 evaluates eight domains: physical functioning, role limitations due to physical health, social functioning, pain, vitality, mental health, role limitations due to emotional health, and general health perceptions. The individual scores can be combined to create physical and mental summary scores.

Some generic instruments were developed for use in cancer populations, but have been used with little to no modifications in other patient groups and in the general population (e.g. FACT-G, EORTC-QLC-C30). The Functional Assessment of Cancer Therapy-General (FACT-G) is a

27-item HRQoL questionnaire that assesses physical, social/family, emotional, and functional well-being[6]. The European Organization for Research and Treatment of Cancer Quality of Life Questionnaire (EORTC-QLQ-C30) is a 30-item questionnaire that assesses role, cognitive, emotional, and social functioning, together with individual symptoms (e.g. fatigue, nausea and vomiting, pain) and global health status [7].

A new generation of generic tools has been developed using extensive qualitative and psychometric methods under the Patient Reported Outcomes Measurement Information System (PROMIS) cooperative group funded by the United States National Institutes of Health[8,9]. These tools enable clinical researchers to experience the advantages of generic assessment with the heightened precision usually reserved for targeted QoL tools.

Targeted health-related quality of life tools

Targeted measures ask questions that tend to be more specific to a given disease, symptom, or treatment. Disease-specific instruments focus on the concerns, symptoms, and treatment side effects associated with a particular disease (e.g. head and neck cancer). Symptom-specific measures focus on a specific symptom or problem that is common across many different diseases (e.g. fatigue, depression). Treatment-specific measures focus on concerns that are associated with a particular treatment (e.g. radiotherapy/radiation therapy). Specific instruments are often more sensitive, but do not capture all aspects of health. For this reason, many clinicians and researchers prefer a combined approach, administering both generic and specific measures.

Disease-specific

1. The FACT-Head and Neck (FACT-HN) scale is a self-report instrument consisting of the FACT-G and a head and neck cancer-specific subscale[10]. The 10 items of the head and neck cancer-specific subscale measure ability to eat, dry mouth, ability to breath, voice quality and strength, concerns regarding appearance, ability to swallow, and mouth, throat, and neck pain.

2. The FACT-HN Symptom Index (FHNSI) is comprised of 10 items from the FACT-HN that have been selected by experts as the most important symptom targets when treating patients with advanced head and neck cancer[11]. The 10 items include pain, lack of energy, ability to swallow, face/neck pain, trouble breathing, ability to communicate, nausea, ability to eat solid foods, worrying condition will worsen, and contentment with current QoL.

3. The EORTC QLQ-H&N35 assesses QoL associated with head and neck cancer and its treatment, and consists of scales measuring pain, swallowing, speech, special senses, social eating, social contact, and sexuality[12]. The EORTC QLQ-H&N35 is applicable to all head and neck cancers, and to all modalities of treatment.

4. The University of Washington Quality of Life scale (UW-QOL) is designed for use in head and neck cancer patients, and measures 12 domains of HRQoL (i.e. pain, appearance, activity, recreation, swallowing, chewing, speech, shoulder problems, taste, saliva, mood, and anxiety) as well as global HRQoL and QoL[13].

Symptom-specific

1. The EORTC oral symptom and function scale is an addendum to the QLQ-C30 that measures four domains: face and mouth pain, tooth pain, mouth function (e.g. chewing, swallowing), and changes following radiation[14]. This scale has been shown to be responsive to change during treatment and subsequent follow-up[15].

2. The Oral Mucositis Daily Questionnaire (OMDQ) is a 10-item questionnaire designed for daily administration. The questions assess mouth and throat soreness and related functional

limitations (i.e. sleeping, swallowing, drinking, eating, and talking), together with overall health[4].

3. The Oral Mucositis Weekly Questionnaire – Head and Neck Cancer (OMWQ-HN) is based on the OMDQ (and similarly assesses mouth and throat soreness and related functional limitations)[16].

Treatment-specific

1. The McMaster University Head and Neck Radiotherapy Questionnaire (HNRQ) consists of 22 items that evaluate symptoms in six domains: oral cavity, throat, skin, digestion, energy, and psychosocial[17].

2. The Quality of Life-Radiation Therapy Instrument/Head and Neck companion module (QOL-RTI/H&N) is both disease and treatment specific. The QOL-RTI/H&N is a 39-item self-report questionnaire consisting of the 25 general items of the QOL-RTI plus a 14-item head and neck module that assesses pain, saliva, mucus, taste, chewing, swallowing, speech, appearance, and cough. This questionnaire was designed to be specifically relevant to the head and neck radiotherapy patient[18].

What are the quality of life outcomes of oral complications?

Quality of life and head and neck radiotherapy

Numerous studies describe the symptom and HRQoL experience of head and neck cancer patients undergoing radiotherapy. In general, oral symptoms and impaired HRQoL are already present prior to radiotherapy, worsen while on treatment, and sometimes recover to pretreatment, but not necessarily healthy, levels. The following paragraphs detail some relevant studies.

One-hundred-thirty-eight head and neck cancer patients undergoing radiotherapy participated in a randomized, double-blind, controlled trial of an oral antimicrobial lozenge versus a placebo lozenge to prevent/treat oral mucositis[19]. Patients completed the EORTC QLQ-C30 and a trial-specific checklist during the study. Patients reported mild problems with emotional and social functioning prior to radiotherapy, as well as specific problems of fatigue, pain, and sleep disturbance. Global QoL was also impaired prior to treatment. During radiotherapy, patients experienced moderate worsening of chewing, marked worsening of mouth/throat pain, and mouth soreness on eating food. Dryness of the mouth rapidly worsened on radiotherapy, and did not recover following the radiotherapy. Moreover, patients experienced a moderate decrease in role-functioning scores following the radiotherapy.

In another sample of head and neck cancer patients, global QoL, as measured by the EORTC QLQ-C30, worsened during radiation therapy and only partially recovered in the 6 months following the treatment[15]. A similar pattern of change was observed for other domains of the EORTC QLQ-C30.

Seventy-five patients with head and neck cancer who were receiving radiation therapy with or without chemotherapy completed the OMWQ-HN and the FACT-HN 5 times during the course of the treatment[16]. There was a steady worsening of scores over time on all scales, and a corresponding increase in specific functional limitations.

As discussed, HRQoL deficits often persist for months following the completion of radiotherapy. Epstein et al.[14] studied 65 patients with primary head and neck cancers who had completed radiotherapy over 6 months earlier. The EORTC QLQ-C30 plus the EORTC oral symptom and function scale was used to measure HRQoL. Dry mouth was by far the most common symptom reported, with 92% of patients experiencing this complication. Other patient-reported oral symptoms included change in taste (75%), difficulty swallowing (63%), difficulty chewing (43%), and sore mouth when eating (40%). The majority of patients experienced some pain (58%), with 17% reporting moderate or severe pain. Approximately half of the patients reported tension, worrying, irritability, or depression. In addition, patients reported problems in functioning, including difficulty taking long walks or performing other strenuous activities (43%), and limitations with work or household jobs (42%). Indeed, 15% patients were unable to work. The cancer or its treatment also had effects on the patients' families (45%), on social activities (60%), and on personal finances (57%).

Quality of life and chemotherapy

Oral mucositis and other domains of HRQoL have been assessed in other groups of oncology patients. Sonis et al.[20] found that fatigue was more common in cycles with mucositis (9%) versus those without mucositis (5%) amongst patients with solid tumours who received myelo-suppressive chemotherapy.

Cella et al.[3] described subjective and objective measures of oral mucositis in 323 acute leukaemia, chronic leukaemia, lymphoma, and multiple myeloma patients randomized to iseganan or placebo for the treatment of chemotherapy-related oral mucositis. Patients were evaluated 3 times per week for the first 3 weeks of therapy. Objective measures consisted of clinician scoring of stomatitis and dysphagia using the National Cancer Institute Common Toxicity Criteria. Oral mucositis, by both objective and subjective measures, increased and then decreased over the course of the study. Most patients reported their peak mouth pain within 2 days of their peak stomatitis (57%). However, several patients did not experience any increase in mouth pain (29%), stomatitis (19%), and/or dysphagia (24%). Peak mouth-pain scores correlated with peak stomatitis ($r = 0.69$).

Quality of life and haematopoietic stem-cell transplantation

Another common setting for the evaluation of oral mucositis and its impact on HRQoL is haematopoietic stem-cell transplantation (HSCT). In a placebo-controlled trial of palifermin for oral mucositis, the OMDQ and FACT-G questionnaires were administered to patients[4]. There was a 38% reduction in mouth and throat soreness in the palifermin group. Similar reductions were also seen in terms of swallowing, drinking, eating, talking, and sleeping. The FACT physical and functional well-being scores were higher with palifermin, but there was no difference in the FACT emotional and social/family well-being scores.

What is health economics?

Health economics is the study of how healthcare resources are allocated within a society[21,22].

After a new healthcare technology has been shown to be both safe and effective, decision-makers typically ask themselves the following two questions: (1) Can they afford the new technology?; and (2) Is the new technology worth the additional costs? The field of health economics has developed specific methods to answer these questions, and so allow decision-makers to make rational assessments on how to deliver the most appropriate healthcare, given their limited budget.

Health economics is becoming increasingly important as healthcare spending continues to consume a larger percentage of the gross domestic product in many countries around the world. Indeed, many governments have established formal bodies to assess the cost-effectiveness of health technologies, such as the National Institute for Health and Clinical Excellence (NICE) in the United Kingdom.

How do you assess health economics?

Health economists first need to understand from what perspective the analysis should be taken. Typically, analyses are performed from the hospital, payer, or societal perspectives. The hospital and payer perspectives are generally only concerned about direct healthcare costs. Direct healthcare costs are those that the payer incurs, such as costs for a hospitalization or supportive care provided (i.e. nutritional support, drug treatment). The societal perspective is typically taken when decisions are being made at the national government level. Here, both direct healthcare costs and indirect productivity costs, such as lost wages due to disability or premature death, are assessed. Of note, direct costs from the societal perspective are best documented as costs borne by the payer, not what is charged by the hospital or physician[21].

Initially, a burden of illness study is conducted to determine the costs associated with the current standard of care in a disease state. These studies are typically retrospective analyses of patient records within a hospital's or an insurer's claim database. However, it is possible to prospectively collect this type of information.

After one has demonstrated the present burden of illness, and identified that a new medical technology would fulfill an unmet need, health economists will then want to assess the possible budget impact of this new health technology. Budget impact models can be developed to estimate number of patients who may benefit from the new treatment, and if the new additional costs will offset costs elsewhere in the system.

If the new treatment will be more costly than the present standard of care, the decision-maker will want to understand if the new treatment is 'worth' the additional cost. Costs can be evaluated against a variety of different metrics:

1. Cost–effectiveness analysis (CEA) – assesses cost compared to a particular outcome, such as cases prevented, hospital admissions prevented, and life years saved (LYS). These measures of effectiveness are typically easy for stakeholders to understand, and allow for comparison of medical technologies within the same disease state. A drawback to CEA is that it does not allow for easy comparisons across disease states (where different metrics of effectiveness may be used).

2. Cost–utility analysis (CUA) – uses a common metric of health that can be used to compare new treatments across disease states. This metric is called a quality-adjusted life year (QALY). A QALY is a measure of both the quality and quantity of life. The quality weight for 1 year of life has a value of 1 for perfect health and 0 for death. Hence, 5 years in perfect health would be considered 5 QALYs. If being in a particular health state is given a 0.5 quality weight, then 5 years in that health state would be considered to be 2.5 QALYs. Traditionally, therapies costing <$50 000/QALY have been deemed cost-effective, although the level of this threshold has been debated.

3. Cost–benefit analysis (CBA) – assesses both costs and benefits in monetary units. Benefits are valued in dollars (or other currencies) by assessing willingness to pay for that benefit. CBA is not used that much, because of the difficulties involved in valuing health benefits in monetary units.

What are the economic outcomes of oral complications?

Cost of oral cancer

A number of studies have examined the cost of treating oral cancer (see below). In general, the research shows that treating oral cancer is costly, that costs increase as tumour stage increases, and that costs are influenced by complications of cancer treatment.

It should be noted that cost of care analyses in cancer patients that are determined by review of patient care records are expected to underestimate the total cost of such care, as the estimated costs will be affected by the detail of recording/coding of complications, and the fact that some care may have been administered by other providers (e.g. dental/oral care).

Dutch researchers calculated that the average cost of diagnosis, treatment, and 2-year follow-up care in head and neck cancer patients was €21 858 (1996 Euros) within two Dutch university hospitals between 1994 and 1996[23]. The cost of treating head and neck cancer patients will be much higher, at present, as a result of inflation.

Funk and colleagues [24] used patient billing records from one university hospital system to determine that the median 1-year cost of treating oral cancer was approximately $32 000 (1983 US Dollars). The most significant factor in predicting healthcare costs in this sample was type of treatment modality used, followed by the stage of tumour.

Zavras et al.[25] also found that tumour stage was associated with treatment costs. They reviewed hospital records and reported the mean direct inpatient costs of treating Stage I, II, III, and IV oral cancer was $3662, $5867, $10 316, and $11 467 (2001 US Dollars), respectively. The relatively low cost of care figures found in this study may be attributable to the vagaries of the Greek healthcare system.

Similarly, a retrospective review of medical records within two UK hospitals revealed that the average 3-year cost of treating oral cancer patients increased with the stage of the disease[26]. Thus, costs for treating pre-cancer, stages 1, 2, 3, and 4 were £1869, £4914, £8535, £11 883, and £13 513, respectively.

The above studies were all conducted by reviewing the medical records of patients within one or two hospitals. Hence, these studies were unable to account for differences in care delivered at other hospitals, or healthcare received outside a hospital (i.e. primary care costs, social care costs). Another limitation of assessing costs within a hospital is that researchers typically use hospital charges rather than reimbursed costs, which are a better estimate of opportunity costs.

Lang et al.[27] showed that average Medicare payments (1998 US dollars) within the first year following diagnosis of head and neck cancer were $22 589 higher than age- and sex-matched patients without cancer. They also demonstrated the relationship of tumour stage and 5-year costs (i.e. $37 434, $42 698, $58 387, and $53 741 for *in situ*, localized, regional, distant disease, respectively). Furthermore, they estimated that the burden of head and neck cancer to Medicare over a 5-year timeframe could be more than $250 million. It should be noted that pharmaceuticals were not covered under Medicare during the study period, and so this study was unable to account for these additional costs.

Epstein et al.[28], using the Medicaid claims database, determined the median 1-year cost of medical care (including prescription drugs) for those treated for late-stage oral and pharyngeal cancer was $27 665, while those treated for early-stage disease was only $22 658. The actual costs may be higher than reported in this study, because Medicaid payments may be lower than private commercial plans, and direct costs paid by the patient were not included in the evaluation.

The above studies assessed costs from a hospital or insurers perspective. In order to assess costs from a societal perspective, the costs incurred by the patient must also be assessed. Yabroff and colleagues[29] estimated that, on average, the value of time head and neck cancer patients spend traveling to receive medical care, waiting for appointments, and receiving care within the first year following diagnosis was $2268. Furthermore, a report from the Centers for Disease Control and Prevention calculated that cancers of the lip, oral cavity, and pharynx were responsible for 82 863 years of potential life lost, which corresponded to $1.8 billion in productivity losses, between 1997 and 2001[30].

Cost-effectiveness of oral cancer screening

Oral cancer screening programmes are advocated due to the morbidity, mortality, and costs associated with oral cancer. They are particularly relevant in follow-up of previously treated patients with upper aerodigestive tract cancers, who are at highest risk of recurrence of original tumour and/or development of a new primary tumour.

The UK National Health Service R&D Health Technology Assessment programme developed a very comprehensive cost effectiveness model of various oral cancer-screening strategies[26]. These researchers determined that screening high-risk patients (tobacco and alcohol users) for oral cancer in the age range of 40 and 60 would be cost-effective (i.e. £18 919/QALY).

Cost-effectiveness of head and neck cancer therapy

Cost-effectiveness models can also be used to inform the most cost-effective therapy for cancer patients. A Japanese study [31] assessed sentinel lymph node radiolocalization as a navigation tool during surgery in 11 patients with early-stage head and neck cancer and determined that this technique would not only prevent seven surgical deaths per 1000 patients, but it would also save $1218 in costs as compared with ipsilateral neck dissection.

Hopper et al.[32] demonstrated the cost-effectiveness of using Foscan-mediated photodynamic therapy (Foscan-PDT) when compared to 'no treatment' for patients with advanced head and neck cancer (i.e. £14 206/LYS). Foscan-PDT was the better strategy when compared with either palliative chemotherapy or palliative surgery as Foscan-PDT was both more effective and cheaper (£5741 vs. £9924 vs. £16 912, respectively).

Proton therapy has been shown to be cost-effective compared with conventional radiotherapy amongst head and neck cancer patients[33]. Thus, researchers estimated the cost-effectiveness ratio was SEK 35 000 per QALY in patients ≥65 years of age.

Cost of prevention and management of oral complications of cancer therapy

Oral mucositis due to cancer therapy may require new hospitalization, prolonged hospital stay, and generally increased resource utilization. Studies have shown that the incremental cost associated with oral mucositis may be significantly higher for HSCT patients than those receiving radiation or chemotherapy, and that higher costs are associated with increased severity of oral mucositis.

Peterman and colleagues [34] retrospectively reviewed the medical charts of 45 head and neck cancer patients treated with radiation or chemotherapy. The costs of healthcare resources linked to managing oral mucositis were estimated by examining both hospital charges and Medicare reimbursement rates. The low and high estimates of the mean incremental costs due to mucositis were $2949 and $4037. Total costs were greater for patients experiencing more severe mucositis. These incremental costs described above can quickly add up, since most patients receive multiple chemotherapy cycles.

Elting et al.[35] reported similar results in a retrospective study of the cost of chemotherapy-induced mucositis in 599 solid-tumour patients. During an average chemotherapy cycle, patients who developed oral mucositis were hospitalized for 2 more days compared to those who did not develop oral mucositis. Mean US Medicare payments were used to estimate that the average hospitalization cost was $3893 per cycle without oral mucositis and $6277 per cycle with oral mucositis. Additionally, the incremental costs of National Cancer Institute (NCI) grade 1–2 mucositis was $2725, while those of NCI grade 3–4 mucositis was $5565.

A more recent study found even higher costs associated with mucositis. Nonzee et al.[36] performed a chart review of 99 head and neck cancer patients receiving chemoradiotherapy within three large referral hospitals. Resource utilization was recorded for the 2 months following chemoradiotherapy, and costs were estimated by applying standard rates. The researchers estimated that the median incremental medical costs for those patients who developed mucositis were $17 244.

A multinational study of 92 HSCT patients [37] showed that patients who developed oral mucositis had a $43 000 increase in hospital charges compared to patients who did not develop oral mucositis. This study also used multivariate regression to identify that a one-point increase in peak Oral Mucositis Assessment Scale (OMAS) score was associated with double the risk of significant infection, 2.7 additional days of total parenteral nutrition (TPN), 2.6 additional days of injectable narcotic therapy, 2.6 additional days in hospital, and $25 405 in additional hospital charges.

Vera-Llonch et al.[38] provided a more comprehensive assessment of the cost of oral mucositis by performing a retrospective chart review of 281 patients receiving allogeneic HSCT. Mean total inpatient hospital charges including professional, pharmacy, and laboratory fees ranged from $213 995 to $437 421 for patients without and those with the highest grade oral of mucositis. Again, they found statistically significant positive relationships between the highest recorded grade of oral mucositis and days of TPN, days of injectable narcotic therapy, length of hospital stay, and total inpatient charges.

The high costs of oral mucositis should be considered in decision-making about prevention/management of oral mucositis. Elting and colleagues [39] estimated hospitalization costs using the results from a trial of 212 HSCT patients randomized to either palifermin or placebo for the prevention of oral mucositis[40]. The mean estimated hospitalization costs in the clinical trial were $73 938 for patients receiving palifermin and $77 533 for patients receiving placebo. Although this cost difference was not significant ($p = 0.39$), the authors concluded that cost savings from reduced hospitalizations can offset the cost of palifermin prophylaxis (approximately $8250 per patient at the time of publication).

One study assessed the impact of amifostine during radiation therapy in 54 head and neck cancer patients[41]. No significant antitoxic benefit was observed for amifostine, and the costs of treatment were greater for the amifostine group than the no-amifostine group.

References

1 Cella D, Nowinski CJ (2002). Measuring quality of life in chronic illness: the Functional Assessment of Chronic Illness Therapy measurement system. *Arch Phys Med Rehabil*, 83(12Suppl 2), S10–7.

2 Cella DF (1995). Measuring quality of life in palliative care. *Semin Oncol*, 22 (2 Suppl 3), 73–81.

3 Cella D, Pulliam J, Fuchs H, et al. (2003). Evaluation of pain associated with oral mucositis during the acute period after administration of high-dose chemotherapy. *Cancer*, 98(2), 406–12.

4 Stiff PJ, Emmanouilides C, Bensinger WI, et al. (2006). Palifermin reduces patient-reported mouth and throat soreness and improves patient functioning in the hematopoietic stem-cell transplantation setting. *J Clin Oncol*, 24(33), 5186–93.

5 Ware JE, Snow KK, Kosinski M (2000). *Sf-36 Health Survey: Manual and Interpretation Guide*. Quality Metric Incorporated, Lincoln.

6 Cella DF, Tulsky DS, Gray G, et al. (1993). The Functional Assessment of Cancer Therapy scale: development and validation of the general measure. *J Clin Oncol*, 11(3), 570–9.

7 Aaronson NK, Ahmedzai S, Bergman B, et al. (1993). The European Organization for Research and Treatment of Cancer QLQ-C30: a quality of life instrument for the use in international trials in oncology. *J Natl Cancer Inst*, 85(5), 365–76.

8   Cella D, Yount S, Rothrock N, et al. (2007). The Patient-Reported Outcomes Measurement Information System (PROMIS): progress of an NIH Roadmap cooperative group during its first two years. *Med Care*, 45(5 Suppl 1), S3–11.

9   Reeve BB, Hays RD, Bjorner JB, et al. (2007). Psychometric evaluation and calibration of health-related quality of life items banks: plans for the Patient-Reported Outcome Measurement Information System (PROMIS). *Med Care*, 45(5 Suppl 1), S22–31.

10 List MA, D'Antonio LL, Cella DF, et al. (1996). The Performance Status Scale for Head and Neck Cancer Patients and the Functional Assessment of Cancer Therapy – Head and Neck Scale. A study of utility and validity. *Cancer*, 77(11), 2294–301.

11 Cella D, Paul D, Yount S, et al. (2003). What are the most important symptom targets when treating advanced cancer? A survey of providers in the National Comprehensive Cancer Network (NCCN). *Cancer Invest*, 21(4), 526–35.

12 Bjordal K, Hammerlid E, Ahlner-Elmqvist M, et al. (1999). Quality of life in head and neck cancer patients: validation of the European Organization for Research and Treatment of Cancer Quality of Life Questionnaire – H&N35. *J Clin Oncol*, 17(3), 1008–19.

13 Rogers SN, Gwanne S, Lowe D, Humphris G, Yueh B, Weymuller EA (2002). The addition of mood and anxiety domains to the University of Washington quality of life scale. *Head Neck*, 24(6), 521–9.

14 Epstein JB, Emerton S, Kolbinson DA, et al. (1999). Quality of life and oral function following radiotherapy for head and neck cancer. *Head Neck*, 21(1), 1–11.

15 Epstein JB, Robertson M, Emerton S, Phillips N, Stevenson-Moore P (2001). Quality of life and oral function in patients treated with radiation therapy for head and neck cancer. *Head Neck*, 23(5), 389–98.

16 Epstein JB, Beaumont JL, Gwede CK, et al. (2007). Longitudinal evaluation of the Oral Mucositis Weekly Questionnaire – Head and Neck Cancer, a patient-reported outcomes questionnaire. *Cancer*, 109(9), 1914–22.

17 Browman GP, Levine MN, Hodson DI, et al. (1993). The Head and Neck Radiotherapy Questionnaire: a morbidity/quality-of-life instrument for clinical trials of radiation therapy in locally advanced head and neck cancer. *J Clin Oncol*, 11(5), 863–72.

18 Trotti A, Johnson DJ, Gwede C, et al. (1998). Development of a head and neck companion module for the Quality of Life – Radiation Therapy Instrument (QOL-RTI). *Int J Radiat Oncol Biol Phys*, 42(2), 257–61.

19 Duncan GG, Epstein JB, Tu D, et al. (2005). Quality of life, mucositis, and xerostomia from radiotherapy for head and neck cancers: a report from the NCIC CTG HN2 randomized trial of an antimicrobial lozenge to prevent mucositis. *Head Neck*, 27(5), 421–8.

20 Sonis ST, Elting LS, Keefe D, et al. (2004). Perspectives on cancer therapy-induced mucosal injury: pathogenesis, measurement, epidemiology, and consequences for patients. *Cancer*, 100(9 Suppl), 1995–2025.

21 Gold MR, Siegel JE, Russell LB, Weinstein MC (1996). *Cost-effectiveness in health and medicine*. Oxford University Press, New York.

22 Drummond MF, Sculpher MJ, Torrance GW, O'Brien BJ, Stoddart GL (2005). *Methods for the economic evaluation of health care programmes*. Oxford University Press, New York.

23 Van Agthoven M, van Ineveld BM, de Boer MF, et al. (2001). The costs of head and neck oncology: primary tumours, recurrent tumours and long-term follow-up. *Eur J Cancer*, 37(17), 2204–11.

24 Funk GF, Hoffman HT, Karnell LH, et al. (1998). Cost-identification analysis in oral cavity cancer management. *Otolaryngol Head Neck Surg*, 118(2), 211–20.

25 Zavras A, Andreopoulos N, Katsikeris N, Zavras D, Cartsos V, Vamvakidis A (2002). Oral cancer treatment costs in Greece and the effect of advanced disease. *BMC Public Health*, 2, 12–20.

26 Speight PM, Palmer S, Moles DR, et al. (2006). The cost-effectiveness of screening for oral cancer in primary care. *Health Technol Assess*, 10(14), 1–144.

27 Lang K, Menzin J, Earle CC, Jacobson J, Hsu MA (2004). The economic cost of squamous cell cancer of the head and neck. *Arch Otolaryngol Head Neck Surg*, 130(11), 1269–75.

28 Epstein JD, Knight TK, Epstein JB, Bride MA, Nichol MB (2008). The cost of care for early and late stage oropharyngeal cancer in the California Medicaid population. *Head Neck*, 30(2), 178–86.

29 Yabroff KR, Davis WW, Lamont EB, et al. (2007). Patient time costs associated with cancer care. *J Natl Cancer Inst*, 99(1), 14–23.

30 Centers for Disease Control and Prevention (2005). Annual smoking-attributable mortality, years of potential life lost, and productivity losses – United States, 1997–2001. MMWR Morb Mortal Wkly Rep, 54(25), 625–8. Last accessed on 11/3/2008 at: http://www.cdc.gov/mmwr/preview/mmwrhtml/mm5425a1.htm

31 Kosuda S, Kusano S, Kohno N, et al. (2003). Feasibility and cost-effectiveness of sentinel lymph node radiolocalization in stage N0 head and neck cancer. *Arch Otolaryngol Head Neck Surg*, 129(10), 1105–9.

32 Hopper C, Niziol C, Sidhu M (2004). The cost-effectiveness of Foscan mediated photodynamic therapy (Foscan-PDT) compared with extensive palliative surgery and palliative chemotherapy for patients with advanced head and neck cancer in the UK. *Oral Oncol*, 40(4), 372–82.

33 Lundkvist J, Ekman M, Ericsson SR, Jonsson B, Glimelius B (2005). Proton therapy of cancer: potential clinical advantages and cost-effectiveness. *Acta Oncol*, 44(8), 850–61.

34 Peterman A, Cella D, Glandon G, Dobrez D, Yount S (2001). Mucositis in head and neck cancer: economic and quality of life outcomes. *J Natl Cancer Inst Monogr*, (29), 45–51.

35 Elting LS, Cooksley C, Chambers M, Cantor SB, Manzullo E, Rubenstein EB (2003). The burdens of cancer therapy. Clinical and economic outcomes of chemotherapy-induced mucositis. *Cancer*, 98(7), 1531–9.

36 Nonzee NJ, Dandade NA, Markossian T, et al. (2008). Evaluating the supportive care costs of severe radiochemotherapy-induced mucositis and pharyngitis: results from a Northwestern University Costs of Cancer Program pilot study with head and neck and nonsmall cell lung cancer patients who received care at a county hospital, a Veterans Administration hospital, or a comprehensive cancer care center. *Cancer*, 113(6), 1446–52.

37 Sonis ST, Oster G, Fuchs H, et al. (2001). Oral mucositis and the clinical and economic outcomes of hematopoietic stem cell transplantation. *J Clin Oncol*, 19(8), 2201–5.

38 Vera-Llonch M, Oster G, Ford CM, Lu J, Sonis S. (2007). Oral mucositis and outcomes of allogeneic hematopoietic stem-cell transplantation in patients with hematologic malignancies. *Support Care Cancer*, 15(5), 491–6.

39 Elting LS, Shih YC, Stiff PJ, et al. (2007b). Economic impact of palifermin on the costs of hospitalization for autologous hematopoietic stem-cell transplant: analysis of phase 3 trial results. *Biol Blood Marrow Transplant*, 13(7), 806–13.

40 Spielberger R, Stiff P, Bensinger W, et al. (2004). Palifermin for oral mucositis after intensive therapy for hematologic cancers. *N Engl J Med*, 351(25), 2590–8.

41 Braaksma M, van Agthoven M, Nijdam,W, Uyl-de Groot C, Lavendag P (2005). Costs of treatment intensification for head and neck cancer: concomitant chemoradiation randomised for radioprotection with amifostine. *Eur J Cancer*, 41(14), 2102–11.

Chapter 30

Sources of information

Andrew Davies and Joel Epstein

"Learning is like rowing upstream; not to advance is to drop back"
Chinese proverb

Introduction

The editors aimed to produce an up-to-date textbook on the oral complications of cancer and its management. However, one of the major drawbacks of textbooks is that although they are 'up-to-date' when written, they may become 'out-of-date' within a relatively short period of time. The purpose of this chapter is to discuss the main sources of information, recommend some specific sources of information, and provide some advice with regard to keeping abreast of new developments in the area of interest. It should be noted that the potential sources of information are numerous, and that the (limited) recommended sources of information reflect the personal preferences/experiences of the editors.

Textbooks

Textbooks remain an important source of healthcare information (Box 30.1). It is important that the reader accesses the most relevant type of textbook (e.g. generic oncology, generic supportive care, generic dentistry/oral medicine, specific textbook). Equally, for the reasons discussed above, it is important that the reader accesses the most recent edition of the textbook, and takes into account the date of publication of that edition (and so the likelihood of developments in clinical practice). It should be noted that many textbooks are written with a specific audience in mind (e.g. healthcare professionals in developed countries), and so the content may not be appropriate/relevant for other types of audiences (i.e. healthcare professionals in developing countries).

Journals

Journals are an important source of state-of-the-art healthcare information. However, it can be difficult to keep up-to-date with the literature, due to the number/variety of relevant journals. Indeed, articles on oral complications commonly appear in oncology, supportive care, and dentistry/oral medicine journals. Nevertheless, by adopting a number of simple strategies, it is possible to keep relatively up-to-date with the literature (Box 30.2):

1. Regular searching of relevant databases (see below).
2. Subscribing to automatic database search updates (e.g. My NCBI section of PubMed).
3. Subscribing to automatic journal content lists.
4. Attending relevant in-house/local journal clubs.

Box 30.1 Recommended textbooks

Generic oncology textbooks

- DeVita VT Jr, Lawrence TS, Rosenberg SA, DePinho RA, Weinberg RA (2008). DeVita, Hellman, and Rosenberg's cancer: principles and practice of oncology, 8th edn. Lippincott Williams & Wilkins, Philadelphia
- Halperin EC, Perez CA, Brady LW (2007). Perez and Brady's principles and practice of radiation oncology, 5th edn. Lippincott Williams & Wilkins, Philadelphia

Generic supportive care textbooks

- Berger A, Shuster JL Jr, Von Roenn JH (2006). Principles and practice of palliative care and supportive oncology, 3rd edn. Lippincott Williams & Wilkins, Philadelphia
- Doyle D, Hanks G, Cherny N, Calman K (2005). Oxford textbook of palliative medicine, 3rd edn. Oxford University Press, Oxford

Generic dental/oral medicine textbooks

- Greenberg MS, Glick M, Ship JA (2008). Burket's oral medicine, 11th edn. BC Decker Inc, Hamilton
- Little JW, Falace DA, Miller CS, Rhodus NL (2007). Dental management of the medically compromised patient, 7th edn. Mosby, St. Louis

Specific textbooks

- Davies A, Finlay I (2005). Oral care in advanced disease. Oxford University Press, Oxford

Box 30.2 Recommended peer review journals

Generic oncology journals

- Journal of Clinical Oncology
- Lancet Oncology
- British Journal of Cancer
- Cancer

Generic supportive care journals

- Journal of Pain and Symptom Management
- Supportive Care in Cancer

Generic dental/oral medicine journals

- Oral Diseases
- Journal of the American Dental Association
- Journal of Oral Pathology and Medicine
- Oral Surgery Oral Medicine Oral Pathology Oral Radiology and Endodontology
- British Dental Journal
- Special Care Dentistry

Specific journals

- Oral Oncology
- Head and Neck

Databases

A variety of health-related databases have been developed, with each one having a somewhat different focus of attention (and including somewhat different sources of information). The choice of database(s) to be searched will depend on the nature of the problem being researched. Table 30.1 presents details of some of the more important health-related databases. Similarly, the choice of search strategy to be used will depend on the nature of the problem being researched. It is important to use a search strategy that is sensitive (i.e. relevant papers are identified), is specific (i.e. irrelevant papers are not identified), and, in most cases, produces a manageable number of references. Nevertheless, even the 'best' search strategy will not identify all of the relevant papers, and will identify numerous irrelevant papers. Indeed, inexperienced database searchers should seek advice/training from more experienced database searchers (e.g. medical librarians, established researchers).

Internet

An increasingly important source of information is the World Wide Web component of the Internet. The Internet has a number of advantages, especially the relative ease of access to information (i.e. information is available at any time and is accessible from anywhere). However, the

Table 30.1 Recommended databases

Database	Content	Comments
PubMed http://www.ncbi.nlm.nih.gov/pubmed/	Subject areas – varied including medicine, nursing and dentistry Dates – 1950 to present Content – References, abstracts, (full text articles)	Co-ordinated by National Library of Medicine (USA). PubMed is based on the Medline database, and incorporates the CancerLit database. PubMed/Medline are the pre-eminent medical databases. Contains links to articles in 'free access' journals.
CINAHL (Cumulative Index to Nursing and Allied Health Literature)	Subject areas – emphasis on literature relating to nursing and professions allied to medicine Dates – 1981 to present Content - References, abstracts	Useful source of additional information (from Medline) on stated subject areas.
EMBASE (Excerpta Medica Database)	Subject areas – emphasis on literature relating to biomedical sciences and pharmacology Dates – 1974 to present Content - References, abstracts	Useful source of additional information (from Medline) on stated subject areas.
The Cochrane Collaboration http://www.cochrane.org/	Subject areas – systematic reviews of all aspects of healthcare. Content – References, abstracts, (full text reviews)	Several reviews relating to oral complications of cancer and its treatment. Abstracts available for free throughout world, whilst full text available for free in certain parts of world (e.g. UK). The reviews are regularly updated.

Internet also has a number of disadvantages, including the relative lack of regulation of websites (i.e. anyone can develop their own website, can promote their own viewpoint). Moreover, the ever-increasing number websites can make searching the Internet an evermore time-consuming activity.

The Health On the Net Foundation is an independent organization, which has developed a code of practice for healthcare websites, and which maintains a searchable database of approved healthcare websites (http://www.hon.ch/). Furthermore, the use of this specific 'search engine' can be much more productive than the use of a generic search engine (e.g. Google, Yahoo). Thus, the search term 'oral complications of cancer and its treatment' yielded a manageable 405 hits using The Health On the Net Foundation search engine, but an unmanageable >2.25 million using the Google search engine (Table 30.2).

Table 30.2 Recommended websites

Organisation	Website address	Website content	Comments
National Cancer Institute (USA)	http://www.cancer.gov/	Comprehensive website dedicated to all aspects of cancer, including sections on oral cancer and the oral complications of cancer treatment	Information provided for both health care professionals and patients and carers.
National Institute of Dental and Craniofacial Research (USA)	http://www.nidcr.nih.gov/	Comprehensive website dedicated to all aspects of oral health, including sections on oral cancer and the oral complications of cancer treatment	Information provided for both health care professionals and patients and carers.
National Cancer Center Network (USA)	http://www.nccn.org/	Guidelines on the management of cancer, including head and neck cancer	Information for health care professionals.
The Cochrane Collaboration	http://www.cochrane.org/	Systematic reviews of various treatments, including those for cancer and complications of cancer/cancer treatment	See Table 30.1. Reviews have 'Plain language summaries' for patients and carers.
Cancer Index	http://www.cancerindex.org/	A 'gateway' site to internet resources about cancer and its treatment	Links provided for both health care professionals and patients and carers.
Multinational Association for Supportive Care in Cancer	htttp://www.mascc.org/	Guidelines on the management of cancer complications, including oral mucositis	Information for health care professionals.
American Academy of Oral Medicine	http://www.aaom.com/	Information about various oral problems, including oral problems secondary to cancer treatment	Information for patients and carers (and health care professionals).
(Oral supportive care website)	http://www.oral supportivecare.com/	Site still under development	Site contains template for oral supportive care plan for 'cancer survivors'

Index

AC+T regimen 142
aciclovir 198
acinic cell tumour 66
Actinomyces naeslundii 186, 187
Actinomyces viscosus 186, 187
acupuncture 214–15
adenoid cystic carcinoma 66
adjuvant analgesics 247
advanced cancer patients, oral problems
    in 279–87
  aetiology 281
  assessment 283–4
  clinical features 281–3
  epidemiology 279–81
  management 284–7
    multidisciplinary working 285
    palliative care 285, 286, 287
    terminal phase 285–6
  severity of symptoms 282
aetiology 2–7
  oral cancer 54–7
  see also different conditions
age, and cancer incidence/mortality 2
  geriatric patients 272
ageusia 228
agglutinin 167
airway complications 82–3
  chronic aspiration and pneumonia 83
  tracheal stenosis 82–3
  tracheo-innominate artery erosion 83
  tracheo-oesophageal fistula 83
  tracheomalacia 83
alcohol, and oral cancer 55
alemtuzumab, oral effects 6
alveolar processes 11–12
ameloblastic carcinoma 69
ameloblastoma 68–9
amifostine 94, 131, 211
  cost-effectiveness 298
amphotericin 181, 182
ampicillin-sulbactam 191
anaemia 132
analgesic ladder 246
angular cheilitis 24
angular stomatitis 174
antiemetics 247
aphthous ulcers 29–31
areca nut, and oral cancer 55
artificial saliva 215–16
ascorbic acid 213
aspergillosis 175–6
  management 181
Aspergillus fumigatus 175
aspiration, chronic 83
atropine 255

autoimmune polyendocrinopathy-candidiasis-
    ectodermal dystrophy (APECED) 56

bacteraemia 188
bacterial infections 23, 185–92
  aetiology 185
  children 263
  clinical features 185–9
    bacteraemia and sepsis 188
    deep-space infections 188
    necrotizing gingivitis/stomatitis 187
    odontogenic infections 186
    oral mucositis 188
    periodontal disease 186–7
    sialoadenitis 187–8
  investigation 190
  management 190–2
Bacteroides spp. 186
Bacteroides loescheii 233
betel leaves, and oral cancer 55
bevacizumab, oral effects 6
biofilm 163–4
biological therapy, oral cancer 60–1
biperiden 212
bisphosphonate-related osteonecrosis
    of jaw 135, 151–60
  aetiology 152–4
    duration of treatment 153
    potency of bisphosphonate 152–3
    route of administration 153
  case study 157–60
  clinical features 154
  epidemiology 151–2
  ground glass appearance 155
  investigations 154–5
  management 156–7
  prevention 155–6
  staging 154
black hairy tongue 28
Blastomyces dermatitidis 176
blastomycosis 176
  management 181
blood supply of oral cavity 18
bone tumours 71–2
bortezomib, oral effects 5
brachytherapy 92
BRON *see* bisphosphonate-induced
    osteonecrosis of jaw
bullae 22
bullous pemphigoid 2
burning mouth syndrome 245
butyric acid 235

cadaverine 235
calcium phosphate 131

Candida albicans 56, 171
Candida glabrata 171
Candida guilliermondii 171
Candida krusei 171
Candida parapsilosis 171
Candida tropicalis 171
candidosis 171–5
    advanced cancer patients 281
    chronic erythematous 174
    chronic hyperplastic 172–3
    chronic mucocutaneous 174
    classification 171–2
    clinical features 172–4
    erythematous 24
    erythematous (atrophic) 172
    laboratory diagnosis 174
    management 175
    predisposing factors 173
    pseudomembranous 24, 172
carbamazepine 245
carcinoma ex pleomorphic adenoma 66–7
caries 186
    children 265
    management 191
    post-HSCT 135
caspofungin 181
cathelicidin 167
cefotaxime 191
cefoxitin 191
ceftizoxime 191
Centipeda periodontii 235
cervical lymph nodes, enlargement 58
cetuximab 60
    oral effects 6
cevimeline 213–14
cheilitis, angular 174
chemical plaque control 45
chemotherapy
    complications 3, 4, 5–6, 123–7
        aetiology 123
        clinical features 124–7
        epidemiology 123
    cost-effectiveness of 297
    oral cancer 60
    and quality of life 294
    and taste disturbance 227
chewing gum 212–13
children 261–8
    oral complications
        caries 265
        haemorrhage 263–4
        infections 262–3
        mucositis 262
        oral graft-versus-host disease 266–7
        salivary gland dysfunction 263
        second tumours 267
        skeletal/dental malformation 126, 264–5, 266
        taste disturbance 263
        trismus 266
    role of paediatric dental professionals 267–8
    types of cancer in 261, 262
chlorhexidine 45, 156
    oral effects 4, 45
CHLORIDE menmonic 21

chondrosarcoma 71
citric acid 213
clear cell odontogenic carcinoma 69
clindamycin 191
clinical features 7
cloxacillin 191
co-existent conditions
    oral 7
    physical 7
    psychological/psychiatric 7
Coccidioides immitis 176
coccidioidomycosis 176
    management 181
cold sores 197
commensal microbiota 165–6
competitive inhibition 166
Comprehensive Geriatric Assessment (CGA) 273
cost-benefit analysis 295
cost-effectiveness analysis 295
cost-utility analysis 295
coumarin/toroxutin 212
Coxsackie group A viruses 196
cryotherapy 147
cryptococcosis 176
    management 182
cystatins 167
cytokines 134
cytomegalovirus 24, 196, 200

dasatinib, oral effects 5
deep-space infections 188
    management 191
defensins 167
dental abscess 38
dental care 44–6
    chemical plaque control 45
    children 267–8
    interdental cleaning 45
    toothbrushing 44–5
dental caries *see* caries
dental developmental abnormalities 126, 264–5, 266
    agenesis 264, 265
    microdontia 264
    shortened roots 265
    V-shaped roots 266
dental malformation 126
dental plaque 165
denture care 46–7
denture stomatitis 174
    advanced cancer patients 279
dentures
    complete 46–7, 48
    hygiene 47, 49–50
    partial 47–50
    problems in advanced cancer patients 279
developmental abnormalities 137
    dental 126, 264–5, 266
diet, and oral cancer 56
dimethyl sulphide 235
dipyrone 247
distigmine 213–14
Down's syndrome 27
doxycycline 191
drooling 253–5

dysgeusia 228
dysphagia 80
  geriatric patients 274

ecological plaque hypothesis 163
edentulous patients 50
effects of cancer 2–3
Eikenella corrodens 235
electron therapy 92
Enterobacteriaceae 188, 233
EP-GP 167
epidemiology 1–2
  oral cancer 53–4
Epstein-Barr virus 24, 196, 199–200
erlotinib 60
  oral effects 5
erosion 22
erythema 22
erythema migrans 28
Eubacterium spp. 163, 186
European Organization for Research and Treatment
  of Cancer Quality of Life Questionnaire
  (EORTC-QLQ-C30) 292
Ewing sarcoma 71–2
examination
  extraoral 22–3
  intraoral 23
external beam radiotherapy 91–2
extramedullary plasmacytoma 70
extraoral examination 22–3

facial aesthetics 81–2
facial nerve (VII), marginal mandibular branch 85
FACT-Head and Neck (FACT-HN) scale 292
FACT-HN Symptom Index (FHNSI) 292
famciclovir 198
fissured tongue 27
fistulae 22
  chronic 82
  tracheo-oesophageal 83
floor of mouth 14
fluconazole 182
flucytosine 182
foetor ex ore 233
foetor oris 233
FOLFOX regimen 142
foramen caecum 14
Foscan photodynamic therapy 297
Functional Assessment of Cancer Therapy-General
  (FACT-G) 291
fungal infections 24, 171–83
  aspergillosis 175–6
  blastomycosis 176
  cancer patients 178–83
  Candida spp. 171–5
  children 263
  coccidioidomycosis 176
  cryptococcosis 176
  differential diagnosis 179
  geotrichosis 177
  histoplasmosis 177
  laboratory investigations 180
  management 181–2
  mucormycosis (zygomycosis) 177

  paracoccidioidomycosis 177–8
  penicilliosis 178
  sporotrichosis 178
Fusobacterium nucleatum 186, 187
Fusobacterium nucleatum polymorphum 235
Fusobacterium nucleatum vincentii 235
Fusobacterium periodontium 235

gag reflex 11
gel carriers 41–2
genetic factors in oral cancer 55
geographic tongue 28
geotrichosis 177
geriatric dentistry/oncology 271–3
geriatric patients 271–6
  cancer mortality 272
  oral supportive care 273–4
    barriers to 274–6
  personal issues related to care 275–6
  societal/institutional barriers to care 275–6
ghost cell odontogenic carcinoma 69
gingival crevicular fluid 168
gingivitis 13
  management 191
  necrotizing 187
gingivostomatitis, primary herpetic 196–7
glossitis
  benign migratory 28
  median rhomboid 174
glycopyrronium bromide 255
graft-versus-host disease, oral 131–2, 133
  children 266–7

haematological tumours 70–1
  lymphomas 71
  plasma cell disorders 70–1
haematopoietic stem cell transplantation 129–37
  high dose conditioning 129
  oral complications 129–37
    dental/periodontal tissues 135
    developmental abnormalities 137
    haemorrhage 136
    infection 135–6
    musculoskeletal tissues 135
    nervous tissues 135
    oral mucosa 130–4
    salivary glands 134–5
    secondary malignancies 136
  and quality of life 294
  reduced-intensity conditioning 129
haemorrhage 255–8
  causes 256
  chemotherapy-induced 125
  children 263–4
  post-HSCT 136
  treatment 256, 257
halitosis 233–8
  aetiology 233–5
    oral causes 233–5
    systemic causes 235
  chemotherapy-induced 126–7
  clinical features 236
  definition 233
  epidemiology 233

halitosis (*cont.*)
  investigation 236–7
  odiferous agents 235
  organolpetic score 346
  treatment 237–8
head and neck, examination 36
health economics
  assessment 295
  cost of oral cancer 295–6
  cost of oral cancer screening 297
  definition 294
  prevention/management of oral
    complications 297–8
health-related quality of life *see* quality of life
herpes labialis 197
herpes simplex virus 24, 195–8
  clinical features
    primary herpetic gingivostomatitis 196–7
    secondary infection 197
  diagnosis 197
  epidemiology 195
  management 197–8
herpesviruses 187, 195
histatins 167
Histoplasma capsulatum 177
histoplasmosis 177
  management 181
history 21–2
HSCT *see* haematopoietic stem cell transplantation
human herpes virus 6 196
human herpes virus 7 196
human herpes virus 8 196, 200–1
human immunodeficiency virus 196
human papillomavirus 196, 201
human recombinant keratinocyte-growth factor
  see palifermin
hydrogen sulphide 235
hyoscine hydrobromide 255
hyperbaric oxygen 157
hypodontia 13
hypogeusia 225, 228
hypoglossal nerve (XII) 84

imaging 37
  radiography 23, 37
imatinib, oral effects 5
imipenem 191
immune system 168
immunodeficiency 168
immunoglobulins 167
implants 40
incidence, age-related 2
incidence of oral cancer 1
infection 163–8
  advanced cancer 279
  bacterial *see* bacterial infections
  chemotherapy-related 125
  children 263
  colonization of oral cavity 163–5
  dental plaque 165
  fungal *see* fungal infections
  maintenance of oral microbiota 165–8
    commensal 165–6

gingival crevicular fluid 168
  immune system 168
  oral mucosa 165
  saliva 166–7
  oral microorganisms 164
  post-HSCT 135–6
  viral *see* viral infections
information sources 301–4
  databases 303
  Internet 303–4
  journals 301, 302
  textbooks 301, 302
intensity-modulated radiation therapy 40
interdental cleaning 45
International Classification of Diseases (ICD-9) 141
intraoral examination 23
intraosseous carcinoma 69
investigations 23–5
  oral cancer 58–9
iseganan 131
isotope therapy 92
itraconazole 181, 182

Kaposi's sarcoma 73
Kaposi's sarcoma associated herpes virus 200–1
ketoconazole 181, 182

lactoferrin 167
lactoperoxidase 167
laryngeal nerve
  recurrent 85
  superior 85
laxatives 247
Lemierre syndrome 188
lingual nerve (V3) 84
lingual thyroid 14
Ludwig's angina 188
lymphatic drainage of oral cavity 18
lymphomas 71
lymphoproliferative disorder,
  post-transplantation 136
lysozyme 167

McMaster University Head and Neck Radiotherapy
  Questionnaire (HNRQ) 293
malic acid 213
management 7–8
  ongoing 41–2
  pretreatment 38–41
Mandibular Function Impairment Questionnaire
  (MFIQ) 106
masticatory insufficiency 80–1
measles virus 196
median rhomboid glossitis 174
Medical Outcomes Study 36-item Short Form
  Health Survey (SF-36) 291
Melkersson-Rosenthal syndrome 27
melphalan, and oral mucositis 142
meropenem 191
methyl mercaptan 235
metronidazole 191
microbial homeostasis 163, 166
microbial testing 23–4

microorganisms
  oral 164
  and oral cancer 56
minocycline 191
mortality
  age-related 2
  oral cancer 54
mouth *see* oral cavity
mouth opening 106
moxifloxacin 191
mUC5B 167
MUC7 167
mucocoeles 134
mucoepidermoid carcinoma 66
mucormycosis (zygomycosis) 177
  management 181
mucositis 141–8, 245
  aetiology 141–3
  bacterial 188
  chemotherapy-induced 125, 144
  children 262–3
  clinical features 144–5
  cost of treatment 298
  epidemiology 141
  following HSCT 130–1
  genetics of 143
  geriatric patients 273
  management 131, 145–8
  pathophysiology 143
  post-radiation 141
  risk of 142
  scoring systems 145
multidisciplinary working 7, 285
multiple myeloma 70–1
mumps virus 196

nafcillin 191
necrotizing gingivitis 187
  management 191
necrotizing stomatitis 187
  management 191
nefopam 247
nerve supply 15–16, 18
neurologic dysfunction 84–5
  facial nerve (VII), marginal mandibular branch 85
  hypoglossal (XII) and lingual (V3) nerves 84
  phrenic nerve 84
  spinal accessory nerve (XI) 84
  sympathetic trunk 85
  vagus (X), recurrent laryngeal and superior
    laryngeal nerves 85
neurotoxicity 125–6
neutron therapy 92
neutropenic ulcers 31, 134
non-opioid analgesics 247
non-steroidal anti-inflammatory drugs 247
nuclear factor κB 143
nutrition 81
nutritional compromise 236

odontoblasts 13
odontogenic tumours 68–9
  benign, ameloblastoma 68–9

malignant
  ameloblastic carcinoma 69
  clear cell odontogenic carcinoma 69
  ghost cell odontogenic carcinoma 69
  intraosseous carcinoma 69
oncocytoma 65
oral assessment 21–5
  examination 22–3
  history 21–2
  investigations 23–5
  tools 25
Oral Assessment Guide 24, 25
oral cancer 53–61
  aetiology 54–7
    alcohol 55, 56
    betel leaves and areca nut 55
    diet 56
    genetic factors 55
    microorganisms 56
    oral health 56, 57
    radiation 57
    socioeconomic status 56
    systemic health 56
    tobacco 54–5, 56
  clinical features 57–8
  cost of 295–6
  epidemiology 53–4
  geographical factors 53
  investigations 58–9
  management 59–61
    biological therapy 60–1
    chemotherapy 60
    radiotherapy 60
    surgery 59–60
  mortality 54
  staging 58
oral cancer screening 297
oral care *see* oral hygiene
oral cavity 11–18
  alveolar processes 11–12
  examination 36–7
  floor of mouth 14
  lymphatic drainage 18
  nervous innervation 15–16, 18
  palate 11, 12
  pillars of fauces 11, 12
  salivary glands 15
  teeth 12–14
  tongue 14–15
  vasculature 18
oral health, and oral cancer 56, 57
oral hygiene 8, 43–51, 245–6
  care of oral mucosa 51
  children 267–8
  dental care 44–6
  denture care 46–7
  edentulous patients 50
  maintenance of 43–4
  partial dentures, removal/insertion 47–50
oral mucosa 165
  care of 51
Oral Mucositis Daily Questionnaire
  (OMDQ) 292

Oral Mucositis Weekly Questionnaire – Head and Neck Cancer (OMWQ-HN) 293
oral surgery, complications 79–86
  airway-related 82–3
  chronic fistulae 82
  donor site problems 86
  facial aesthetics 81–2
  hardware failure 85–6
  masticatory insufficiency/trismus 80–1
  neurologic 84–5
  nutrition 81
  quality of life 86
  speech and swallowing impairment 80
  treatment failure 79–80
oral symptoms 22
oral varicosities 27
organolpetic score 346
orofacial pain 241–8
  aetiology 242–4
    direct effect of tumour 242–3
    effect of cancer therapy 243–4
  anatomy and physiology 241–2
  clinical features 244–5
    burning mouth syndrome 245
    oral mucositis 245
    temporomandibular disorder 244
    trigeminal neuralgia 244–5
  epidemiology 242
  management 245–8
oropharynx, examination 36
osteonecrosis of jaws
  bisphosphonate-induced 135, 151–60
  geriatric patients 274
  post-radiation 117–20
    aetiology 117–18
    clinical features 118
    epidemiology 117
    geriatric patients 274
    investigation 118
    management 118–20
    treatment 120
osteosarcoma 71

p53 143
paediatric *see* children
pain *see* orofacial pain
palate 11, 12
palifermin 131, 147
  cost-effectiveness 298
  oral effects 4
palliative care 285, 286, 287
pamidronate, and BRON 152
papillary cystadenoma lymphomatosum 65
papilloma virus 196
papules 22
paracetamol 247
Paracoccidioides brasiliensis 177
paracoccidioidomycosis 177–8
  management 182
paramyxoviruses 196
paraneoplastic syndromes 2
partial dentures 47–50
Patient Reported Outcomes Measurement Information System (PROMIS) 292

penciclovir 198
penicillin G 191
penicilliosis 178
Penicillium marneffei 178
Peptostreptococcus micros 186
pericoronitis 186
periodontal disease 186–7
  management 191
  post-HSCT 135
phrenic nerve 84
picornaviruses 196
pillars of fauces 11, 12
pilocarpine 212, 213–14
piperacillin-tazobactam 191
plaques 22
plasma cell disorders 70–1
pleomorphic adenoma 65
pneumonia 83
polymorphous low-grade adenocarcinoma 66
Porphyromonas endodontalis 186, 233
Porphyromonas gingivalis 187, 233
posaconazole 181
pretreatment
  management 38–41
  screening 35–8
Prevotella (Bacteroides) melaninogenica 233
Prevotella intermedia 187, 233
proline-rich glycoprotein 167
prophylaxis 8
propionic acid 235
proton therapy 92
pulpal infection 186
putrescine 235
pyogenic granuloma 134
pyridostigmine 213–14

quality of life 86
  chemotherapy 294
  definition of 291
  head and neck radiotherapy 293–4
  HSCT 294
  measurement 291–3
    generic tools 291–2
    targeted tools 292–3
Quality of Life-Radiation Therapy Instrument/Head and Neck companion module (QOLRTI/H&N) 293

racial pigmentation 27
radiation, and oral cancer 57
radiation caries 35
radiobiology 89–91
radiography 23
  supplementary 37
radioprotectors 94, 211–12
radiosensitivity 91
radiotherapy
  complications 94–5
    osteonecrosis of jaws 117–20
  definition 89
  modalities 91–3
    brachytherapy 92
    electron therapy 92
    external beam radiotherapy 91–2

isotope therapy 92
  proton/neutron therapy 92
  total body irradiation 93
oral cancer 60
oral complications 4
regimens 93–4
  altered fractionation 93
  radioprotectors 94
  tissue-sparing techniques 93–4
  treatment gaps 94
salivary gland dysfunction 211
and taste disturbance 227
red lesions 32
redistribution 90
remineralization 41–2
reoxygenation 91
repair 90
repopulation 90–1
restorations 40–1
retromolar pad 12
retroviruses 196
rhabdomyosarcoma 72
rituximab, oral effects 6
Rothia mucilaginosa 163

saliva
  excessive secretion *see* sialorrhoea
  protection of commensal microbiota 166
  proteins 167
  thick (tenacious) 255
saliva stimulants 212–15
  acupuncture 214–15
  chewing gum 212–13
  organic acids 213
  parasympathomimetic drugs 213–14
saliva substitutes 215–16
  in palliative care 287
salivary flow-rate measurement 24–5, 38
salivary gland dysfunction 2, 203–17
  aetiology 205
  assessment 208–9, 210
  chemotherapy-induced 125
  children 263
  clinical features 206–7
  complications 206
    prevention of 216–17
    treatment 217
  epidemiology 204
  geriatric patients 274
  management 209, 211
  pathophysiology 205–6
  post-HSCT 134
  prevention 211–12
    radioprotectors 211–12
    radiotherapy 211
    surgical transfer of salivary glands 211
  symptomatic treatment 212–16
    saliva stimulants 212–15
    saliva substitutes 215–16
  treatment of cause 212
salivary gland tumours 65–8
  benign
    oncocytoma 65
    pleomorphic adenoma 65

    Warthin's tumour 65
  malignant
    acinic cell tumour 66
    adenoid cystic carcinoma 66
    carcinoma ex pleomorphic
      adenoma 66–7
    mucoepidermoid carcinoma 66
    polymorphous low-grade adenocarcinoma 66
  minor 67–8
salivary glands 15
  anatomy 16, 17
  major 203
  minor 203–4
  radioiodine-induced effects 94–5
  stimulation 203
  surgical transfer 211
sarcomas 71–3
  bone tumours 71–2
  Kaposi's sarcoma 73
  soft-tissue 72–3
scopolamine 255
scrotal tongue 27
sepsis 188
shoulder syndrome 84
sialoadenitis
  bacterial 187–8
    management 191
sialochemistry 24
sialorrhoea 253, 254
sinuses 22
skeletal malformation 126
snuff, and oral cancer 54
socioeconomic status, and oral cancer 56
solid tumours 136
solitary plasmacytoma of bone 70
sorafenib, oral effects 5
speech impairment 80
spinal accessory nerve (XI) 84
Sporothrix schenkii 178
staging, oral cancer 58
Staphylococcus aureus 188
stomatitis
  angular 174
  denture 174, 279
  necrotizing 187
Streptococcus anginosus 187
Streptococcus mitis 163
Streptococcus mutans 186
Streptococcus oralis 163
Streptococcus salivarius 163, 237
Streptococcus sanguis 187
Streptococcus sobrinus 186
sunitinib, oral effects 5
supportive care interventions 3
surgery
  oral cancer 59–60
  pain after 243–4
swallowing impairment *see* dysphagia
sympathetic trunk 85
systemic health, and oral cancer 56

Tannerella forsynthensis (Bacteroides forsythus) 233
Tannerella forsythia 187
taste buds 225

taste disturbance 225–30
  aetiology 226–7
    chemotherapy 227
    drug therapy 227
    radiotherapy 227
    zinc deficiency 227
  assessment 228–9
  chemotherapy-related 126
  children 263
  clinical features 228
  epidemiology 225
  geriatric patients 274
  management 229–30
    dietary therapy 229
    zinc therapy 229–30
  post-HSCT 135
teeth 12–14
  care of 44–6
  extractions 39–40
temporomandibular disorder 244
tenacious (thick) saliva 255
terminal phase, oral care in 285–7
tetracycline 191
TheraBite 108, 112
ticarcillin-clavulanate 191
tobacco, and oral cancer 54–5, 56
tongue 14–15
  black hairy 28
  fissured/scrotal 27
  geographic 28
  innervation 15
tonsils 11
toothbrushing 44–5, 46
toothpastes 45
total body irradiation 93, 134
tracheal stenosis 82–3
tracheo-innominate artery erosion 83
tracheo-oesophageal fistula 83
tracheomalacia 83
trastuzumab, oral effects 6
treatment effects 3, 4, 5
treatment failure 79–80
treatment gaps 94
trench mouth 187
Treponema denticola 187, 233
Treponema pallidum 56
triclosan 237
trigeminal neuralgia 244–5
trismus 81, 99–112
  aetiology 100–1
  children 266
  clinical features 101–6
  definition 99
  epidemiology 99–100
  investigations 106–7
  prevention 107–8
  treatment 108–12

ulcers 22, 28–9
  neutropaenic 31
  oral cancer 57
  recurrent aphthous 29–31
University of Washington Quality of Life scale
  (UW-QOL) 292

vagus nerve (X) 85
valaciclovir 198
valeric acid 235
vancomycin 191
varicella zoster virus 24, 196, 198–9
varices 27
venous lakes 27
vesicles 22
Vincent's angina 187
viral infections 24, 195–201
  children 263
  cytomegalovirus 200
  Epstein-Barr virus 199–200
  herpes simplex virus 195–8
  herpesviruses 187, 195
  human herpes virus 8 200
  human papillomavirus 201
  varicella zoster virus 198–9
voriconazole 181

Warthin's tumour 65
white lesions 31, 32
wound healing, compromised 126

xerostomia 204, 207
  advanced cancer patients 282
  clinical features 207
  epidemiology 204

zinc deficiency, and taste disturbance 227
zinc supplements 229–30
zoledronate, and BRON 152